The MMPI: A Practical Guide

The MMPI: A Practical Guide

by John R. Graham, Ph.D.

Professor of Psychology
Kent State University

New York
OXFORD UNIVERSITY PRESS

Library of Congress Cataloging in Publication Data
Graham, John Robert, 1940-
The MMPI.
Bibliography: p.
Includes index.
1. Minnesota multiphasic personality inventory.
I. Title. [DNLM: 1. MMPI. WM145   G739m]
BF698.8.M5G72   155.2'83   76-56854   ISBN 0-19-502304-8

Printed in the United States of America

Dedication

TO
Grant Dahlstrom —
an eminent psychologist, a stimulating mentor, and a good friend.

Foreword

by
James N. Butcher

About 20 years ago, Paul Meehl evaluated the status of clinical prediction and advanced some compelling arguments for the relative merits of actuarial versus clinical prediction. Meehl's ideas began a movement aimed at removing clinical assessment decisions from the realm of the subjective by imposing a more rigorous objective scientific framework. Subsequent developments on actuarial prediction have been impressive: a clinician or a clerk can now generate a personality description with a simple, casual thumbing through of a reference book (often called "cookbook" in the trade) using only a series of scores obtained from an MMPI profile, or even obtain a complete diagnostic narrative report from an electronic computer!

It may seem to the neophyte in the field that we have arrived at the actuaries' promised land. It may appear that the task of clinical assessment, with which the psychologist gained entry into the mental health field, may now conveniently be relegated to the computer, allowing psychologists to perform more "interesting" and complex tasks such as therapy, consultation, etc. Can we really, at this point, dispense with the clinician's "integrative clinical function" in the assessment task and rely upon automatically combined, actuarially derived data as the sole basis for our diagnostic decisions? Have we, at last, arrived at the "center city" of Meehl's (1956) forward vision?

The answer must be a somewhat woeful, although definite, negative. Although considerable gains in the empirical description of abnormal behavior were made in the 10 years after Meehl's challenge, recent progress has been disappointing. It is uncertain whether this present lull is asymptotic or simply a resting period before a great surge forward. However, it is clear that advances in methodology as well as growth in new knowledge have pretty much ended. Because empirical research and methodological advances have stopped short of the promised goal, where does this leave the clinicians who have been awaiting the master cookbook? Reliance upon contemporary automated outputs for important clinical decisions is careless psychological practice.

I believe that it will always be necessary for clinicians to mange clinical assessment personally. This means that it is important for clinicians to be prepared in traditional assessment skills. Jack Graham's clinical guide to MMPI interpretation will find an important place in the process of teaching MMPI interpretation skills and will serve as a basic clinician's reference book that every experienced practitioner will find invaluable.

With over 9,000 books and articles already published on the MMPI, including some excellent interpretation manuals, why another MMPI book? I am impressed with the fact that Graham's volume is not just a thorough presentation of all of the important information, including the well founded empirical bases, the clinical lore, and the master clinician's tips on approaching MMPI data that cannot be found elsewhere in the published literature. Graham goes well beyond the usual didactic approach of associating personality descriptors for MMPI code types and presents a clear, step-by-step approach to MMPI interpretation that teaches rather than lists. In addition, this volume presents a wide range of new, useful information on the MMPI clinical scales and the special scales that are becoming more widely used. The book is well written; its organization is excellent — presenting both administrative and interpretative material in a manner that introduces students or newcomers to the field to the complex task of clinical interpretation without overwhelming them.

Graham, a second generation "multer" who is well grounded in the strong tradition of empirical research, presents clinical MMPI interpretation in a unique way. His approach to clinical problems shows both the flexible sensibleness required in real life clinical assessment situations and the rigorous demand for objectivity — the sine qua non of MMPI intervention.

Preface

As its title suggests, this book is intended for anyone who uses or is interested in learning how to use the MMPI. For the student in psychology, medicine, counseling, social work, and related fields it represents an efficient way to become acquainted with a vast amount of information about the MMPI, its methodology, and its uses. For the practicing clinician (psychologist, counselor, psychiatrist, physician, social worker, etc.) it can serve as a source book to which he or she can make continuing reference as MMPIs are interpreted in clinical work. It is likely to be especially useful in preparing written reports which are based, at least in part, on the MMPI.

In Chapter 1 the rationale underlying the MMPI is discussed, and the methodology utilized in constructing the basic scales is presented. Chapter 2 contains detailed information about various forms of the MMPI, scoring the MMPI protocol, and coding the profile. Chapter 3 is devoted to consideration of the validity scales. In addition to discussion of the construction of each validity scale, information relevant to the identification of response sets and to the interpretation of the scales singly and in configuration is presented. Each of the 10 standard clinical scales is discussed in Chapter 4, and interpretive information is presented for high and low scores on each scale. The interpretation of frequently occurring two-point code types is discussed in Chapter 5. Chapters 6 and 7 cover some of the more frequently used special scales. For each special scale, construction procedures, reliability, validity, and interpretation of high and low scores are discussed. Chapter 8 presents the author's general strategy for interpreting MMPIs, and the strategy is illustrated with an actual case. This section should be especially beneficial to beginning MMPI users who have not yet developed their own interpretive approaches. Chapter 9 briefly discusses six of the most commonly used computerized interpretation services. A special feature of this chapter is that the illustrative case discussed in Chapter 8 was sent to the services and the resulting reports are included.

A guiding principle throughout the preparation of this book was that material should be presented in a way that will be most useful to the practicing clinician and the clinical student. No attempt has been made to include all of the technical information and research data concerning the MMPI. Other sources, such as the MMPI *Manual* (Hathaway & McKinley, 1967) and the two-volume *MMPI Handbook* (Dahlstrom, Welsh, & Dahlstrom, 1972, 1975), are readily available to those who require these kinds of information. In order to present material in the most useful way, specific sources are not cited for individual interpretive statements. Instead, the sources consulted in formulating the descriptive material are listed at the ends of the appropriate chapters.

Although the author is painfully aware of the limitations of the MMPI, it is his sincere belief that the MMPI is the best personality assessment technique currently available. If used appropriately the MMPI is a tool that can make assessment tasks more efficient and more fruitful. It is hoped that this book will help the clinician better to understand and utilize the MMPI in clinical assessment.

Acknowledgments

Many persons have supported the preparation of this book. I am indebted to the authors and publishers who have granted permission to reproduce their works. Specific recognition is given as the works appear in the book. Behaviordyne Corporation, Clinical Psychological Services, Inc., Institute of Clinical Analysis, Psychological Corporation, Roche Psychiatric Service Institute, and Veterans Administration MMPI Research Laboratory permitted portions of their interpretive reports for the illustrative case included in Chapter 9. W. Grant Dahlstrom deserves thanks for providing some materials that were difficult to locate. Roy S. Lilly wrote a computer program for generating T-scores from raw score data. The following individuals contributed clerical assistance: Jeffrey Buck, Adele Davis, Becky Graham, Cindy Orlasky, and Patricia White. Special appreciation is expressed to Joseph D. Matarazzo for his encouragement and his helpful editorial comments and to Leonard A. Pace of Williams & Wilkins for his continuing support. Finally, thanks go to Becky, John, Mary, and David Graham who contributed to this book by tolerating my preoccupation with its preparation for the past year and a half.

Table of Contents

1
Introduction

GENERAL DESCRIPTION OF THE MMPI

The Minnesota Multiphasic Personality Inventory (MMPI) consists of 566 self-reference statements. The person taking the test responds to each statement as true as applied to him, as false as applied to him, or as not applying to him. The relatively unambiguous stimuli and the structured response format qualify the MMPI for classification as an objective technique of personality assessment. Traditionally, great importance has been placed on the differences between objective and projective assessment procedures. In addition to the differences in stimulus ambiguity and the extent to which response format is structured, it also has been suggested that objective and projective techniques differ in terms of the involvement of a skilled clinician in the interpretation of test results. It has been suggested that whereas a skilled clinician is an integral part of the interpretation of projective test protocols, objective test results can be interpreted by less skilled individuals by reference to appropriate norms. In clinical practice, this distinction does not exist. As Matarazzo (1972) has stated, interpretation of both objective and projective techniques is "a highly subjective art which requires a well-trained and experienced practitioner to give such 'scores' predictive meaning in the life of any given human being" (p. 11).

After individual or group administration of the test, using any of several available forms and answer sheets, an individual's responses are scored objectively either by hand or with machine scoring equipment. The scoring procedures yield scores for 4 validity scales and 10 basic clinical or personality scales. Numerous additional scales and indices also have been developed, and some of these are discussed later in this *Guide*. The raw scores from the standard validity and clinical scales are transformed to T-scores (mean = 50; SD = 10) using data provided in the *Manual* (Hathaway & McKinley, 1967). The responses of the Minnesota normal group provide the basis for the T-score conversions. Separate norms are available for males and females. The T-scores are utilized to construct a profile on a standard profile sheet. This profile serves as the basis for generating inferences about the individual who was examined.

1

ORIGINAL PURPOSE

The MMPI was first published in 1943 by the Psychological Corporation. The test authors, Starke Hathaway, PhD, and Jovian McKinley, MD, were working in the University of Minnesota Hospitals and hoped that the MMPI would be useful for routine diagnostic assessments. During the late 1930's and early 1940's a primary goal of the clinical psychologist and the psychiatrist was to assign appropriate psychodiagnostic labels to individual cases. An individual interview or mental status examination and individual psychological testing usually were done of each patient. It was hoped that a group-administered paper-and-pencil personality inventory would provide a more efficient way of arriving at appropriate psychodiagnostic evaluation.

RATIONALE

Hathaway and McKinley utilized the empirical keying approach in the construction of the various MMPI scales. This approach, which requires that one empirically determine items that differentiate between groups of subjects, is a common technique today. However, it represented a significant innovation at the time of the MMPI construction. Most prior personality inventories had been constructed according to a logical keying approach. With this earlier approach, test items were selected or generated rationally according to face validity, and responses were keyed according to the subjective judgment of the test author concerning what kinds of responses were likely to be indicative of the attributes being measured. Both clinical experience and research data seriously questioned the adequacy of this logical keying approach. Increasingly, it became apparent that subjects could falsify or distort their responses to items in order to present themselves in any particular way they chose. Further, empirical studies indicated that the subjectively keyed responses often were not consistent with differences actually observed between groups of subjects. In the newly introduced empirical keying procedure, responses to individual test items are treated as unknowns, and empirical item analysis is utilized to identify test items that differentiate between criterion groups. Such an approach to the item responses overcomes many of the difficulties associated with the earlier, subjective approaches.

CLINICAL SCALE DEVELOPMENT

The first step in the construction of the basic MMPI scales was to collect a large pool of potential inventory items.* Hathaway and McKinley selected a wide variety of personality-type statements from such sources as psychological and psychiatric case histories and reports, textbooks, and earlier published scales of personal and social attitudes. From an initial pool of about 1,000 statements the test authors selected a pool of 504 statements that they judged to be reasonably independent of each other.

The next step was to select appropriate criterion groups. One criterion group, hereafter referred to as the Minnesota normals, consisted primarily

---

* Information concerning clinical and validity scale development is abstracted from a series of articles by Hathaway (1956, 1965), Hathaway & McKinley (1940, 1942), McKinley & Hathaway (1940, 1944), McKinley, Hathaway, & Meehl (1948), and Meehl & Hathaway (1946).

of relatives and visitors of patients in the University of Minnesota Hospitals. This group was augmented by several other groups of normal subjects. These included a group of recent high school graduates who were attending precollege conferences at the University of Minnesota, a group of Work Progress Administration workers, and some medical patients at the University of Minnesota Hospitals. The second major group of subjects, hereafter referred to as clinical subjects, was made up of psychiatric patients at the University of Minnesota Hospitals. This second group included patients representing all of the major psychiatric diagnostic categories being utilized clinically at the time of the test construction. Clinical subjects were divided into subgroups of discrete diagnostic samples according to their clinically arrived at diagnostic labels. Whenever there was any doubt about a patient's clinical diagnosis or when more than one diagnosis was present, the patient was not included in this clinical reference group. The different subgroups of clinical subjects formed were: hypochondriasis, depression, hysteria, psychopathic deviate, paranoia, psychasthenia, schizophrenia, and hypomania.

The next step in scale construction was to administer the original 504 test items to the Minnesota normals and to the patients in each of the clinical groups. For each of the clinical groups, separately, an item analysis was conducted to identify those items in the pool of 504 that differentiated significantly between the clinical group and a group of normal subjects. Individual MMPI items that were identified by this procedure were included in the resulting MMPI scale for that clinical group.

In an attempt to cross-validate such a clinical scale (e.g., the depression scale), new groups of normal subjects and clinical subjects with that particular clinical diagnosis were selected and the scale was administered to each. If significant differences were found between scores for the normal group and the clinical group in question, the clinical scale was considered to have been adequately cross-validated and thus was ready for use in the differential diagnosis of new patients whose diagnostic features were unknown.

At a somewhat later time two additional clinical scales were constructed. First, the Masculinity-Femininity (Mf) scale originally was intended to distinguish between homosexual males and heterosexual males. Because of difficulty in identifying adequate numbers of items that differentiated between these two groups, Hathaway and McKinley subsequently broadened their approach in the construction of the Mf scale. In addition to the all too few items that did discriminate between homosexual and heterosexual males, other items were identified that were differentially endorsed by normal male and female subjects. Also, a number of items from the Terman and Miles I scale (1936) were added to the original item pool and included in the Mf scale. Second, the Social Introversion (Si) scale was developed by Drake (1946) and has come to be included as one of the basic MMPI scales. Although this scale initially was constructed by identifying items from the original item pool that differentiated successfully between female college students who tended to participate in many extracurricular activities and female college students who were not very socially participative, its use now has been extended to males as well as females.

VALIDITY SCALE DEVELOPMENT

Hathaway and McKinley at the outset also developed four scales, here-after referred to as the validity scales, whose purpose was to detect deviant test-taking attitudes. The "Cannot Say" scale or category is simply the total number of items in the MMPI omitted or responded to as both true and false by the individual taking the test. Obviously, the omission of large numbers of items, which tends to lower the scores on the clinical scales, calls into question the interpretability of the whole resulting pro-file.

The L scale, originally called the "Lie" scale of the MMPI, was designed to detect a rather unsophisticated and naive attempt on the part of an individual to present himself in an overly favorable light. The L scale items were rationally derived and cover everyday situations in order to assess the strength of the person's unwillingness to admit even very minor weaknesses in character or personality. An example of an L scale item is "I do not read every editorial in the newspaper every day." Most people would be quite willing to admit that they do not read every editorial every day, but a person determined to present himself in a very favorable light might not be willing to admit to such a perceived shortcoming.

The F scale of the MMPI was designed to detect individuals who are approaching the test-taking task in a way different from that intended by the test authors. F scale items were selected by examining for each item the endorsement frequency of the Minnesota normal group and identifying those items endorsed in a particular direction by fewer than 10% of the normals. Obviously, because few normal people endorse an item in that direction, a person who does endorse the item in that direction is exhibit-ing a deviant response.

The K scale of the MMPI was designed to identify clinical defensiveness. Items in the K scale were selected empirically by comparing the responses of a group of patients who were known to be clinically deviant but who produced normal MMPI profiles with a group of people producing normal MMPI profiles and for whom there was no indication of psychopathology. It was intended that a high K score be indicative of defensiveness and call into question the person's responses to all of the other items. The K scale also was later utilized to develop a correction factor for some of the clinical scales. Hathaway and McKinley reasoned that, if the effect of a defensive test-taking attitude as reflected by a high K score is to lower scores on the clinical scales, perhaps one might be able to determine the extent to which the scores on the clinical scales should be raised in order to reflect more accurately a person's behavior. By comparing the efficiency of each clinical scale with various portions of the K scale added as a correction factor, McKinley et al. determined the appropriate weighting of the K scale score for each clinical scale to correct for the defensiveness indicated by the K scale. Some clinical scales are not K-corrected at all, because the simple raw score on those clinical scales seemed to produce the most accurate prediction about a person's clinical condition. Other scales have propor-tions of K, ranging from .2 to 1.0, added in order to elevate appropriately the clinical scales.

CURRENT APPROACH TO MMPI UTILIZATION

After a decade of clinical use and additional validity studies it became apparent that the MMPI was not adequately successful for the purpose for which it originally was developed, namely, the valid psychodiagnosis of a new patient. Although patients in any particular clinical category (e.g., depression) were likely to obtain high scores on the corresponding clinical scale, they also often obtained high scores on other clinical scales. Also, many normal subjects also obtained high scores on one or more of the clinical scales. Clearly, the clinical scales are not pure measures of the symptom syndromes suggested by the scale names.

A number of different reasons have been suggested for the MMPI's failure to fulfill its original purpose. From further research it became apparent that many of the clinical scales of the MMPI are highly intercorrelated, making it highly unlikely that only a single scale would be elevated for an individual. Also, the unreliability of specific psychiatric diagnoses themselves contributes to the failure of the MMPI scales to differentiate among clinical groups.

Although the failure of the MMPI scales to differentiate among clinical groups might have been bothersome in the 1940's, this failure is not particularly critical today. Currently, practicing clinicians place less emphasis on diagnostic labels per se. Accumulating evidence suggests that psychiatric nosology is not as useful as is medical diagnosis. Information in a psychiatric chart that a patient's diagnosis is schizophrenia, for example, does not tell us much about the etiology of the disorder for that individual or about recommended therapeutic procedures.

For this reason, the MMPI currently is used in a way quite different from the way in which it originally was intended to be used. It is assumed that the clinical scales are measuring something, because reliable differences in scores are found among individuals from different clinical reference groups. The new approach treats each MMPI scale as an unknown and, through clinical experience and empirical research, the correlates of each scale are identified. When a person obtains a score on a particular scale, the clinician attributes to that person the characteristics and behaviors that through previous research and experience have been identified for other individuals with similar scores on that scale. To lessen the likelihood that excess meaning will be attributed because of the clinical scale names, the following scale numbers have been assigned to the original clinical scales, and today they replace the clinical labels:

Present Scale Number	Discarded Scale Name
1	Hypochondriasis
2	Depression
3	Hysteria
4	Psychopathic Deviate
5	Masculinity-Femininity
6	Paranoia
7	Psychasthenia
8	Schizophrenia
9	Hypomania
0	Social Introversion

Thus, for example, when discussing a patient among themselves, MMPI experts will refer to him or her as a "four-nine" or a "one-two-three," descriptive phrases in shorthand which communicate to the listener the particular behavior descriptions associated with the "4-9" or "1-2-3" syndrome.

In addition to identifying empirical correlates of high scores on each of the above numbered scales, it also is possible to identify empirical correlates for low scores and for various combinations of scores on the scales (e.g., highest scale in the profile, two highest scales in the profile, etc.). Some investigators have developed very complex rules for classifying individual MMPI profiles and have identified behavioral-empirical correlates of profiles which meet these criteria. Thus, even though the MMPI has not been successful in terms of its original purpose (differential diagnosis of clinical group believed in the 1930's to be discrete psychiatric types), it has proved possible subsequently to use the test to generate descriptions of and inferences about individuals (normals and patients) on the basis of their own MMPI profiles. It is this new behavioral description approach to the utilization of the MMPI in everyday practice that has led to the instrument's great popularity among practicing clinicians.

2
Administration and Scoring

One appealing feature of the MMPI is that although it takes an experienced clinician to interpret it, it can be administered easily to individual subjects or groups of subjects by nonprofessional examiners. The availability of a number of different MMPI test forms increases the number and range of potential subjects. In addition, the test can be scored objectively by hand or by machine. Because of these factors, MMPI users sometimes become careless in the administration and scoring of the test. It must be emphasized that the same caution and attention to standardized procedures that are appropriate for other psychological tests also must be followed with the MMPI. Persons who administer the test should be familiar with all of the material presented in the *Manual* (Hathaway & McKinley, 1967). Also, Chapter 1 of *An MMPI Handbook,* Vol. 1 (Dahlstrom, Welsh, & Dahlstrom, 1972) discusses additional administrative problems and considerations.

The *Manual* indicates that individuals 16 years of age or older with at least 6 years of schooling should be able to complete the MMPI satisfactorily. Experience suggests that if they are properly motivated and carefully supervised, and if appropriate forms of the test are employed, people with even less than 6 years of education may be able to take the test. Reading level seems to be the primary consideration in determining who can take the test. Some examiners have individuals read aloud some of the MMPI items to determine whether they can read well enough to take the test. Other test users have found it useful to administer some brief measure of reading ability, such as the Kent Emergency Scales (Kent, 1946), before administering the MMPI.

Age is another important factor in determining who can take the MMPI. As long as visual handicaps or other physical problems do not interfere, there is no upper age limit on who can take the test. There are, however, several considerations in determining the youngest age for which the test is appropriate. Although the *Manual* (Hathaway & McKinley, 1967) indicates 16 as the youngest age for which the test is appropriate, the MMPI has been administered successfully to persons as young as 13 or 14 years of age. Younger individuals, even if they can read well enough and can maintain their attention and motivation long enough to complete the test, may not have a range of experience wide enough to make the content of many items meaningful to them. Separate norms for adolescents are presented in Tables 6 through 9 of Appendix H of the *Handbook* (Dahlstrom et al., 1972). Whereas specialized norms may be useful in comparing the level of a person's scores with his specific reference group, the generating by a practicing clinician of inferences from profiles constructed from such norms is questionable, because most interpretative data are based on profiles derived from the adult norms.

Clinical condition of potential examinees is another important consideration. Completion of the entire MMPI is a lengthy and tedious task for most subjects. Persons who are very anxious or agitated often find the task almost unbearable. It frequently is possible to break the testing session into several shorter periods for such individuals. Persons who are very confused may not be able to understand or to follow the standard instructions. Such individuals sometimes can complete the test satisfactorily if it is administered individually using either the box or auditory tape form in contrast to the booklet form. Some examiners find it useful to read the items to the subject, with either the examiner or the subject recording the responses.

For most individuals the test can be administered either individually or in groups, using the forms of the test and answer sheet most convenient for the examiner. For persons of average or above average intelligence, without complicating factors, the testing time typically is between 1 and 1¹/₂ hr. For less intelligent individuals, or those with other complicating factors, the testing time may exceed 2 hr. Although it sometimes is more convenient to have the subject take the MMPI home to complete and return to the examiner, whenever possible it is preferable to have the MMPI completed in the professional atmosphere of the clinician's office.

It is important in administering the MMPI to anyone in any setting to communicate clearly to them the purpose(s) for which the test is being given and to assure them of the confidentiality of the test results. A person who knows why he is taking the test, who knows who will see the test results, and who knows how the results will be used on his or her behalf is more likely to be cooperative and to approach the task in a manner that will make the resulting data meaningful.

TEST FORMS

The availability of several basic forms of the MMPI ensures that the test can be administered to a broad spectrum of people in a manner that is most convenient to both subjects and examiner. Forms are available for individual administrations, for group administrations, for blind individuals or others who cannot read the printed items, and for subjects who have limited facility with the English language. Researchers also have developed experimental forms of the test in which reading difficulty has been reduced, in which items are presented in an oral interrogative form, in which items are presented in the second person, and so forth. In this section only those forms most often utilized by the practicing clinician are discussed. For other forms the reader is referred to Chapters 2 and 3 of the *Handbook,* Vol. 1 (Dahlstrom et al., 1972).

Individual (Box) Form

In the box form (Catalog no. 5F023)* each of the 550 items† is printed on a 3^{1}/$_{2}$-in. by 2^{1}/$_{4}$-in. card. The cards are presented in random order in a wooden box which includes instructions inside the cover. The box also contains three dividers labeled TRUE, FALSE, and CANNOT SAY. The examinee is instructed to read each item and to decide whether it is true as applied to him or false as applied to him and to place the card behind either the TRUE or FALSE divider. For items that do not apply to him or that deal with something that he does not know aobut, the cards are placed behind the CANNOT SAY divider. The instructions indicate that fewer than 10 cards should be placed behind the CANNOT SAY divider.

The box form is especially useful for individuals of limited ability and/or education who might have difficulty completing the booklet forms. It also is easier than the booklet forms for disturbed or confused persons who might get mixed up in marking answers on a separate sheet.

It is a good idea to place at the front of the box a few items that have easy vocabulary and that are free of content that might be especially upsetting to the person taking the test. Also, many examiners include instructions to limit the use of the CANNOT SAY category even more than is indicated in the standard instructions. If a person places many items in the CANNOT SAY category, he should be encouraged to reconsider the items and to try to place them into either the TRUE or FALSE category. With this prodding most people will leave no items or only a few items in the CANNOT SAY category.

The first step in scoring the box form is for the examiner to transfer the responses to the box form answer sheet (Catalog no. SF217). This answer sheet has 550 blanks arranged in columns labeled A through J and rows numbered 1 through 55. Each card is identified by a column letter and a row number. CANNOT SAY responses are entered as question marks in the appropriate blanks of the answer sheet. The examiner next identifies those cards in the TRUE category that have the lower right-hand corner cut off. For these items a red X is placed in the appropriate blanks of the answer sheet. Cards in the FALSE category with the lower left-hand corner cut off are identified and each is recorded as a red X in the appropriate blank of the answer sheet. It should be noted that items in the TRUE and FALSE categories that have been recorded on the answer sheet indicate infrequent responses and not necessarily abnormal one.

After the appropriate entries are made on the answer sheet, the responses are scored for the 4 validity indicators and the 10 basic clinical scales. The CANNOT SAY score simply is the number of question marks on the record form. The L score is obtained by counting the number of red

---

* MMPI materials are available only from the Psychological Corporation, 757 Third Avenue, New York, New York 10017. Catalog numbers are indicated in parentheses.
† Although the original MMPI item pool consisted of 504 items, 46 items were added when the Mf Scale was constructed, bringing the total number of items to 550.

X's among the last 15 items (numbers J41 through J55). For the F and K scales and for the 10 clinical scales, transparent scoring templates (Catalog no. 5F413) are used for hand scoring. For each of these scales the appropriate template is placed over the record form. The raw score is determined by counting the number of blanks that contain a red X next to an X on the scoring template, plus the number of blank cells on the record form that correspond to the O's on the template. The raw scores are recorded in the appropriate blanks along the right edge of the record form.

Group (Booklet) Form

The group form consists of 566 items printed in a reusable paper booklet (Catalog no. 5F061). To obtain a more economical method of scoring the answer sheets, 16 items are duplicated in the booklet and on the answer sheet. Instructions, which are printed on the front of the booklet, direct the person being examined to read each statement and to decide whether it is true as applied to him or false as applied to him and to mark his answers on a separate answer sheet. Although he is told to make no mark for a statement that does not apply to him or that is something that he does not know about, he is cautioned not to leave any blank spaces if he can avoid it.

Several different types of answer sheets are available for use with the group form. The most commonly utilized answer sheet is one that was designed for use with the IBM 805 scoring machine (Catalog no. 5F255). This sheet has true or false blanks numbered 1 to 566, and the person being examined blackens in the space corresponding to his response. This sheet may be machine scored or may be scored by hand using a set of scoring templates (Catalog no. 5F437). In hand scoring, the CANNOT SAY score is determined by counting the number of items left blank or marked as both TRUE and FALSE. The L score is the number of FALSE responses to the following items: 15, 45, 75, 105, 135, 165, 195, 225, 255, 285, 30, 90, 120, 150. It should be noted that these items are easily identified by their location on the answer sheet. Raw scores for the F and K scales and for the 10 basic clinical scales are determined by placing the appropriate templates over the answer sheet and counting the number of blackened spaces. There are two scoring templates (front and back) for the K, Pa, Pt, Sc, and Si scales and one template for the other scales. There are different templates for male and female subjects for the Mf scale. Commercial machine scoring is not available for the IBM 805 answer sheet.

The Hankes answer sheet (Catalog no. 5F310) also is intended for use with the group form. The sheet contains numbered boxes for each item in the booklet. A person indicates a true response to an item by blackening in an oval within the box above the item number, whereas a false response is indicated by blackening in an oval within the box below the item number. No hand scoring keys are available for the Hankes answer sheets, but many clinicians have constructed templates for scoring them. They may be machine scored by sending them to TESTSCOR, 309 Snelling Avenue, Minneapolis, Minnesota 55404. The Psychological Corporation Test Catalog should be consulted for costs and other details concerning this scoring service.

The NCS answer sheet (Catalog no. 5F281) also may be used with the group form. On this sheet a response to each of the 566 items is indicated by blackening in a circle containing either T or F. As with the Hankes answer sheet, no hand scoring keys are available for the NCS sheets. They must be machine scored by sending them to National Computer Systems, 4401 West 76th Street, Minneapolis, Minneapolis   55435.

The IBM 1230 answer sheet also is designed for use with the group form. This sheet is intended for scoring with the IBM 1230 or IBM 1232 scoring machines. Examiners interested in this answer sheet should write to the Psychological Corporation, 757 Third Avenue, New York, New York   10017 for costs and other information.

Form R

In Form R the 566 items contained in the booklet form are printed in a hard cover, spiral-bound booklet with step-down pages (Catalog no. 5F114). Instructions appear on the first page of the booklet. A Form R answer sheet (Catalog no. 5F346) is inserted over two pegs in the back of the booklet. As a person works through the booklet, each item is aligned with the appropriate space on the answer sheet. A response is indicated by blackening in an oval containing either T or F.

A major advantage of Form R is that the hard cover permits the test to be completed even when a desk or table space is not available. Also, for many persons the alignment of items and appropriate spaces on the answer sheet makes the task easier than with the group form. A further advantage is that the items have been rearranged from the group form order in such a way that all items required for scoring the standard validity and clinical scales appear in the first 399 items. One disadvantage of Form R is that because no item numbers appear on the answer sheet, responses to particular items cannot be identified unless the answer sheet is reinserted into a test booklet.

The Form R answer sheet may be machine scored or hand scored. For machine scoring, answer sheets should be sent to National Computer Systems, 4401 W. 76th Street, Minneapolis Minnesota   55435. Details concerning costs are presented in the Psychological Corporation Test Catalog. Hand scoring of the Form R answer sheet requires a special set of scoring templates (Catalog no. 5F425). The CANNOT SAY score is determined by counting the number of items left blank or answered as both TRUE and FALSE. Raw scores for the L, F, and K scales and for the 10 basic clinical scales are obtained by placing the transparent templates over the answer sheet and counting the number of blackened ovals that appear in the boxes on the template. Because all 566 item responses appear on one side of the answer sheet, only one template is needed for each scale, with the exception of the Mf scale, which has different templates for male and female subjects. All raw scores are recorded at the bottom of the answer sheet beneath arrows on the scoring templates.

Tape Recording Form

There is a standard tape recording of MMPI items (Catalog no. 5F035) available for administration to semiliterates and persons with other disabilities that make completion of other forms difficult or impossible. The tape is played to the person, and during a pause after each item, the response is recorded either by the person being examined or by the examiner. The items appear on the tape in the same order as in the group form; therefore, the same answer sheets and scoring procedures utilized for the group form also are appropriate for the tape form.

Short Forms

Because the length of time required to complete the MMPI is sometimes prohibitive, numerous efforts have been made to develop short or abbreviated forms of the test. The utilization of short forms always leads to a loss of information. Many of the additional scales that were subsequently developed cannot be scored if all of the MMPI items are not administered. Before deciding to utilize a short form, the examiner should carefully think about whose time is being saved. Because the MMPI typically is not administered by the clinician personally, the time saved by utilizing a short form is that of the person being examined and/or of a clerical worker. In most situations, there is no compelling reason to shorten the time of test administration. However, it is recognized that in some instances where testing time is quite limited, the examiner may have to consider using a short form of the test.

The most acceptable abbreviated form involves the administration of only those items that are scored for the validity scales and the basic clinical scales. With the group form of the test, a person is instructed to complete the first 366 items and 33 additional items that are scattered throughout the remainder of the test booklet. The booklet form numbers for these additional items are: 371, 374, 377, 383, 391, 397, 398, 400, 406, 411, 415, 427, 436, 440, 446, 449, 450, 451, 455, 461, 462, 469, 473, 479, 481, 482, 487, 502, 505, 521, 547, 549, 564. Some individuals become confused with these directions, so some examiners type the 33 additional items on a separate sheet, number them consecutively, and insert the sheet into a standard test booklet. Such a procedure requires that the scoring templates for scales K and Si be modified appropriately. In the Form R test booklet, all of the items scored on the validity and basic clinical scales appear as the first 399 items in the booklet. Thus, a persn can be instructed simply to complete only the first 399 items in the booklet. Several of the other more promising short forms are summarized in Appendix A of this *Guide*.

CONSTRUCTING THE PROFILE

For the box form and for Form R the reverse side of the record form contains profiles for males and females. For the IBM 805 answer sheet, which is used with the group form, a separate profile sheet, with a male profile on one side and a female profile form on the other side, is used. These profiles are included with IBM 805 answer sheets, and they also may be purchased separately (Catalog no. 5F712).

A first step in constructing the profile is to transfer the raw scores from the answer sheet or record form to appropriate blanks at the bottom of the profile form, making sure that the profile is the appropriate one for the person's sex. At this time it also is important to be certain that identifying data (name, age, date, education, etc.) are recorded on the profile sheet.

At this point a K-correction is added to the raw scores for the Hs, Pd, Pt, Sc, and Ma scales. The proportion of a person's K scale raw score that is to be added to each of these scales is indicated on the profile form. There has been some discussion in the literature concerning the possibility that profiles without the K-correction added might be more appropriate in some settings. However, because the standard profile form is based on K-corrected scores and because virtually all of the data concerning interpretation of scores are derived from K-corrected scores, it is recommended that the K-correction be used routinely.‡

For each scale the examiner then should refer to the T-score related numbers in the column above the scale label. The number in the column corresponding to the raw score (K-corrected if appropriate) on the scale is marked by the examiner either with a small x or a small dot. Standard procedure calls for raw scores of less than 30 on the CANNOT SAY (?) scale to be plotted as 30. Many examiners find it less confusing if raw scores less than 30 are indicated in the appropriate blank but are not plotted as part of the profile. After a dot or x has been entered in the column above each scale label, the MMPI profile for the person examined is completed by connecting the plotted dots or x's with each other. Traditionally, the 3 validity scales are joined to each other but are not connected with the 10 clinical scale scores.

Because a T-score scale is printed on each side of the profile sheet, by plotting the scores in the above manner on the profile sheet, the raw scores for each scale can be converted visually to T-scores. A T-score has a mean of 50 and a standard deviation of 10. The T-score conversions provided on the profile sheet are based on the responses of the Minnesota normal standardization group which was described in Chapter 1 of this *Guide*. Thus, a T-score of 50 for any particular scale indicates that a person's score is equal to the average or mean score for the normal standardization group examined by Hathaway and McKinley. Scores greater than 50 indicate scores higher than the average for the standardization group, and scores below 50 indicate scores lower than average for the standardization group.

CODING THE PROFILE

Although it is possible to derive some useful information by interpreting an examinee's T-score on a single scale in isolation, much of the information relevant to interpretation of MMPI protocols is *configural* in nature. In addition to interpreting individual scales, it is necessary to consider the pattern of the scales in relation to each other. To facilitate profile interpretation, coding is a procedure for recording most of the essential information about a profile in a concise form and for reducing the possible number of different profiles to a manageable size. Coding conveys information about

---

‡ One exception is when using the Marks, Seeman, and Haller codebook for adolescents (1974). This codebook utilizes noncorrected scores that must be converted to T-scores with special tables provided by the authors.

the scores on scales relative to each other and also indicates an absolute range within which scores fall. Coding also permits easy grouping of similar profiles, using all or only part of the code.

Two major coding systems have been utilized in the MMPI literature: Hathaway's (1947) original system and a more complete system developed by Welsh (1948). Because much of the information relevant to interpretation has been presented in both systems, the MMPI user is advised to become acquainted with both systems. Although in the following chapters of this *Guide* only the Welsh code will be utilized, the procedure for coding profiles using both the Hathaway and Welsh systems will be described in the next section.

Hathaway Code

Step 1

Utilize the number instead of the name of each clinical scale:

Hs − 1	Pa − 6
D − 2	Pt − 7
Hy − 3	Sc − 8
Pd–4	Ma − 9
Mf − 5	Si − 0

Step 2

Record in descending order of T-score values the numbers of any clinical scales having T-scores greater than 54.

Step 3

Insert a prime (′) after the last scale number in the code which has a T-score of 70 or more.

Step 4

Underline the adjacent scale numbers that are within one T-score point of each other. When two scale numbers have the same T-score, place in the ordinal sequence found on the profile sheet and underline.

Step 5

Use a dash (−) and then record the number of the lowest scale on the profile if that scale has a T-score of less than 46. If no scales have T-score values less than 46, no numbers appear to the right of the dash. After the number of the lowest scale, record in ascending order of T-scores the numbers of any scales whose T-score lie between the lowest scale and a T-score of 46.

Step 6

Follow the same rule for underlining these low scores as presented in Step 4 above for high scores.

Step 7

To the right of and separated from the clinical scales, record the *raw scores* for L, F, and K in that order and separate them by colons (:).

Step 8

If the raw score of L is equal to or greater than 10 or if the raw score of F is equal to or greater than 16, a capital X is placed immediately after the code for the clinical scales to suggest that the profile may be invalid.

An example of the Hathaway code is presented in Table 2.1.

Welsh Code

Step 1

Utilize the number instead of the name of each clinical scale:

Hs – 1	Pa – 6
D – 2	Pt – 7
Hy – 3	Sc – 8
Pd – 4	Ma – 9
Mf – 5	Si – 0

Step 2

Record the 10 numbers of the clinical scales in order of T-scores, from the highest on the left to the lowest on the right.

Step 3

To the right of and separated from the clinical scales, record the four validity scales (?, L, F, K) in order of T-scores with the highest on the left and the lowest on the right. The set of clinical scales and the set of validity scales are coded separately.

Step 4

When adjacent scales are within one T-score point, they are underlined. When adjacent scales have the same T-score, place in the ordinal sequence found on the profile sheet and underline.

Step 5

To indicate scale elevations, appropriate symbols are inserted after scale numbers as follows:

90 & greater	*
80–89	"
70–79	'
60–69	—
50–59	/
40–49	:
30–39	#
29 & less	to the right of #

If a 10-point T-score range does not contain any scale, the appropriate symbol for that elevation must be included. It is not necessary to include a symbol to the left of the scale with the highest score or to the right of the scale with the lowest score.

Step 6

Repeat Steps 4 and 5 for the validity scales. An example of the Welsh

Table 2.1 Examples of Hathaway and Welsh codes

Scale name	Scale no.	Raw score	T-score
Cannot Say		5	50
L		7	60
F		13	73
K		7	40
Hypochondriasis	1	20	64
Depression	2	41	92
Hysteria	3	21	54
Psychopathic Deviate	4	16	43
Masculinity-Femininity	5	23	57
Paranoia	6	3	35
Psychasthenia	7	46	84
Schizophrenia	8	44	83
Hypomania	9	8	28
Social Introversion	0	4	28

Hathaway code: 278'15 − 9064   7:13:7
Welsh code: 2*78" '1 − 53/4:6#90   F'L − ?/K

code also is presented in Table 2.1. As a practice exercise, the reader might wish to cover the codes at the bottom of Table 2.1 and himself code the T-scores into first the Hathaway code and then the Welsh code using the instructions given above.

3

The Validity Scales

For the MMPI to yield maximally accurate and useful information, it is necessary that the person examined approach the test-taking task in the manner intended by the test authors. After carefully reading each item and considering its content, he or she should give a direct and, as far as possible, honest response utilizing the response format provided. To the extent that deviations from this procedure occur, the resulting profile either should be considered invalid and not interpreted further or should be interpreted in the context of the test-taking attitude of the person. Early inventories were criticized for being succeptible to distortion and for not including any index of test-taking attitude. Although it was hoped that the empirical keying procedure utilized in developing the MMPI would make such distortions less likely, subsequently four validity indicators were developed specifically to detect deviant test-taking attitudes. In addition to providing important information about test-taking attitudes, in common with the clinical scales, the validity scales themselves have come to be used as sources of inferences about extra-test behaviors. Both aspects of the validity scales will be considered in this chapter. The items included in each validity scale and the keyed response for each item are presented in Appendix N of this *Guide*.*

CANNOT SAY (?) SCALE

The Cannot Say score simply is the number of omitted items (including items answered both true and false). There are a number of reasons why people omit items on the MMPI. Occasionally, items are omitted because of carelessness or confusion. Omitted items also can reflect an attempt to avoid admitting undesirable things about oneself without directly lying. Indecisive people, who cannot decide between the two response alternatives, may leave many items unanswered. Some items are omitted because of a lack of information or experience necessary for a meaningful response. For example, if an individual has never read *Alice in Wonderland,* he may

---

* Item numbers in Appendix N and elsewhere in this *Guide* are for the booklet (group) form of the MMPI.

not feel that he can respond meaningfully to the item "I liked *Alice in Wonderland* by Lewis Carroll."

Regardless of the reasons for omitting items, a large number of such items can lead to lowered scores on other scales. Therefore, the validity of a resulting protocol with many omitted items should be questioned. Traditionally, Cannot Say raw scores greater than 30 have been interpreted as indicating profile invalidity. As indicated in Chapter 2, however, the best procedure probably is to ensure that few or no items are omitted. If encouraged before beginning the MMPI to answer all items, most people usually will use the Cannot Say response category infrequently. Also, if the examiner scans answer sheets at the time that the test is completed and encourages individuals to try to answer previously omitted items, most people will complete all or most of the items. If it is not possible to return protocols with instructions to try to answer omitted items, protocols with more than 30 items omitted should not be interpreted further.

L SCALE

As indicated in Chapter 1, the L scale originally was constructed to detect a deliberate and rather unsophisticated attempt on the part of the subject to present him- or herself in a favorable light (Meehl & Hathaway, 1946). The 15 rationally derived L scale items deal with rather minor flaws and weaknesses to which most people are willing to admit. However, individuals who deliberately are trying to present themselves in a very favorable way are not willing to admit even such minor shortcomings. The result is that such people produce high L scale scores.

Although most L scale items are not answered in the scored direction (false) by most people, many normal individuals do endorse several of the items in the scored direction. The average raw score for the MMPI standardization group was 4. However, subsequent research revealed that scores on the L scale are related to educational level, intelligence, socioeconomic status, and psychological sophistication. Better educated, brighter, more sophisticated people from higher social classes score lower on the L scale. The typical L scale score for college students, for example, is 0 or 1.

High Scores on L Scale

Because of the relationship between L scale scores and demographic variables, such variables must be taken into account when deciding if a score should be considered high. Whereas a raw score of 4 or 5 on the L scale would be about average for a lower middle class laborer of average or below average intelligence, such a score would be considered as moderately high for a college educated person from an upper middle class background.

When the L scale score is higher than would be expected when appropriate demographic variables are taken into account, one should entertain the possibility that the person is not being honest and frank in answering all of the other MMPI items. The result of such a test-taking attitude is, inferentially, that the individual's scores on most or all of the clinical scales have been lowered (distorted) in the direction of appearing better adjusted psychologically.

In addition to thus suggesting a defensive test-taking attitude, high L scale scores have been found empirically to be associated with some other important extra-test attitudes and behaviors. Thus, high scorers tend to be overly conventional and socially conforming. They are unoriginal in their thinking and inflexible in their approaches to problems. In addition, they have a poor tolerance for stress and pressure. They are rigid and moralistic and overevaluate their own worth. They utilize repression and denial excessively, and they appear to have little or no insight into their own motivations. Also, they have little awareness of the consequences to other people of their behavior. In some rare cases, an extremely high L scale score may be suggestive of a full blown clinical confusion that may be either organic or functional in nature.

Low Scores on L Scale

On the other hand, low scores on the L scale suggest that the person responded frankly to the items and was confident enough about himself to be able to admit to minor personal faults and shortcomings. Low scorers have been described by Gough, McKee, and Yandell (1955) as perceptive, socially responsive, self-reliant, and independent. They also appear to be strong, natural, and relaxed, and they function effectively in leadership roles. They are able to communicate their ideas effectively, although at times they impress others as somewhat cynical and sarcastic.

Summary of Descriptors*

A high L scale score is indicative of an individual who (is)

1. trying to create a favorable impression by not being honest in responding to the items
2. conventional; socially conforming
3. unoriginal in thinking; inflexible in problem solving
4. has poor tolerance for stress and pressure
5. rigid, moralistic
6. overevaluates own worth
7. utilizes repression and denial excessively
8. manifests little or no insight into own motivations
9. shows little awareness of consequences to other people of his/her own behavior
10. may be confused

A low L scale score is indicative of a person who (is)

1. responded frankly to the items
2. confident enough about self to be able to admit minor faults and shortcomings
3. perceptive, socially reliant

---

* The reader should recognize that the descriptors listed in this and subsequent summaries are *modal* ones and that all descriptors will not apply necessarily to all individuals with a given score or configuration of scores. The descriptors should be viewed as hypotheses to be validated by reference to the individual's history, to his behavior, and to his performance on other psychological tests.

4. self-reliant, independent
5. strong, natural, relaxed
6. functions effectively in leadership role
7. communicates ideas effectively
8. described by others as cynical, sarcastic

F SCALE

The F scale originally was developed to detect deviant or atypical ways of responding to the test items (Meehl & Hathaway, 1946). The 64 items in the F scale are ones that were answered in the scored direction by fewer than 10% of adult normal subjects. Thus, if the person who was just examined endorses many F scale items in the scored direction, he or she is said to be not responding as most normal people do. A subsequent factor analysis of the 64 F scale items by Comrey (1958) identified 19 content dimensions, tapping such diverse characteristics as paranoid thinking, antisocial attitudes or behavior, hostility, and poor physical health. A person can obtain a high F scale score by endorsing items in some, but not necessarily all, of these 19 content areas. In general, and because the scales of the MMPI are intercorrelated, high scores on the F scale are associated with elevated clinical scales, especially scales 6 and 8. Scores on the F scale also have been found to correlate with age and with race, with adolescents and blacks typically scoring higher on the F scale than other groups.

As used by the practicing clinician, the F scale serves three important functions. First, it is an index of test-taking attitude and is useful in detecting deviant response sets. Second, if one can rule out profile invalidity, the F scale is a good indicator of degree of psychopathology, with higher scores suggesting greater psychopathology. Finally, scores on the F scale allow inferences about extra-test behaviors.

High Scores on F Scale

When T-scores on the F scale are equal to or greater than 100 (raw score ≥ 26), a deviant response set that can invalidate the profile should be considered. For example, random responding, all true responding, and deliberate attempts to fake bad responses all result in F scale scores in this 100 range (see discussion of profile invalidity below for details about these deviant response sets). Seriously disturbed persons rarely produce such elevated F scale scores. However, Gynther, Altman, and Warbin (1973) have demonstrated reliable and potentially important correlates for psychiatric patients who do have F scale T-scores equal to or greater than 100. Such patients display delusions of reference, visual and auditory hallucinations, reduced speech, withdrawal, and poor judgment. In addition, they are likely to be monosyllabic, to have a short attention span, and to be disoriented for place. They may not know why they are in the hospital; they are likely to be diagnosed as psychotic; and there may be evidence of organic etiology.

In a T-score range of 80 to 99 (raw score = 16 to 25), F scale scores may be indicative of all false responding or of malingering (see discussion of profile invalidity below for details about these two response sets). It also is possible that the person is using the test to exaggerate his problems as a plea for help. Also, some individuals who are very resistant to the testing procedure produce scores in this range. If a deviant response set can be ruled out, F scale scores in this range are suggestive of very serious psychopathology. Many clearly psychotic individuals earn F scale scores at this level.

Psychotic persons and those labeled as severe neurotics often have F scale scores in a T-score range of 65 to 79 (raw score = 10 to 15). Also, individuals with very deviant social, political, or religious convictions have been found to score at this level. In such cases, examination of the actual items may be useful in detecting such convictions. Gough et al. (1955) have demonstrated that among people who are relatively free of serious psychopathology, scores in this range may indicate moodiness, restiveness, affection, restlessness, and dissatisfaction. In addition, such people may be changeable, unstable, curious, complex, opinionated, and opportunistic.

When F scale scores fall within a T-score range of 50 to 64 (raw score = 3 to 9), the person usually has endorsed items relevant to some particular content area (e.g., relationship with family, sexual concerns, health concerns, antisocial beliefs). Although such individuals may be experiencing difficulties in a specific area, they may be functioning effectively in other aspects of their life situations. The clinical practitioner who is interested in knowing such information about an examinee need simply write out on a sheet of paper each F scale item endorsed by him and scan these items for the content categories or information.

Low Scores on F Scale

T-scores in the 45 to 49 range (raw score = 0 to 2) indicate that the individual is answering items as most normal people do and thus is likely to be socially conforming in his everyday, extra-test behavior. Low scores obtained from subjects known to have significant psychopathology indicate that they are denying turmoil and psychological problems. Scores in this range also are found for people who deliberately are faking good responses on the test (see discussion of profile invalidity below for details about the faking good response set).

Summary of Descriptors

High F scale scores

A T-score equal to or greater than 100 (Raw score ≥ 26) is indicative of a person who (is):
1. may have responded to the MMPI items in a random way
2. may have answered all of the MMPI items true
3. may have been faking bad responses when he took the MMPI
4. if a hospitalized psychiatric patient, may manifest
   a. delusions of reference
   b. visual and/or auditory hallucinations
   c. reduced speech
   d. withdrawal

e. poor judgment

f. monosyllabic speech

h. short attention span

i. lack of knowledge of why he/she was hospitalized

j. a clinically arrived at diagnosis of psychosis

k. some extra-test signs of organic etiology

A T-score in a range of 80 to 99 (raw score 16 to 25) is indicative of a person who (is):

1. may have answered all MMPI items false

2. may be malingering

3. exaggerates symptoms as a plea for help

4. may be quite resistant to testing procedure

5. may be clearly psychotic by the usual criteria

A T-score in a range of 65 to 79 (raw score 10 to 15) is indicative of a person who (is):

1. has very deviant social, political, or religious convictions

2. may manifest clinically a severe neurotic or psychotic condition

3. if relatively free of serious psychopathology, is described as:

    a. moody

    b. restive

    c. affected

    d. restless

    e. dissatisfied

    f. changeable, unstable

    g. curious

    h. complex

    i. opinionated

    j. opportunistic

A T-score in a range of 50 to 64 (raw score 3 to 9) is indicative of an individual who (is):

1. has endorsed items relevant to some particular problem area

2. typically functions effectively in most aspects of his life situation

Low F scale scores

A T-score in a range of 45 to 49 (raw score 0 to 2) is indicative of an individual who (is):

1. answered items as most normal people do

2. socially conforming

3. free of disabling psychopathology

4. may have tried to fake a good profile

K SCALE

When early experience with the MMPI indicated that the L scale was quite insensitive to several kinds of test distortion, the K scale was developed as a more subtle and more effective index of attempts by the examinee to deny psychopathology and to present himself in a favorable light or, conversely, to exaggerate psychopathology and to try to appear in a very unfavorable light (Meehl & Hathaway, 1946; McKinley et al., 1948). High scores on the K scale thus were thought to be associated with a defensive approach to the test, whereas low scores were indicative of unusual frankness and self-criticality. In addition to identifying these deviations in test-taking attitudes, a statistical procedure also was developed for correcting scores on some of the clinical scales (see discussion of the K-correction in Chapter 2). The K scale was developed empirically by contrasting specific item responses of abnormal individuals who produced normal profiles with responses to the same items of a group of normals.

Subsequent research and experience with the MMPI have indicated that the K scale is much more complex than was intended originally. Scores on the K scale are related to socioeconomic status, with higher socioeconomic status individuals obtaining higher K scale scores. There has been little research to support the routine use of the K-correction to the clinical scales. Although the K-correction may lead to better discriminative power for each clinical scale, it does not necessarily improve the accuracy of the overall profile configuration. However, because the K-correction was adopted as a standard part of the MMPI scoring, and because virtually all information about profile interpretation is based on K-corrected scores, it is recommended that the K-correction be used routinely unless separate norms and interpretive data are available for uncorrected scores. Marks et al. (1974) have used such an approach in utilizing uncorrected scores in their codebook for adolescents, but they are a notable exception within the ranks of users of the MMPI.

The 30 items in the K scale cover several different content areas in which a person can deny problems (e.g., hostility, suspiciousness about motivations of other people, family dissension, lack of self-confidence, excessive worry). The K scale items tend to be much more subtle than items in the L scale; therefore, it is less likely that a defensive person will recognize the purpose of the items and will be able to avoid detection.

In interpreting K scale scores, it is essential that a person's socioeconomic status be taken into account. For college students and college-educated people, K scale scores in a T-score range of 55 to 70 should be considered average. Thus, scores must be greater than 70 to be considered high and less than 55 to be considered low for such people. For lower middle and upper lower class individuals, T-scores typically range from 40 to 60. Thus, for a score to be treated as a high score, it must exceed 60, whereas a score must be below 40 to be considered as a low score for such individuals.

High Scores on K Scale

When a K scale score is higher than is typically expected for a person's socioeconomic status, the possibility of a deliberate attempt to deny problems and psychopathology and thereby to appear in a favorable light or the possibility of all false responding should be considered (see discussion of profile invalidity below for details about these two response sets). High K scale scorers may be trying to maintain an appearance of adequacy, control, and effectiveness. High scorers tend to be shy and inhibited, and they are hesitant about becoming involved emotionally with other people. In addition, they are intolerant and unaccepting of unconventional beliefs and behavior in other people. They lack self-insight and self-understanding. Delinquency is unlikely among people with high scores on the K scale. When high K scale scores are accompanied by marked elevations on the clinical scales, it is likely that the person is quite seriously disturbed psychologically but has little or no awareness of his problems.

Average Scores on K Scale

When K scale scores fall within the range that is expected for a person's socioeconomic status, he is maintaining a healthy balance between positive self-evaluation and self-criticism. Such people tend to be well adjusted psychologically and to manifest few signs of emotional disturbance. They are independent, self-reliant, and capable of dealing with problems in their daily lives. They tend to have high intellectual abilities, to have wide interests, and to be ingenious, enterprising, versatile, and resourceful. They are clear thinking, and they approach problems in a reasonable and systematic way. In social situations, they mix well with other people, are enthusiastic and verbally fluent, and tend to take an ascendant role.

Low Scores on K Scale

When a person earns a K scale score lower than is expected for his socioeconomic status, the possibility of all true responding or of his deliberate attempt to present himself in an unfavorable light should be considered (see discussion of profile invalidity below for details about these two response sets). Low scores also may indicate that the subject is exaggerating his problems as a plea for help or that he is experiencing confusion that may be either organic or functional in nature.

Low scorers tend to be very critical of themselves and of others and to be quite self-dissatisfied. They may be quite ineffective in dealing with problems in their daily lives, and they tend to have little insight into their own motives and behavior. They are socially conforming and tend to be overly compliant with authority. They are inhibited, retiring, and shallow, and they have a slow personal tempo. They tend to be rather awkward socially and to be blunt and harsh in social interactions. Their outlook toward life is characterized as cynical, skeptical, caustic, and disbelieving, and they tend to be quite suspicious about the motivations of other people.

Summary of Descriptors

A high K scale score is indicative of an individual who (is)

1. may have tried to fake a good profile
2. may have responded false to most of the MMPI items
3. trying to give an appearance of adequacy, control, and effectiveness
4. shy, inhibited
5. hesitant about becoming emotionally involved with other people
6. intolerant, unaccepting of unconventional attitudes and beliefs in other people

7. lacks self-insight and self-understanding
8. not likely to display overt delinquent behavior
9. if clinical scales also are elevated, may be seriously disturbed psychologically but has little awareness of this

An average K scale score is indicative of an individual who (is)

1. maintained a healthy balance between positive self-evaluation and self-criticism in responding to the MMPI items
2. psychologically well adjusted
3. shows few overt signs of emotional disturbance
4. independent, self-reliant
5. capable of dealing with problems in daily life
6. has high intellectual ability
7. exhibits wide interests
8. ingenious, enterprising, versatile, resourceful
9. clear thinking, approaches problems in reasonable and systematic way
10. a good mixer
11. enthusiastic, verbally fluent
12. takes ascendant role

A low K scale score is indicative of an individual who (is)

1. may have responded true to most of the MMPI items
2. trying to fake a bad profile
3. may be exaggerating problems as a plea for help
4. exhibits either overt acute psychotic or organic confusion
5. critical of self and others, self-dissatisfied
6. ineffective in dealing with problems of daily life
7. shows little insight into own motives and behavior
8. socially conforming
9. overly compliant with authority
10. inhibited, retiring, shallow
11. has a slow personal tempo
12. socially awkward
13. blunt, harsh in social situations
14. cynical, skeptical, caustic, disbelieving
15. suspicious about motivations of other people

PROFILE INVALIDITY

Some MMPI users label as invalid and uninterpretable any protocol with more than 30 omitted items or with a T-score greater than 70 on one or more of the validity scales (L, F, K). Although this practice is a very conservative one and is not likely to result in labeling as valid profiles that are in fact invalid, it represents an oversimplified view of profile validity and causes many valid profiles to be discarded. For example, Dahlstrom and Welsh (1960) have indicated that F scores in a T-score range of 65 to 80 are more likely to be produced by psychotic and severely neurotic persons than by others. Gynther et al. (1973) have demonstrated that profiles with F scale scores equal to or greater than 100 can have reliable extra-test personality and behavioral correlates (e.g., disorientation, hallucinations, delusions, short attention span, etc.). In addition, the experienced clinician is not very surprised to encounter a K scale score greater than 70 among college-educated persons. Thus, it appears that a more sophisticated approach to profile validity is indicated.

Deviant Response Sets

To produce a valid protocol a person must read and consider the content of each MMPI item and respond to the item as true or false. Occasionally individuals respond in a stylistic way (e.g., false to *each* item) without reference to item content. Such behavior usually occurs among people who lack adequate reading skills, who are too confused to follow directions, or who have a very negativistic attitude toward the assessment procedure. Obviously, the examiner should try to be aware of such factors before administering the test, but sometimes, particularly in situations where large numbers of people are tested at once, such individuals do complete the test.

Random responding

One deviant response set involves a random or near random response to

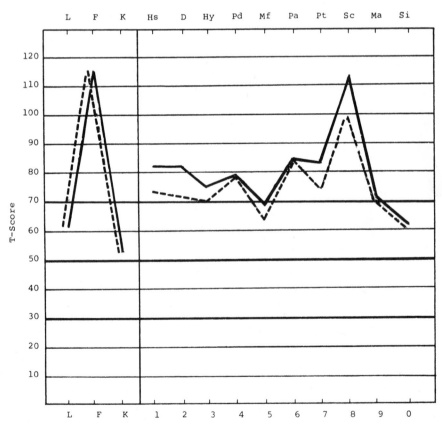

Fig. 3.1. K-corrected profiles indicative of random response set for males (———) and females (– – –).

the test items. A person may respond in a clearly random manner, or he or she may adopt an idiosyncratic response pattern such as marking every block of eight items as true, true, false, false, true, true, false, false, or every block of six items as true, false, true, false, true, false, and repeating this with each such subsequent block. Because the responses are made without regard to item content, the resulting protocol must be considered invalid. The profile configuration resulting from a completely random response set is shown in Figure 3.1. In the random response profile, the F scale is greater than 100 and scales L and K are both at or slightly above 50. The clinical scales are characterized by a *psychotic slope,* usually with a spike on scale 8 and a subspike on scale 6. Scales 5 and 0 remain below 70.

All true responding

If a person answers all items in the true direction, the resulting profile looks like the one presented in Figure 3.2. The salient features of the profile are an extremely elevated F scale score (usually off the top of the profile sheet), scales L and K well below 50, a positive (psychotic) slope, a spike on scale 8, and a subspike on scale 6.

All false responding

The person who responds false to all items will produce a profile like the

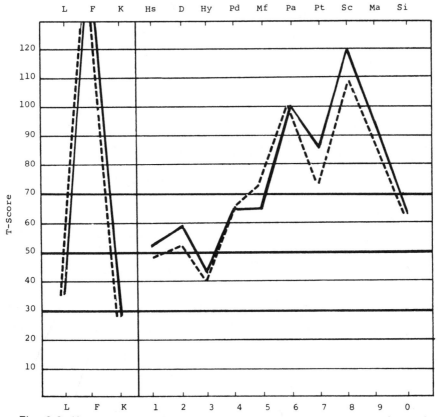

Fig. 3.2. K-corrected profiles indicative of all true response set for males (——) and females (– – –).

one shown in Figure 3.3. Note the simultaneous elevations on scales L, F, and K and the *neurotic-like slope* of the clinical scales.

Faking Bad

Some people (for example, court referrals, involuntary draftees, etc.) complete the MMPI with a desire to appear worse off or more pathological than they really are ("fake bad"). When this attempt is very direct and blatant, the resulting profile may at first glance appear to be suggestive of severe disturbance. A typical profile for a person who is faking bad is presented in Figure 3.4. Such a profile is characterized by a very elevated F scale score (often above 100) and L and K scale scores at or slightly below the mean. Except for scale 5, the clinical scales usually are quite elevated, with scales 6 and 8 as the highest two in the profile.

Gough (1950) has found that people who are trying to create the impression of severe psychopathology score considerably higher on the F scale than on the K scale. He has suggested that the difference between the F scale *raw score* and the K scale *raw score* can serve as a useful index for detecting fake bad profiles. Gough (1950) and Meehl (1951) indicated that when such an index number is positive and is greater than 9 it indicates

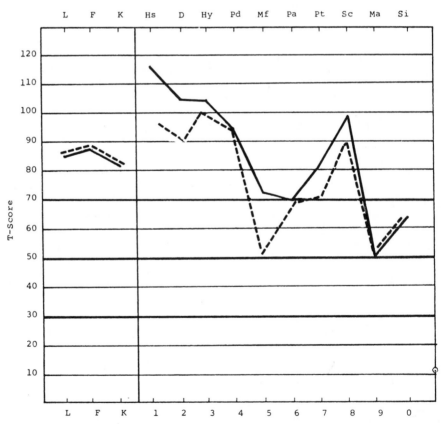

Fig. 3.3. K-corrected profiles indicative of all false response set for males (——) and females (– – –).

that a profile should be considered as a fake bad profile. Carson (1969) has suggested that a cut-off score of +11 yields a more accurate identification of fake bad profiles. Although a single cutoff score cannot be established for all settings, whenever the F scale raw score is greater than the K scale raw score the possibility of faking bad should be considered, and as the difference becomes greater the likelihood of a fake bad profile becomes greater.

The fake bad profile can be differentiated from that of a severely disturbed person in several ways. First, the F scale score is usually higher for the fake bad profile. The usual range of F scale scores in an individual who has been clinically diagnosed as psychotic is 70 to 90, whereas in the fake bad profile the F scale score usually is well above 100. In addition, in a valid profile from a disturbed person the L and K scales typically are elevated along with the F Scale. Finally, in a fake bad profile the clinical scales tend to be more extremely elevated than in a valid profile from a disturbed person.

Fake bad profiles can be differentiated from those resulting from random responding because in the fake bad profile the L and K scales usually are below the mean whereas in the random response profile they are somewhat above the mean. In addition, the random response profile usually has a

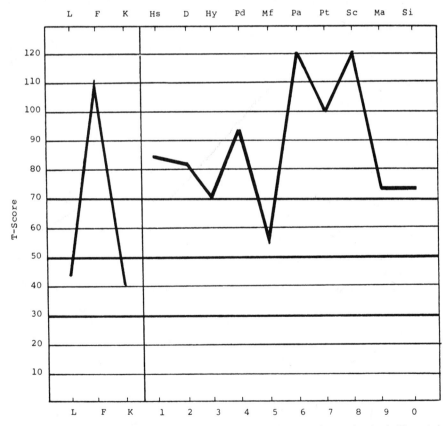

Fig. 3.4. Typical K-corrected profile produced by subject who is deliberately faking bad.

spike on scale 8, whereas the fake bad profile shows simultaneous extreme elevations on scales 6 and 8.

If one compares the fake bad profile with the profile resulting from an all true response set, several differences are obvious. First, in the all true profile the F scale score is much more elevated (greater than 120), and the L and K scale scores are lower than in the fake bad profile. Although both types of profiles show elevations for scales 6 and 8, in the all true profile the slope of the profile is more clearly psychotic-like, with scales 1, 2, and 3 at or near T-scores of 50.

The fake bad profile is easily differentiated from the profile resulting from an all false response set. Whereas the F scale is considerably higher than the L and K scales for the fake bad profile, in the all false profile all three scales are elevated simultaneously. In addition, the all false profile has a clearly negative slope.

If a person tends to exaggerate his symptoms but does not blatantly fake bad responses (malingering), the resulting profile is harder to differentiate from a valid one from a disturbed person. However, in the malingering

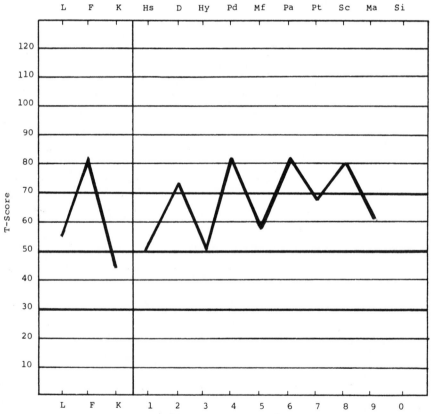

Fig. 3.5. K-corrected saw-toothed profile indicative of malingering. (From W. G. Dahlstrom & G. S. Welsh, *An MMPI Handbook: A Guide to Use in Clinical Practice and Research.* The University of Minnesota Press, Minneapolis. Copyright 1960 by the University of Minnesota. Reprinted with permission.)

profile, the F scale is not as extremely elevated as in the fake bad profile, and scales L and K are usually near 50. The most salient feature of the malingering profile is its *saw-toothed* appearance (Fig. 3.5). This results because the person who is malingering tends to endorse a wide array of the obviously pathological items which appear on scales 2, 4, 6, and 8.

Faking Good

Sometimes people completing the MMPI, including a surprising number of patients voluntarily seeking professional help, are motivated to deny problems and to appear better off psychologically than is in fact the case. In its most blatant form this tendency is referred to as "faking good." A typical profile resulting from such a test-taking attitude is presented in Figure 3.6. The clearest indication of a fake good profile is a *V-shaped* validity scale configuration with simultaneous elevations on scales L and K and an F scale score in a T-score range of 40 to 50. Most of the clinical scales will be in a T-score range of 30 to 50, with scale 5 often the highest of the clinical scales.

Because of the rather obvious nature of the L scale items, individuals who are bright, well educated, and psychologically sophisticated may

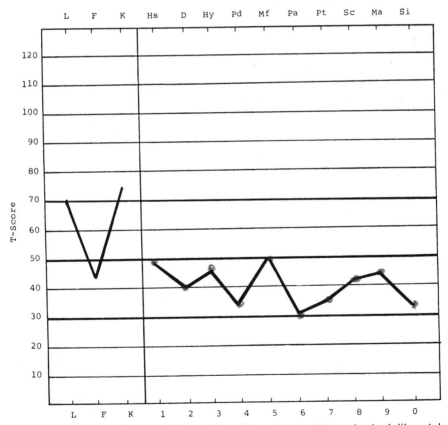

Fig. 3.6. Typical K-corrected profile produced by subject who is deliberately faking good.

detect the purpose of the items and will obtain a lower score on the L scale. However, because the K scale items are not as obvious as those in the L scale, even bright, well educated, and psychologically sophisticated people produce very elevated scores on the K scale if they adopt a fake good attitude toward the test. Before concluding that a high K scale score is indicative of a fake good strategy, the socioeconomic status of the person should be considered. Higher socioeconomic individuals tend to score higher on the K scale than do lower socioeconomic individuals, and scores in a T-score range of 60 to 70 do not necessarily imply faking for the higher socioeconomic individuals.

Some clinicians tend to use the F minus K index to identify fake good profiles as well as fake bad profiles. If the F scale *raw score* minus the K scale *raw score* is negative (K greater than F) and large, it may be that a fake good attitude is present. Whereas it is clear that a fake good profile does have a higher K scale than F scale score, it is not as easy to determine a cutoff score as is the case with fake bad profiles. The F minus K index is especially inappropriate for higher socioeconomic people, who tend to produce high K scale scores even if they are not faking good.

GENERAL SOURCES CONSULTED IN PREPARING CHAPTER 3

Carson, R. C. Interpretive manual to the MMPI. In J. N. Butcher (Ed.), *MMPI: Research Developments and Clinical Applications*. New York: McGraw-Hill, 1969.

Dahlstrom, W. G., Welsh, G. S., & Dahlstrom, L. E. *An MMPI Handbook: Volume I. Clinical Interpretation*. Minneapolis: University of Minnesota Press, 1972.

Duckworth, J. C., & Duckworth, E. *MMPI Interpretive Manual for Clinicians and Counselors*. Muncie, Ind.: Accelerated Development, Inc., 1975.

Lachar, D. *The MMPI: Clinical Assessment and Automated Interpretation*. Los Angeles: Western Psychological Services, 1974.

4

The Clinical Scales

A primary goal of this chapter is to discuss the nature of each clinical scale in an attempt to help the MMPI user understand the dimensions being reflected in and tapped by the scale. In addition, descriptive material is presented for high scorers and low scorers on each scale. In order to present information in a way that is most directly useful to the clinician, sources are not cited for each descriptor. The general approach utilized has been to examine all previously reported descriptive data for each scale, to augment these data from the author's own research and experience, and to present a meaningful synthesis of all data. The sources consulted in preparing this chapter are listed at the end of the chapter. The items included in each clinical scale and the keyed response for each item are presented in Appendix N of this *Guide*.

The definition of a high score on the clinical scales has varied considerably in the literature. Some writers consider a T-score above 70 as a high score. Others have defined high scores in terms of the upper quartile in a distribution. Still others have presented descriptors for several T-score levels. Another approach has been to identify the highest scale in the profile (high point) irrespective of its T-score value. A careful examination of the literature suggests that basically the same general picture of high scoring individuals emerges regardless of which of the above definitions is utilized. In his own clinical practice the author considers a T-score of 70 as a high score.

The individual clinician may make, if he or she wishes, whatever subjective adjustments are required to take into account a particular examinee's actual T-score level on a scale. In general, the higher the scores, the more likely it is that the descriptors discussed below will apply to an examinee. In addition, the intensity and salience of the inferred extra-test symptoms or behaviors are likely to increase as the elevation of a scale increases. Whenever the data clearly indicate that different descriptors are appropriate for different levels of high scores, the differences are discussed.

Limited information is available concerning the meaning of low scores on the clinical scales. Although it often has been assumed that low scorers on a scale are characterized by the absence of traits and/or behaviors that are present for high scorers, this is not always the case. Although low scores have been defined in several different ways in the literature, it generally is acceptable to consider T-scores below 45 as low scores. Whenever a low score is understood differently in this chapter, specific notation to that effect is made.

SCALE 1 (HYPOCHONDRIASIS)

Scale 1 originally was developed to identify patients who manifested a pattern of symptoms associated with the label of hypochondriasis. The syndrome is characterized in clinical terms by preoccupation with the body and concomitant fears of illness and disease. Although such fears are not of delusional quality, they are quite persistent.

Of all of the clinical scales of the MMPI, scale 1 seems to be the most clearly unidimensional in nature. All of the 33 items in the scale deal with somatic concerns or with general physical competence. Factor analytic studies have indicated that much of the variance in scale 1 scores is accounted for by a single factor, one that is characterized by the denial of good health and the admission of a variety of somatic symptoms.

High Scores on Scale 1

As might be expected, high scorers are characterized by excessive bodily concern. They tend to have generally vague, nonspecific complaints, particularly as scores become more elevated. When specific symptoms are elicited, they tend to be epigastric in nature. Chronic fatigue, pain, and weakness also tend to be characteristic of high scorers. Although medical patients with bona fide physical problems generally show somewhat elevated scores on scale 1, their scores are considerably lower than those obtained by psychiatric patients with somatization reactions. That high scores on scale 1 tend to be associated with neurotic conditions is suggested by the presence of clinical diagnoses such as hypochondriasis, neurasthenia, depression, or anxiety in psychiatric patients who score high on this scale. Psychopathic acting out is rare.

High scale 1 scorers in both psychiatric and nonpsychiatric samples tend to be characterized by a rather distinct set of personality attributes. They are likely to be selfish, self-centered, and narcissistic. Their outlook toward life tends to be pessimistic, defeatist, and cynical. They are generally dissatisfied and unhappy and are likely to make those around them miserable. They complain a great deal and communicate in a whiny manner. They are demanding of others and are very critical of what others do. Hostility is likely to be expressed in rather indirect ways. Scores on scale 1 seem to correlate negatively with intellectual ability, and high scorers often are described as dull, unenthusiastic, unambitious, and lacking ease in oral expression.

High scorers generally do not exhibit much manifest anxiety, and in general they do not show signs of major incapacity. Rather, they appear to be functioning at a reduced level of efficiency. Problems are much more likely to be long-standing than situational or transient in nature.

Because of their lack of insight and their generally cynical outlook, high scorers are not very responsive to psychotherapy or counseling. They tend to be very critical of their therapists and to terminate a relationship when the therapist is perceived as not giving them enough support and attention.

Low Scores on Scale 1

Because scale 1 is unidimensional in nature, low scorers tend to be very much the opposite of high scorers. In addition to being free of somatic preoccupation, they seem to be optimistic, alert, sensitive, insightful, and generally effective in their daily lives.

Summary of Descriptors for Scale 1

A high scale 1 score indicates an individual who (is)

1. has excessive bodily concern
2. has somatic symptoms that generally are vague, but if specific are likely to be epigastric in nature
3. complains of chronic fatigue, pain, and weakness
4. likely to have been given a neurotic diagnosis (hypochondriacal, neurasthenic, depressive)
5. lacks manifest anxiety
6. selfish, self-centered, narcissistic
7. has pessimistic, defeatist, cynical outlook
8. dissatisfied, unhappy
9. makes others miserable
10. complains
11. whiny
12. demanding and critical of others
13. expresses hostility indirectly
14. rarely acts out in psychopathic manner
15. dull, unenthusiastic, unambitious
16. ineffective in oral expression
17. has long-standing problems
18. in extra-test behavioral adjustment gives no indication of major incapacity but rather seems to be functioning at a reduced level of efficiency
19. not very responsive in psychotherapy or counseling because of lack of insight and cynical outlook
20. critical of therapist
21. tends to terminate therapy when therapist is perceived as not giving enough attention and support

A low scale 1 score indicates an individual who (is)

1. free of somatic preoccupation
2. optimistic
3. sensitive
4. insightful
5. generally effective in daily life

SCALE 2 (DEPRESSION)

Scale 2 was developed originally to assess symptomatic depression. The primary characteristics of symptomatic depression are poor morale, lack of hope in the future, and a general dissatisfaction with one's own life situation. Many of the 60 items in the scale deal with various aspects of depression such as denial of happiness and personal worth, psychomotor retardation and withdrawal, and lack of interest in one's surroundings. Other items in the scale cover a variety of other symptoms and behaviors, including physical complaints, worry or tension, denial of impulses, difficulty in controlling one's own thought processes, and religious fervor. Scale 2 seems to be an excellent index of an examinee's discomfort and dissatisfaction with his life situation. Whereas very elevated scores on this scale may be suggestive of clinical depression, more moderate scores tend to be indicative of a general attitude or life style characterized by poor morale and lack of involvement.

High Scores on Scale 2

High scorers on this scale (particularly if the T-scores exceed 80) often display depressive symptoms. They may report feeling depressed, blue, unhappy, or dysphoric. They tend to be quite pessimistic about the future in general and more specifically about the likelihood of overcoming their problems and making a better adjustment. Self-depreciation and guilt feelings are common. Behavioral manifestations may include refusal to speak, crying, and psychomotor retardation. Patients with high scores often receive depressive diagnoses, with depressive neurosis (reactive depression) being the most common. Other symptoms often found in high scorers include physical complaints, weakness, fatigue or loss of energy, agitation, and tension. They also are described as irritable, high-strung, and prone to worry.

High scorers also show a marked lack of self-confidence. They report feelings of uselessness and inability to function in a variety of situations. They see themselves as having failed to achieve adequately in school and at their jobs.

A lifestyle characterized by withdrawal and lack of intimate involvement with other people is common. High scorers tend to be described as introverted, shy, retiring, timid, seclusive, and secretive. Also, they tend to be aloof and to maintain psychological distance from other people. They often have a severely restricted range of interests and may withdraw from activities in which they previously have participated. They are very cautious and conventional in their activities.

High scorers may have great difficulty in making even simple decisions, and they may be overwhelmed when faced with major life decisions such as vocation, marriage, etc. They tend to be very overcontrolled and to deny their own impulses. They are likely to try to avoid unpleasantness and will make concessions in order to avoid confrontations.

Because a high scale 2 score is suggestive of great personal distress, it may indicate a good prognosis for psychotherapy or counseling. There is some evidence, however, that high scorers may tend to terminate treatment when the immediate crisis passes.

Low Scores on Scale 2

Low scorers on Scale 2 tend to be much more comfortable than high scorers. They indicate that they do not experience tension, anxiety, guilt, and depression and that they feel relaxed and at ease. They tend to be self-confident and generally are emotionally stable and capable of effective functioning in most situations. They are cheerful and optimistic and have little difficulty in verbal expression. They are alert, active, and energetic. They tend to seek out additional responsibilities and are seen as quite competitive by others.

Low scorers feel at ease in social situations and are rather quick to assume a leadership role. They appear to be clever, witty, and colorful, and they generally create very favorable first impressions.

Low scorers also tend to be somewhat impulsive and undercontrolled. Their lack of inhibitions leads them to be somewhat show-offish and exhibitionistic, and they may arouse hostility and resentment in other people. Also, they often find themselves in conflict with authority figures.

Summary of Descriptors for Scale 2

A high scale 2 score indicates a person who (is)

1. feels blue, depressed, unhappy, dysphoric
2. pessimistic about the future
3. self-depreciatory
4. harbors guilt feelings
5. refuses to speak
6. cries
7. slow moving, sluggish
8. depressive diagnosis (usually depressive neurosis or reactive depression)
9. has somatic complaints
10. complains of weakness, fatigue, loss of energy
11. agitated, tense
12. irritable, high-strung
13. prone to worry
14. lacks self-confidence
15. feels useless and unable to function
16. feels like a failure at school or on the job
17. introverted, shy, retiring, timid, seclusive, secretive
18. aloof
19. maintains psychological distance; avoids interpersonal involvement
20. cautious, conventional
21. difficulty in making decisions
22. nonaggressive
23. overcontrolled, denies impulses
24. avoids unpleasantness

25. makes concessions in order to avoid confrontations
26. because of discomfort, likely to be motivated for psychotherapy
27. may terminate treatment when immediate stress subsides

A low scale 2 score indicates a person who (is)

1. free of tension, anxiety, guilt, and depression
2. feels relaxed and at ease
3. self-confident
4. emotionally stable
5. functions effectively in most situations
6. cheerful, optimistic
7. has little difficulty in verbal expression
8. alert, active, energetic
9. competitive
10. seeks out responsibilities
11. at ease in social situations
12. assumes leadership role
13. clever, witty, colorful
14. creates favorable first impression
15. impulsive, undercontrolled
16. uninhibited, show-offish, exhibitionistic
17. arouses hostility and resentment in others
18. has conflict with authority figures

SCALE 3 (HYSTERIA)

This scale was developed to identify patients who were utilizing hysterical reactions to stress situations. The hysterical syndrome is characterized by involuntary psychogenic loss or disorder of function.

The 60 items comprising scale 3 are of two general types. Some of the items deal with a general denial of physical health and a variety of rather specific somatic complaints, including heart or chest pain, nausea and vomiting, fitful sleep, and headaches. Another group of items involves a rather general denial of psychological or emotional problems and of discomfort in social situations. Although these two clusters of items are reasonably independent in normal subjects, subjects utilizing hysterical defenses seem to score high on both clusters. In fact, it is not possible to obtain a T-score above 70 on scale 3 without endorsing both kinds of items.

Scores on scale 3 are related to intellectual ability, educational background, and social class. Brighter, better educated, and higher social class subjects tend to score higher on the scale. In addition, high scores, particularly when scale 3 is the highest point in the profile, are much more common for women than for men in both normal and psychiatric populations.

As an exception to the general statement made earlier in this chapter, it is important to take into account the level of scores on scale 3. Whereas marked elevations (T > 80) suggest a pathological condition characterized by classical hysterical symptomatology, moderate levels are associated with a number of characteristics that are consistent with hysterical disorders but which do not include the classical hysterical symptoms.

High Scores on Scale 3

Marked elevations on scale 3 may be suggestive of persons who react to stress and avoid responsibility by developing physical symptoms. The extra-test symptoms usually do not fit the pattern of any known organic disorder. They may include, in some combination, headaches, chest pains, weakness, tachycardia, and acute anxiety attacks. Nevertheless, such persons may be symptom-free most of the time, but under stress the symptoms appear suddenly; and they are likely to disappear just as suddenly when the stress subsides.

Except for the physical symptoms, high scorers tend to be relatively free of other symptoms. Although they sometimes describe themselves as prone to worry, they are not likely to report anxiety, tension, or depression. Hallucinations, delusions, and suspiciousness are rare. In fact, a psychotic diagnosis is almost never found among high scorers on scale 3. The most frequent diagnosis among psychiatric patients is hysterical neurosis (conversion hysteria).

A salient feature of the day-to-day functioning of high scorers is a marked lack of insight concerning the possible underlying causes of their symptoms. In addition, they show little insight concerning their own motives and feelings.

High scorers are often described as extremely immature psychologically, and at times even childish or infantile. They are quite self-centered, narcissistic, and egocentric, and they expect a great deal of attention and affection from others. They often use indirect and devious means to get the attention and affection they crave. When others do not respond appropriately, they may become hostile and resentful, but these feelings are likely to be denied and not expressed openly or directly.

High scale 3 scorers tend to be emotionally involved, friendly, talkative, enthusiastic, and alert. Although their needs for affection and attention drive them into social interactions, their interpersonal relationships tend to be rather superficial and immature. They are interested in other people primarily because of what they can get from them rather than because of a sincere interest in others.

Occasionally high scorers will act out in a sexual or aggressive manner with little apparent attention to or understanding of what they are doing. When confronted with the realities of their behavior, they may act surprised and feel resentful and persecuted.

Because of their needs for acceptance and affection, high scorers may initially be quite enthusiastic about counseling or psychotherapy. They often respond quite well to direct suggestion and advice. However, they are slow to gain insight into the underlying causes of their behavior, and they are quite resistant to psychological interpretations. Problems presented by high scorers frequently include worry about failure in school or work, marital unhappiness, lack of acceptance by their social groups, and problems with authority figures. Histories often include a rejecting father to whom females reacted with somatic complaints and males reacted with rebellion or overt hostility.

Low Scores on Scale 3

Low scorers on scale 3 tend to be rather constricted, conventional, and conforming in their everyday behaviors. They are described by others as unadventurous, as lacking industriousness, and as having a narrow range of interests.

They are cold and aloof and may display blunted affect. They are very limited in social interests and participation, and they tend to avoid leadership responsibilities. They often are seen as unfriendly and tough minded, and they are hard to get to know. They may have difficulties trusting other people, and in general they seem to be rather suspicious.

They are realistic, logical, and level headed in their approach to problems and are not likely to make impulsive decisions. They seem to be content with what others would judge to be a rather dull, uneventful life situation.

Summary of Descriptors for Scale 3

A high scale 3 score indicates an individual who (is)

1. reacts to stress and avoids responsibility through development of physical symptoms
2. has headaches, chest pains, weakness, tachycardia, anxiety attacks
3. has symptoms which appear and disappear suddenly
4. lacks insight concerning causes of symptoms
5. lacks insight concerning own motives and feelings
6. prone to worry
7. lacks anxiety, tension, and depression
8. rarely reports delusions, hallucinations, and suspiciousness
9. unlikely to be given a psychotic diagnosis
10. if a psychiatric patient, most frequently diagnosed as hysterical neurosis (conversion hysteria)
11. psychologically immature, childish, infantile
12. self-centered, narcissistic, egocentric
13. expects attention and affection from others
14. uses indirect and devious means to get attention and affection
15. does not openly express hostility and resentment
16. socially involved
17. friendly, talkative, enthusiastic, alert
18. has superficial and immature interpersonal relationships
19. interested in other people because of what he/she can get from them
20. occasionally acts out in sexual and aggressive manner with little apparent insight into his/her actions
21. initially enthusiastic about treatment
22. responds well to direct advice or suggestion
23. slow to gain insight into causes of own behavior

24. resistant to psychological interpretations and treatment
25. worries about failure in school or at work
26. experiences marital unhappiness
27. feels unaccepted by his/her social group
28. has problems with authority figures
29. has a history of a rejecting father

A low scale 3 score indicates a person who (is)

1. constricted, conventional, conforming
2. unadventurous; lacks industriousness
3. has a narrow range of interests
4. has limited social participation
5. avoids leadership role
6. unfriendly, tough minded, hard to get to know
7. suspicious, has difficulty trusting other people
8. realistic, logical, and level headed in approach to problems
9. seems content with dull, uneventful life situation

SCALE 4 (PSYCHOPATHIC DEVIATE)

Scale 4 was developed to identify patients diagnosed as psychopathic personality, asocial or amoral type. Whereas subjects included in the original criterion group were characterized in their everyday behavior by such delinquent acts as lying, stealing, sexual promiscuity, excessive drinking, and the like, no major criminal types were included. The 50 items in this scale cover a wide array of topics including absence of satisfaction in life, family problems, delinquency, sexual problems, and difficulties with authorities. Interestingly, the keyed responses include both admissions of social maladjustment and assertions of social poise and confidence.

Scores on scale 4 tend to be related to age. Adolescents and college students often score in a T-score range of 55 to 65. It also has been reported that black subjects tend to score higher than white subjects on scale 4. This latter finding may reflect the tendency of blacks to view many social regulations as unfair and therefore as less important in influencing their behavior.

High Scores on Scale 4

High scorers on scale 4 have great difficulty in incorporating the values and standards of society, and they are likely to engage in a wide array of asocial or antisocial behaviors. These behaviors may include lying, cheating, and stealing. Sexual acting out and excessive use of alcohol and/or drugs are not uncommon. High scorers tend to be rebellious toward authority figures and often are in conflict with authorities of one kind or another. They often have stormy relations with their families, and parents tend to be blamed for their difficulties. Underachievement in school, poor work history, and marital problems are characteristic of high scorers.

High scorers are very impulsive individuals who strive for immediate gratification of their impulses. They often do not plan their behavior very well, and they may act without considering the consequences of their actions. They are very impatient and have a limited frustration tolerance. Their behavior may involve poor judgment and considerable risk taking. They tend not to profit from experiences and may find themselves in the same difficulties time and time again.

High scorers are described by others as immature and childish. They are narcissistic, self-centered, selfish, and egocentric. Their behavior often is ostentatious and exhibitionistic. They are insensitive to the needs and feelings of other people and are interested in others in terms of how they can be used. Although they tend to be seen as likeable and generally create a good impression, their relationships with other people tend to be shallow and superficial. This may be in part due to rejection on the part of the people they mistreat, but it also seems to reflect their own inability to form warm attachments with others.

In addition, high scorers typically are very extroverted and outgoing. They are talkative, active, adventurous, energetic, and spontaneous. They are judged by others to be intelligent and self-confident. Although they have a wide range of interests and may become involved in many activities, they lack definite goals and their behavior lacks clear direction.

High scorers tend to be very hostile and aggressive. Their attitude is characterized by sarcasm and cynicism. They are very resentful and rebellious and are prone to act out their aggressive impulses. They also are described as antagonistic and refractory. Aggressive outbursts, sometimes accompanied by assaultive behavior, are common, and often such behavior is not accompanied by guilt. Whereas the high scorers may feign guilt and remorse when their behaviors get them into trouble, such responses are short-lived, disappearing when the immediate crisis passes.

Generally, high scorers are free from disabling felt anxiety and depression. Likewise, psychotic symptoms are uncommon. Among psychiatric patients, a personality disorder diagnosis is most common, with sociopathic personality or passive-aggressive personality occurring most frequently. However, beneath the facade of a carefree and comfortable person, one is likely to find evidence of worry and dissatisfaction. There may be an absence of deep emotional response, and this lack may produce feelings of boredom and emptiness.

Because of their verbal facility, outgoing manner, and apparent intellectual resources, high scorers often are perceived as good candidates for psychotherapy or counseling. Unfortunately, the prognosis for change is poor. Although they may agree to treatment to avoid something more unpleasant (e.g., jail or divorce), they generally are unable to accept blame for their own problems, and terminate treatment as soon as possible. They tend to utilize intellectualization and to blame others for their difficulties.

Low Scores on Scale 4

Low scorers on scale 4 tend to be very conventional, conforming, and accepting of authority. They are rather passive, submissive, and unassertive. They are concerned about how others will react to them, and they tend to be sincere and trusting in their interpersonal relationships.

Low scorers are characterized by a low level of drive. Although they are concerned about status and security, they do not tend to be very competitive. They have a narrow range of interests, and although they are not creative or spontaneous in their approach to problems, they tend to be very persistent. Low scorers also are seen as moralistic and rigid in their views. Males do not seem to be very much interested in sex, and they may actually be afraid of women.

Low scorers tend to be very critical of themselves, and unwarranted self-dissatisfaction is common. They are accepting of advice and suggestion. Although they may initially respond well to psychotherapy or counseling, they tend to become very dependent on treatment and often are afraid to accept responsibility for their own behavior.

Summary of Descriptors for Scale 4

A high scale 4 score indicates a person who (is)

1. has difficulty in incorporating values and standards of society
2. engages in asocial or antisocial behavior
   a. lying, cheating, stealing
   b. sexual acting out
   c. excessive use of alcohol and/or drugs
3. rebellious toward authority figures
4. has stormy family relationships
5. blames parents for his/her problems
6. has a history of underachievement in school
7. has a poor work history
8. experiences marital problems
9. impulsive; strives for immediate gratification of impulses
10. does not plan well
11. acts without considering consequences of actions
12. impatient, has limited frustration tolerance
13. shows poor judgment, takes risks
14. does not profit from experience
15. immature, childish
16. narcissistic, self-centered, selfish, egocentric
17. ostentatious, exhibitionistic
18. insensitive to others
19. interested in others in terms of how they can be used
20. likeable, creates a good first impression
21. has shallow, superficial relationships
22. unable to form warm attachments
23. extroverted, outgoing
24. talkative, active, adventurous, energetic, spontaneous
25. intelligent, self-confident
26. has a wide range of interests
27. lacks definite goals
28. hostile, aggressive
29. sarcastic, cynical

30. resentful, rebellious
31. acts out
32. antagonistic, refractory
33. has aggressive outbursts, assaultive behavior
34. experiences little guilt over behavior
35. may feign guilt and remorse when in trouble
36. free from disabling anxiety, depression, and psychotic symptoms
37. likely to receive a personality disorder diagnosis (antisocial personality or passive-aggressive personality)
38. prone to worry, dissatisfied
39. has an absence of deep emotional response
40. feels bored, empty
41. has a poor prognosis for change in psychotherapy or counseling
42. tends to blame others for his/her problems
43. uses intellectualization
44. may agree to treatment to avoid jail or some other unpleasant experience but is likely to terminate prematurely

A low scale 4 score indicates a person who (is)

1. conventional, conforming
2. accepting of authority
3. passive, submissive, unassertive
4. concerned about how others will react
5. sincere, trusting
6. has low drive, not competitive
7. concerned about status and security
8. has a narrow range of interests
9. not creative or spontaneous
10. persistent
11. moralistic, rigid
12. if a male, not very interested in sex; afraid of women
13. critical of self, self-dissatisfaction
14. accepting of advice and suggestion
15. may become very dependent in treatment
16. afraid to accept responsibility for own behavior

SCALE 5 (MASCULINITY-FEMININITY)

Scale 5 originally was developed by Hathaway and McKinley to identify homosexual invert males. Because of the heterogeneity of the homosexual sample, the test authors could identify only a very small number of cases characterized by sexual inversion and relatively free of neurotic, psychotic, and psychopathic tendencies. Thus, items also were added to this scale if they differentiated between high and low scoring males on the Terman and Miles Attitude Interest Test or if they were endorsed differentially by normal males and females. Although Hathaway and McKinley considered this scale as a preliminary one, it has come to be used in its original form as a standard clinical scale.

The test authors attempted unsuccessfully to develop a corresponding scale for identifying sexual inversion in females. As a result, the standard procedure is to use scale 5 for both male and female subjects. Fifty-five of the items are keyed in the same direction for both sexes, whereas five of the items, all dealing with frankly sexual material, are keyed in opposite directions for males and females. After obtaining raw scores, T-score conversions are reversed for the sexes, so that a high raw score for males automatically is transformed by means of the profile sheet itself to a high T-score whereas a high raw score for females is transformed to a low T-score. The result is that a high T-score for both sexes is indicative of deviation from one's own sex.

Although some of the 60 items in scale 5 deal with frankly sexual material, most items are not sexual in nature and cover a diversity of topics, including interests in work, hobbies and pastimes, worries, fears, and sensitivities, social activities, religious preferences, and family relationships.

Scores on scale 5 are related to intelligence, education, and socioeconomic level, with brighter, better educated, and higher social class subjects obtaining higher scores. It is not uncommon for college students, or college-educated persons, to obtain scores in a T-score range of 60 to 70. These expected elevations are particularly important in determining whether scores should be considered to be extremely elevated. Although a T-score of 80 would be considered extreme for a person with limited formal education and from a lower social class, it would be only a moderate elevation for a better educated person from a middle or upper middle class.

Because of the reversal of scoring with scale 5, high T-scores have different meanings for males and females. Some writers have suggested that high scores for males are equivalent to low scores for females and that both indicate feminine interests and attitudes. A careful analysis of the data for high scoring males and females indicates that such an understanding is a great oversimplification. Thus, high scores and low scores are discussed separately for males and females.

High Scores on Scale 5 (Males)

Although there has been a great reluctance to infer homosexuality from high scores on scale 5, the possibility of homoerotic trends or homosexual behavior must be considered when extreme elevations are obtained, particularly if the scores deviate markedly from what is expected based on the subject's intelligence, education, and social class. Of course, one would want other confirming data before concluding that a subject was homosexual. High scores also may be indicative of conflicts in sexual identity and insecurity in one's masculine role, and high scorers may display clearly effeminate behavior.

High scores for males on scale 5 are indicative of a lack of stereotyped masculine interests. High scoring males tend to have aesthetic and artistic interests, and they are likely to participate in housekeeping and childrearing activities to a greater extent than do most men.

High scoring males are intelligent, capable persons who value cognitive pursuits. They are characterized as ambitious, competitive, and persevering. They are clever, clear-thinking, organized, and logical, and they show good judgment and common sense. They are very curious and may be creative, imaginative, and individualistic in their approach to problems.

Sociability and sensitivity to others are also characteristic of high scoring males. They are quite tolerant of other people and are capable of expressing warm feelings toward them. In interpersonal situations high scoring males tend to be very passive, dependent, and submissive. They are peace loving and will make many concessions to avoid confrontations.

There is some evidence that high scores for males are indicative of good self-control. Acting out behavior is quite rare among high scorers. Even in subgroups with a high degree of delinquency, high scoring males on scale 5 are not likely to display delinquent behavior.

High Scores on Scale 5 (Females)

The most striking feature of high scoring females on scale 5 is their rejection of the traditional female role. Their interests in sports, hobbies, and other activities tend to be more masculine than feminine, and they tend to choose traditionally masculine occupations or professions. They are described as active, vigorous, and assertive. They also tend to be very competitive, aggressive, and dominating, and they are seen by others as rather coarse, rough, and tough.

High scoring females are very outgoing, uninhibited, and self-confident. They are easy going, relaxed, and balanced. They are rather logical and calculated in their behavior and may be rather unemotional. They are seen as unfriendly by many people.

Among hospitalized psychiatric patients, high scoring females tend to be diagnosed as psychotic. They may exhibit hallucinations, delusions, and suspiciousness, but acting out behavior is uncommon.

Low Scores on Scale 5 (Males)

Males who score low on scale 5 are presenting themselves as extremely masculine. They have clearly masculine preferences in work, hobbies, and other activities. They place an overemphasis on physical strength and prowess. They also are described as aggressive, thrill-seeking, adventurous, and reckless. Coarse, crude, and vulgar talk and behavior are not uncommon. The exaggerated nature of their attitudes and behaviors suggests that they may be covering up basic doubts about their own masculinity.

Low scoring males are seen by others as having limited intellectual ability. They have a narrow range of interests and are rather inflexible and unoriginal in their approach to problems. They prefer action to thought and are practical and nontheoretical.

Other people see low scoring males as easy going, leisurely, and relaxed. They also are described as cheerful, jolly, and humorous. They seem to be reasonably contented and are willing to settle down. However, they seem to be unaware of their social stimulus values and lack insight into their own motives.

Low Scores on Scale 5 (Females)

Comparatively little information is available concerning females who score low on scale 5. However, it is clear that low scoring females are describing themselves in terms of a stereotyped female role. Again, as with low scoring males, the exaggerated nature of their attitudes and behaviors suggest that they may be covering up doubts that their own adequacy as females.

Low scoring females tend to be very passive, submissive, and yielding. They are likely to defer to men in decisionmaking. They may be self-pitying, complaining, and fault finding.

Other people describe low scoring females as constricted, sensitive, modest, and idealistic. Among hospitalized psychiatric patients, low scoring females are not likely to be psychotic and may show more social competence than other female patients.

Summary of Descriptors for Scale 5

A high scale 5 score for males indicates a person who (is)

1. conflicted about his sexual identity
2. insecure in masculine role
3. effeminate
4. has aesthetic and artistic interests
5. intelligent, capable; values cognitive pursuits
6. ambitious, competitive, persevering
7. clever, clear-thinking, organized, logical
8. shows good judgment, common sense
9. curious
10. creative, imaginative, and individualistic in approach to problems
11. sociable; sensitive to others
12. tolerant
13. capable of expressing warm feelings toward others
14. passive, dependent, submissive in interpersonal relationships
15. peace-loving; makes concessions to avoid confrontations
16. has good self-control; acting out is rare
17. may display homoerotic trends or overt homosexual behavior

A high scale 5 score for females indicates a person who (is)

1. rejects the traditional female role
2. has masculine interests in work, sports, hobbies
3. active, vigorous, assertive
4. competitive, aggressive, dominating
5. coarse, rough, tough
6. outgoing, uninhibited; self-confident
7. easy-going, relaxed, balanced
8. logical, calculated
9. unemotional
10. unfriendly

11. if a psychiatric patient, may exhibit hallucinations, delusions, and suspiciousness, but is not likely to act out
12. if a psychiatric patient, likely to be given a psychotic diagnosis

A low scale 5 score for males indicates a person who (is)

1. presents himself as extremely masculine
2. overemphasizes strength and physical prowess
3. aggressive, thrill-seeking, adventurous, reckless
4. coarse, crude, vulgar
5. harbors doubts about his own masculinity
6. has limited intellectual ability
7. has a narrow range of interests
8. inflexible and unoriginal approach to problems
9. prefers action to thought
10. practical, nontheoretical
11. easy-going, leisurely, relaxed
12. cheerful, jolly, humorous
13. contented; willing to settle down
14. unaware of social stimulus value
15. lacks insight into own motives

A low scale 5 score for females indicates a person who (is)

1. describes herself in terms of stereotyped female role
2. has doubts about her own femininity
3. passive, submissive, yielding
4. defers to males in decision-making
5. self-pitying
6. complaining, fault finding
7. constricted
8. sensitive
9. modest
10. idealistic
11. if a hospitalized psychiatric patient, not likely to be psychotic
12. if a hospitalized psychiatric patient, likely to show more social competence than other female patients

SCALE 6 (PARANOIA)

Scale 6 originally was developed to identify patients who were judged to have paranoid symptoms such as ideas of reference, feelings of persecution, grandiose self-concepts, suspiciousness, excessive sensitivity, and rigid opinions and attitudes. Although the scale was considered as preliminary because of problems in cross-validation, a major reason for its retention was that it produces relatively few false positives. Persons who score high on the scale usually have paranoid symptoms. However, some patients with clearly paranoid symptoms are able to achieve average scores on scale 6.

Although some of the 60 items in the scale deal with frankly psychotic behaviors (suspiciousness, ideas of reference, delusions of persecution, grandiosity, etc.), many items cover such diverse topics as sensitivity, cynicism, asocial behavior, excessive moral virtue, rigidity, and complaints about other people. It is quite possible to obtain a T-score greater than 70 without endorsing any of the frankly psychotic items.

Although scores on scale 6 are reasonably independent of age, education, and intelligence, black subjects score consistently higher than white subjects. Rather than suggesting gross psychopathology, these elevated scores may reflect the views of many blacks that they are getting a raw deal in life and their generally suspicious attitudes concerning the motives of whites.

Interpretation of scores on scale 6 is very complicated because the scale clearly is not bipolar in nature. Very deviant scores (T > 75) generally are suggestive of frank paranoid or psychotic behavior. More moderate elevations (T = 65 to 75) are associated with a paranoid predisposition. Mild elevations (T = 55 to 65) generally are obtained by persons who are described in fairly positive terms. Moderately low scores (T = 35 to 45) have different meanings for normal and disturbed subjects. The former are seen in generally positive terms, whereas the latter are described more negatively. When scores on scale 6 are extremely low (T < 35), especially if the scale is the lowest one in the profile, one suspects paranoid or psychotic behavior, but it may not be as obvious as with extreme elevations. Because of the complexity of scale 6, a simple dichotomization into high scores and low scores would be a vast oversimplification.

High Scores on Scale 6

Extreme elevations

When scale 6 is elevated above a T-score of 75, and especially when it also is the highest scale in the profile, subjects may exhibit frankly psychotic behavior. Their thinking may be disturbed, and they may have delusions of persecution and/or grandeur. Ideas of reference also are common. They may feel mistreated and picked on; they may be angry and resentful; and they may harbor grudges. Projection is a common defense mechanism. Diagnoses of paranoid schizophrenia or paranoid state are most frequent.

Moderate elevations

When scale 6 scores are within a T-score range of 65 to 75, frankly psychotic symptoms are not as common. However, subjects within this range are characterized by a variety of traits and behaviors that may suggest a paranoid predisposition. They tend to be excessively sensitive and overly responsive to the opinions of others. They feel that they are getting a raw deal out of life and tend to rationalize and to blame others for their own difficulties. Also, they are seen as suspicious and guarded. Hostility, resentment, and an argumentative manner are common. They tend to be very moralistic and rigid in their opinions and attitudes. Rationality is likely to be overemphasized greatly. Prognosis for psychotherapy is poor, because these subjects do not like to talk about emotional problems and are likely to rationalize most of the time. They have great difficulty in establishing rapport with therapists. In therapy, they are likely to reveal hostility and resentment toward family members.

Mild elevations

Subjects scoring within a T-score range of 55 to 65 generally are seen in rather positive ways, particularly if they are not psychiatric patients. They are described as kind, affectionate, generous, sentimental, soft hearted, and peaceable. They also tend to be sensitive to what is going on around them and to be trusting of other people. Although they are cooperative, they tend to be rather frank. They have a wide range of interests and seem to be energetic and industrious. They display much initiative and become ego-involved in work and activities. They are seen as poised, intelligent, fair minded, rational, clear thinking, and insightful. On the more negative side, they are submissive and dependent in interpersonal relationships, and they tend to lack self-confidence. They describe themselves as high-strung and prone to worry.

Low Scores on Scale 6

Moderately low scores on scale 6 (T = 34 to 45) seem to have somewhat different meanings for normal subjects and for subjects who are psychiatric patients or for whom there is other evidence of maladjustment. For normal subjects, particularly if they are above average in intelligence and/or education, rather positive adjectives, such as cheerful, balanced, serious, orderly, mature, and reasonable, are suggested. They tend to be seen as wise, decisive, and persevering. They are socially interested and tend to face life situations adequately. They are trustful and loyal. They tend to be cautious, conventional, and self-controlled in their approach to problems. Scores in this same range, if obtained by disturbed subjects, are suggestive of negative traits and behaviors. Such subjects are seen as stubborn, evasive, and guarded. They are likely to be self-centered and to show little concern for things that do not affect them directly. Self-dissatisfaction and oversensitivity to the reactions of others are common. These subjects are rather uninsightful and lack social interest and social skills. They have a narrow range of interests and tend to be inflexible in their approach to problems. They do not have very strong consciences and have little regard for principles. Other adjectives applied to such subjects are rough, awkward, undependable, touchy, antagonistic, and underachieving. Among hospitalized psychiatric patients, psychotic symptoms or diagnoses are not common.

Extremely low scores(T < 35) should alert the clinician to the possibility of a frank paranoid disorder. Whereas subjects with scores in this range may have delusions, suspiciousness, and ideas of reference, these may be less obvious to others than is true for extremely high scorers. They tend to be very evasive, defensive, and guarded. Rather than being openly hostile, aggressive, and abrasive, they seem more shy, secretive, and withdrawn.

Summary of Descriptors for Scale 6

An extreme scale 6 elevation (T > 75) indicates an individual who (is)

1. manifests frankly psychotic behavior
2. has disturbed thinking
3. has delusions of persecution and/or grandeur
4. has ideas of reference
5. feels mistreated or picked on
6. angry, resentful; harbors grudges
7. uses projection as a defense mechanism
8. most frequently is given a diagnosis of schizophrenia or paranoid state

A moderate scale 6 elevation (T = 65 to 75) indicates an individual who (is)

1. has a paranoid predisposition
2. sensitive; overly responsive to reactions of others
3. feels he is getting a raw deal from life
4. rationalizes; blames others for own difficulties
5. suspicious, guarded
6. hostile, resentful, argumentative
7. moralistic, rigid
8. overemphasizes rationality
9. has a poor prognosis for psychotherapy
10. does not like to talk about emotional problems
11. has difficulty in establishing rapport with therapist
12. expresses hostility and resentment toward family members

A mild scale 6 elevation (T = 55 to 65) indicates an individual who (is)

1. kind, affectionate, generous
2. sentimental, soft hearted, peaceable
3. sensitive
4. trusting
5. cooperative
6. frank
7. has a wide range of interests
8. energetic, industrious
9. shows initiative, becomes ego-involved in work and other activities
10. poised, intelligent, fair minded, rational, clear thinking, insightful
11. submissive
12. lacks self-confidence
13. high-strung, prone to worry

A moderately low scale 6 elevation (T = 35 to 45) indicates an individual who (is)

1. if not a psychiatric patient and with no other evidence of maladjustment
   a. cheerful
   b. balanced

    c. orderly

    d. serious, mature, reasonable

    e. wise, decisive, persevering

    f. socially interested

    g. faces life situations adequately

    h. trustful, loyal

    i. cautious, conventional, self-controlled

2. if a psychiatric patient or with other evidence of maladjustment

    a. stubborn, evasive, guarded

    b. self-centered

    c. shows little concern for things that do not affect him/her directly

    d. self-dissatisfied

    e. overly sensitive to reactions of others

    f. uninsightful

    g. lacks social interests and social skills

    h. has weak conscience, little regard for principles

    i. rough, awkward

    j. undependable

    k. underachieving

    l. touchy, antagonistic

    m. not likely to manifest psychotic symptoms; psychotic diagnosis not common

An extremely low scale 6 elevation (T < 35) indicates an individual who (is)

1. may have a frankly paranoid disorder
2. may have delusions, exhibits suspiciousness, ideas of reference
3. has symptoms that are less obvious than those of extremely high scorers
4. evasive, defensive, guarded
5. shy, secretive, withdrawn

SCALE 7 (PSYCHASTHENIA)

    Scale 7 originally was developed to measure the general symptomatic pattern labeled psychasthenia. Although this label is not used commonly today, it was popular when the scale was developed. Among currently popular diagnostic categories, the obsessive-compulsive neurosis probably is closest to the original psychasthenia label. Persons diagnosed as psychasthenic had thinking characterized by excessive doubts, compulsions, obsessions, and unreasonable fears. This symptom pattern was much more common among outpatients than among hospitalized patients, so the number of cases available for scale construction was small.

    The 48 items in scale 7 cover a variety of symptoms and behaviors. Many of the items deal with uncontrollable or obsessive thoughts, feelings of fear and/or anxiety, and doubts about one's own ability. Unhappiness, physical complaints, and difficulties in concentration also are represented in the scale.

High Scores on Scale 7

Scale 7 is a good index of psychological turmoil and discomfort. High scorers tend to be very anxious, tense, and agitated. They worry a great deal, even over very small problems, and are fearful and apprehensive. They are high-strung and jumpy and report difficulties in concentrating.

High scorers tend to be very introspective, and obsessive thinking, compulsive and ritualistic behavior, and ruminations are common. The obsessions and ruminations often center around feelings of insecurity and inferiority. They lack self-confidence, are self-critical, self-conscious, and self-degrading, and are plagued by self-doubts. High scorers tend to be very rigid and moralistic and to have high standards of behavior and performance for themselves and others. They are likely to be quite perfectionistic and conscientious; they may feel guilty about not living up to their own standards and depressed about falling short of goals.

In general, high scorers are neat, orderly, organized, and meticulous. They are persistent and reliable, but they lack ingenuity and originality in their approach to problems. They are seen by others as dull and formal. They have great difficulties in decisionmaking, and they may vacillate and be indecisive over very small, routine decisions. In addition, they are likely to distort the importance of problems and to be quite overreactive to stress situations.

High scorers tend to be shy and do not interact well socially. They are described as hard to get to know, and they worry a great deal about popularity and social acceptance. Other people see them as sentimental, peaceable, soft-hearted, trustful, sensitive, and kind. Other adjectives used to describe them include dependent, individualistic, verbal, emotional, and immature.

Some high scorers express physical complaints. These may center around the heart, the gastrointestinal system, or the genitourinary system. Complaints of fatigue, exhaustion, and insomnia are not uncommon.

Although high scorers may be uncomfortable and miserable, they are not very responsive in brief psychotherapy or counseling. In spite of some insight into their problems, they tend to rationalize and to intellectualize a great deal. They often are resistant to interpretations and may express much hostility toward the therapist. However, they tend to remain in therapy longer than most patients, and they may show very slow but steady progress. Problems presented in therapy may include difficulties with authority figures, poor work or study habits, or concern about homosexual impulses.

Low Scores on Scale 7

Low scorers on scale 7 seem to be very capable and well adjusted. They are free of disabling fears and anxieties and are very self-confident. They are perceived as warm, cheerful, and friendly. They have a wide range of interests and are responsible, efficient, realistic, and adaptable. Success, status, and recognition are important to them.

Summary of Descriptors for Scale 7

A high scale 7 score indicates an individual who (is)

1. experiences turmoil and discomfort
2. anxious, tense, agitated
3. worried, apprehensive
4. high-strung, jumpy
5. has difficuties in concentrating
6. introspective, ruminative
7. obsessive in his/her thinking
8. has compulsive behaviors
9. feels insecure and inferior
10. lacks self-confidence
11. has self-doubts; self-critical; self-conscious; self-derogatory
12. rigid, moralistic
13. has high standards for himself/herself and others
14. perfectionistic, conscientious
15. guilty, depressed
16. neat, orderly, organized, meticulous
17. persistent
18. reliable
19. lacks ingenuity and originality in approach to problems
20. dull, formal
21. vascillates, is indecisive
22. distorts importance of problems; overreacts
23. shy
24. does not interact well socially
25. hard to get to know
26. worries about popularity and acceptance
27. sentimental, peaceable, soft-hearted, trustful, sensitive, kind
28. dependent
29. individualistic
30. unemotional
31. immature
32. has physical complaints
    a. heart
    b. genitourinary
    c. gastrointestinal
    d. fatigue, exhaustion, insomnia
33. not responsive to brief psychotherapy
34. shows some insight into problems
35. intellectualizes, rationalizes
36. resistant to interpretations in psychotherapy
37. expresses hostility toward therapist
38. remains in psychotherapy longer than most patients
39. makes slow but steady progress in psychotherapy
40. discusses in therapy problems including difficulties with authority figures, poor work or study habits, and concern about homosexual impulses

A low scale 7 score indicates an individual who (is)

1. capable
2. well adjusted
3. free of disabling fears and anxiety
4. self-confident
5. has a wide range of interests
6. responsible, efficient, realistic, adaptable
7. values success, status, and recognition

SCALE 8 (SCHIZOPHRENIA)

Scale 8 was developed to identify patients diagnosed as schizophrenic. This category included a heterogeneous group of disorders characterized by disturbances of thinking, mood, and behavior. Misinterpretations of reality, delusions, and hallucinations may be present. Ambivalent or constricted emotional responsiveness is common. Behavior may be withdrawn, aggressive, or bizarre.

The 78 items in scale 8 cover a wide array of behaviors. Some of the items deal with such frankly psychotic symptoms as bizarre mentation, peculiarities of perception, delusions of persecution, and hallucinations. Other topics covered include social alienation, poor family relationships, sexual concerns, difficulties in impulse control and concentration, and fears, worries, and dissatisfactions.

Scores on scale 8 are related to age and to race. Adolescents and college students often obtain T-scores in a range of 55 to 65, perhaps reflecting the turmoil associated with that period in life. Black subjects, particularly males, tend to score higher than white subjects. The elevated scores for blacks do not necessarily suggest greater overt psychopathology. They may simply be indicative of the alienation and social estrangement experienced by many blacks. Some elevations of scale 8 can be accounted for by subjects who are reporting a large number of unusual experiences, feelings, and perceptions related to the use of drugs.

High Scores on Scale 8

Although one should be cautious about concluding that a subject is schizophrenic on the basis of only the score on scale 8, T-scores in a range of 80 to 90 suggest the possibility of an extra-test psychotic condition. Confusion, disorganization, and disorientation may be present. Unusual thoughts or attitudes, perhaps even delusional in nature, hallucinations, and extremely poor judgment may be evident. Extreme scores on scale 8 (T > 100) usually are not produced by psychotic subjects. They are more likely to be indicative of an individual who is in acute psychological turmoil or of a less disturbed individual who is endorsing many deviant items as a cry for help.

High scores on scale 8 may suggest a schizoid life style. High scorers tend to feel as if they are not part of their social environments. They feel isolated, alienated, misunderstood, and unaccepted by their peers. They are withdrawn, seclusive, secretive, and inaccessible. They may avoid dealing with people and with new situations. They are described by others as shy, aloof, and uninvolved.

High scorers experience a great deal of very generalized anxiety. They may feel very resentful, hostile, and aggressive, but they are unable to express such feelings. A typical response to stress is withdrawal into daydreams and fantasies, and some subjects may have a difficult time in separating reality and fantasy.

High scorers may be plagued by self-doubts. They feel inferior, incompetent, and dissatisfied. Sexual preoccupation and sex role confusion are not uncommon. Their behavior often is characterized by others as nonconforming, unusual, unconventional, and eccentric. Physical complaints may be present, and they usually are vague and long-standing in nature.

High scorers may at time be very stubborn, moody, and opinionated. At other times they are seen as generous, peaceable, and sentimental. Other adjectives used to describe high scorers include immature, impulsive, adventurous, sharp witted, conscientious, and high-strung. Although they may have a wide range of interests and may be creative and imaginative in approaching problems, their goals generally are abstracted and vague, and they seem to lack basic information that is required for problem solving.

The prognosis for psychotherapy is not good because of the long-standing nature of the high scorer's problems and his reluctance to relate in a meaningful way to the therapist. However, high scorers tend to stay in therapy longer than most patients, and eventually they may come to trust the therapist.

Low Scores on Scale 8

Low scorers on Scale 8 tend to be friendly, cheerful, good natured, sensitive, and trustful. They are seen as well balanced and adaptable, and they are responsible and dependable. However, low scorers tend to be somewhat restrained in their relationships, and they avoid deep, emotional involvement with other people. In interpersonal relationships they are submissive and compliant, and they are overly accepting of authority. Low scorers tend to be cautious, conventional, conservative, and unimaginative in their approach to problems, and they tend to be very practical and concrete in their thinking. They are concerned about success, status, and power, but they are so overcontrolled that they are reluctant to place themselves in clearly competitive situations.

Summary of Descriptors for Scale 8

A high scale 8 score indicates an individual who (is)

1. may manifest blatantly psychotic behavior
2. confused, disorganized, disoriented
3. has unusual thoughts or attitudes; delusions
4. has hallucinations
5. shows poor judgment
6. has a schizoid life style
7. does not feel a part of social environment
8. feels isolated, alienated, misunderstood
9. feels unaccepted by peers

10. withdrawn, seclusive, secretive, inaccessible
11. avoids dealing with people and new situations
12. shy, aloof, uninvolved
13. experiences generalized anxiety
14. feels resentful, hostile, aggressive
15. unable to express feelings
16. reacts to stress by withdrawing into daydreams and fantasies
17. has difficulty separating reality and fantasy
18. plagued by self-doubts
19. feels inferior, incompetent, dissatisfied
20. has sexual preoccupation, sex role confusion
21. nonconforming, unusual, unconventional, eccentric
22. vague, long-standing physical complaints
23. stubborn, moody, opinionated
24. generous, peaceable, sentimental
25. immature, impulsive
26. adventurous
27. sharp witted
28. conscientious
29. high-strung
30. has a wide range of interests
31. creative and imaginative
32. has abstract, vague goals
33. lacks basic information required for problem solving
34. has a poor prognosis for psychotherapy
35. reluctant to relate in meaningful way to therapist
36. stays in psychotherapy longer than most patients
37. may eventually come to trust the therapist

A low scale 8 score indicates an individual who (is)

1. friendly, cheerful, good natured, sensitive, trustful
2. well balanced, adaptable
3. responsible, dependable
4. restrained in relationships; avoids deep emotional involvement
5. submissive, compliant, overly accepting of authority
6. cautious, conventional, conservative, unimaginative in approach to problems
7. practical, concrete in thinking
8. concerned about success, status, power
9. reluctant to become involved in clearly competitive situations

SCALE 9 (HYPOMANIA)

Scale 9 originally was developed to identify psychiatric patients mani-festing hypomanic symptoms. Hypomonia is characterized by elevated mood, accelerated speech and motor activity, irritability, flights of ideas, and brief periods of depression.

Some of the 46 items in scale 9 deal specifically with features of the hypomanic disturbance (e.g., activity level, excitability, irritability, grandiosity). Other items cover topics such as family relationships, moral values and attitudes, and physical or bodily concerns. No single dimension accounts for much of the variance in scores, and the sources of variance represented in the scale are not duplicated in other clinical scales.

Scores on scale 9 clearly are related to age and to race. Younger subjects (e.g., adolescents and college students) typically obtain scores in a T-score range of 55 to 65, and for elderly subjects scale 9 scores below a T-score of 50 are not uncommon. Black subjects typically score higher than white subjects on the scale; scores in a T-score range of 60 to 70 are not uncommon for black subjects.

High Scores on Scale 9

Extreme elevations (T > 90) on Scale 9 may be suggestive of the manic phase of a manic-depressive disorder. Patients with such scores are likely to show excessive, purposeless activity and accelerated speech, and they may have hallucinations and/or delusions of grandeur.

Subjects with more moderate elevations are not likely to exhibit frankly psychotic symptoms, but there is a definite tendency toward overactivity and unrealistic self-appraisal. High scorers are energetic and talkative, and they prefer action to thought. They have a wide range of interests and they are likely to have many projects going at once. However, they do not utilize energy very wisely and often do not see projects through to completion. They may be creative, enterprising, and ingenious, but they have little interest in routine or in details. High scorers tend to become bored and restless very easily, and their frustration tolerance is quite low. They have great difficulty in inhibiting expression of impulses, and periodic episodes of irritability, hostility, and aggressive outbursts are not uncommon. An unrealistic and unqualified optimism is also characteristic of high scorers. They seem to think that nothing is impossible, and they have grandiose aspirations. Also, they have an exaggerated appraisal of their own self-worth and self-importance and are not able to see their own limitations.

High scorers are very outgoing, sociable, and gregarious. They like to be around other people and generally create good first impressions. They impress others as being friendly, pleasant, enthusiastic, poised, and self-confident. Their relationships with other people are usually quite superficial, and as others get to know them better they become aware of their manipulations, deceptions, and unreliability.

In spite of the outward picture of confidence and poise, high scorers are likely to harbor feelings of dissatisfaction concerning what they are getting out of life. They may feel upset, tense, nervous, anxious, and agitated, and they describe themselves as prone to worry. Periodic episodes of depression may occur.

In psychotherapy high scorers may reveal negative feelings toward domineering parents, may report difficulties in school or at work, and may admit to a variety of delinquent behaviors. Female subjects may be rebelling against the stereotyped female role, and some male subjects may be concerned about homosexual impulses. The prognosis for psychotherapy is poor. High scorers are resistant to interpretations, are irregular in their attendance, and are likely to terminate therapy prematurely. They engage in a great deal of intellectualization and may repeat problems in a stereotyped manner. They do not become dependent on the therapist, who may be a target for hostility and aggression.

Low Scores on Scale 9

Low scorers on scale 9, particularly if the scale is the lowest one in the profile, are characterized by low energy and activity levels. They appear to be lethargic, listless, apathetic, and phlegmatic, and they are difficult to motivate. Chronic fatigue and physical exhaustion are not uncommon. Depression, accompanied by tension and anxiety, may be present.

Low scorers are reliable, responsible, and dependable. They approach problems in a conventional, practical, and reasonable way, and they are conscientious and persevering. They may lack self-confidence, and they are seen by others as sincere, quiet, modest, and humble. They also tend to be somewhat withdrawn and seclusive, and they see themselves as not being very popular. They tend to be overcontrolled and are not likely to express their feelings directly or openly.

Low scoring males have home and family interests and seem willing to settle down. For hospitalized psychiatric patients, low scale 9 scores have favorable prognostic implications.

Summary of Descriptors for Scale 9

A high scale 9 score indicates an individual who (is)

1. manifests excessive, purposeless activity
2. has accelerated speech
3. has hallucinations, delusions of grandeur
4. energetic, talkative
5. prefers action to thought
6. has a wide range of interests; involved in many activities
7. does not utilize energy wisely, does not see projects through to completion
8. creative, enterprising, ingenious
9. has little interest in routine or details
10. easily bored, restless; has low frustration tolerance
11. has difficulty in inhibiting expression of impulses
12. has episodes of irritability, hostility, aggressive outbursts
13. unrealistic, unqualified optimism
14. has grandiose aspirations
15. exaggerates self-worth and self-importance
16. unable to see own limitations
17. outgoing, sociable, gregarious
18. likes to be around other people
19. creates good first impression
20. friendly, pleasant, enthusiastic
21. poised, self-confident

22. has superficial relationships
23. manipulative, deceptive, unreliable
24. harbors feelings of dissatisfaction
25. feels upset, tense, nervous, anxious
26. agitated, prone to worry
27. may have periodic episodes of depression
28. has negative feelings toward domineering parents
29. has difficulties at school or work; exhibits delinquent behaviors
30. if female, may be rejecting stereotyped female role
31. if male, may be concerned about homosexual impulses
32. has a poor prognosis for therapy
33. resistant to interpretations in psychotherapy
34. attends psychotherapy irregularly
35. may terminate psychotherapy prematurely
36. repeats problems in a stereotyped manner
37. not likely to become dependent on therapist
38. becomes hostile and aggressive toward therapist

A low scale 9 score indicates an individual who (is)

1. has low energy level, low activity level
2. lethargic, listless, apathetic, phlegmatic
3. difficult to motivate
4. reports chronic fatigue, physical exhaustion
5. depressed, anxious, tense
6. reliable, responsible, dependable
7. approaches problems in conventional, practical, and reasonable way
8. lacks self-confidence
9. sincere, quiet, modest, humble
10. withdrawn, seclusive
11. unpopular
12. overcontrolled; unlikely to express feelings openly
13. if male, has home and family interests; willing to settle down
14. if a hospitalized psychiatric patient, has favorable prognosis

SCALE 0 (SOCIAL INTROVERSION)

Although Scale 0 was developed later than the other clinical scales, it has come to be treated as a standard clinical scale. The scale was designed to assess a subject's tendency to withdraw from social contacts and responsibilities. Items were selected by contrasting high and low scorers on the Social Introversion-Extraversion scale of the Minnesota T-S-E Inventory.

The 70 items of this scale are of two general types. One group of items deals with social participation, whereas the other group deals with general neurotic maladjustment and self-depreciation. High scores can be obtained by endorsing either kind of item, or both.

High Scores on Scale 0

The most salient characteristic of high scorers on scale 0 is social introversion. High scorers are very insecure and uncomfortable in social situations. They tend to be shy, reserved, timid, and retiring. They feel more comfortable when alone or with a few close friends, and they do not participate in many social activities. They may be especially uncomfortable around members of the opposite sex.

High scorers lack self-confidence, and they tend to be self-effacing. They are hard to get to know and are described by others as cold and distant. They are sensitive to what others think of them, and they are likely to be troubled by their lack of involvement with other people. They are quite overcontrolled and are not likely to display their feelings directly. They are submissive and compliant in interpersonal relationships, and they are overly accepting of authority.

High scorers also are described as serious and as having a slow personal tempo. Although they are reliable and dependable, their approach to problems tends to be cautious, conventional, and unoriginal. They are somewhat rigid and inflexible in their attitudes and opinions. They also have great difficulty in making even minor decisions. They seem to enjoy their work and get pleasure from productive personal achievement.

High scorers tend to worry, to be irritable, and to feel anxious. They are described by others as being very moody. Guilt feelings and episodes of depression may occur.

Low Scores on Scale 0

Low scorers on scale 0 tend to be sociable and extroverted. They are outgoing, gregarious, friendly, and talkative. They have a strong need to be around other people, and they mix well with other people. They are seen as intelligent, verbally fluent, and expressive. They are active, energetic, and vigorous. They are interested in power, status, and recognition and they tend to seek out competitive situations.

Low scorers have problems with impulse control, and they may act out without considering the consequences of their actions. They are somewhat immature and self-indulgent. Relationships with other people may be superficial and insincere. A tendency to manipulate other people and to be opportunistic may be evident. Their exhibitionistic and ostentatious styles may arouse resentment and hostility in others.

Summary of Descriptors for Scale 0

A high scale 0 score indicates an individual who (is)

1. socially introverted
2. more comfortable alone or with a few close friends
3. reserved, timid, shy, retiring
4. uncomfortable around members of the opposite sex
5. lacks self-confidence, is self-effacing
6. hard to get to know
7. sensitive to what others think
8. troubled by lack of involvement with other people
9. overcontrolled; not likely to display feelings openly
10. submissive, compliant
11. overly accepting of authority

12. serious, has slow personal tempo
13. reliable, dependable
14. cautious, conventional, unoriginal in approach to problems
15. rigid and inflexible in attitudes and opinions
16. has difficulty making even minor decisions
17. enjoys work; gains pleasure from productive personal achievement
18. tends to worry; is irritable, anxious
19. moody
20. experiences guilt feelings, episodes of depression

A low scale 0 score indicates an individual who (is)

1. sociable, extroverted
2. outgoing, gregarious, friendly, talkative
3. has a strong need to be around other people
4. mixes well
5. intelligent, expressive, verbally fluent
6. active, energetic, vigorous
7. interested in power, status, recognition
8. seeks out competitive situations
9. has problems with impulse control
10. may act without considering consequences of actions
11. immature, self-indulgent
12. has superficial, insincere relationships
13. manipulative, opportunistic
14. arouses resentment and hostility in others

SOURCES CONSULTED IN PREPARING CHAPTER 4

Boerger, A. R., Graham, J. R., & Lilly, R. S. Behavioral correlates of single-scale MMPI code types. *Journal of Consulting and Clinical Psychology, 1974, 42,* 398–402.

Carkhuff, R. R., Barnette, W. L., & McCall, J. N. *The Counselor's Handbook: Scale and Profile Interpreations of the MMPI.* Urbana, Ill.: Parkinson, 1965.

Carson, R. C. Interpretive manual to the MMPI. In J. N. Butcher (Ed.), *MMPI: Research Developments and Clinical Applications.* New York: McGraw-Hill, 1969.

Dahlstrom, W. G., Welsh, G. S., & Dahlstrom, L. E. *An MMPI Handbook. Volume I: Clinical Interpretation.* Minneapolis: University of Minnesota Press, 1972.

Drake, L. E., & Oetting, E. R. *An MMPI Codebook for Counselors.* Minneapolis: University of Minnesota Press, 1959.

Dunbar, J. R., & Rabourn, R. E. *A Working Manual for the MMPI.* Unpublished materials, date unknown.

Gilberstadt, H., & Duker, J. *A Handbook for Clinical and Actuarial MMPI Interpretation.* Philadelphia: Saunders, 1965.

Good, P. K. E., & Brantner, J. P. T*Ahe Physician's Guide to the MMPI.* Minneapolis: University of Minnesota Press, 1961.

Gough, H. *Brief Descriptive and Interpretational Summary of Scales of the Minnesota Multiphasic Personality Inventory.* Unpublished materials, 1954.

Hovey, H. B., & Lewis, E. G. *Semiautomatic Interpretation of the MMPI.* Brandon, Vt.: Clinical Psychology Publishing Co., 1967.

Lachar, D. *The MMPI: Clinical Assessment and Automated Interpretation.* Los Angeles: Western Psychological Services, 1974.

Marks, P. A., & Seeman, W. *Actuarial Description of Abnormal Personality.* Baltimore: Williams & Wilkins, 1963.

Pearson, J. S., & Swenson, W. M. *A User's Guide to the Mayo Clinic Automated MMPI Program.* New York: Psychological Corporation, 1967.

Schubert, H. J. P. *A Wide-Range MMPI Manual.* Unpublished Materials, 1973.

Welsh, G. S., & Dahlstrom, W. G. (Eds.), *Basic Readings on the MMPI in Psychology and Medicine.* Minneapolis: University of Minnesota Press, 1956.

5
Two-Point Code Types

From the MMPI's inception, Hathaway and McKinley made clear that *configural* interpretation of an examinee's scores was diagnostically richer and thus more useful than was an interpretation which utilized examination of single scales without regard for relationships among the scales. Meehl (1951), Meehl and Dahlstrom (1960), Taulbee and Sisson (1957), and others also have stressed configural approaches to MMPI interpretation. Thus, some of the earliest MMPI validity studies (e.g., Black, 1953; Guthrie, 1952; Meehl, 1951) grouped profiles according to the two highest clinical scales in the profile and tried to identify reliable extra-test behaviors that were uniquely related to each such profile type. Other investigators (e.g., Gilberstadt & Duker, 1965; Marks & Seeman, 1963) have developed complex rules for classifying multiscale profiles (i.e., those utilizing all 10 of the MMPI scales) into homogeneous groups and have tried to identify extra-test correlates for each such group. For example, the following criteria must be met in order for a profile to be classified as a 4–9 type in the Gilberstadt and Duker system: (1) Pt and Ma greater than T-score 70; (2) no other scales greater than T-score 70; (3) L less than T-score 60; (4) Ma 15 or more T-scores greater than Sc; and (5) Pd 7 or more T-scores greater than Mf. Although clinicians initially were quite enthusiastic about this complex approach to profile classification, they became disenchanted as accumulating research and clinical evidence indicated that only a small proportion of the MMPI protocols encountered in a typical psychiatric setting could be classified using the complex types currently available (Fowler & Coyle, 1968; Huff, 1965; Meikle & Gerritse, 1970).

Currently, there seems to be a moving away from interest in complex rules for classifying profiles and a resurgence of interest in the simpler two-scale approach to classification of MMPI profiles. Gynther and his colleagues (Gynther, Altman, & Sletten, 1973) and Lewandowski and Graham (1972) have demonstrated that reliable extra-test correlates can be identified for profiles that are classified according to their two highest clinical scales. An obvious advantage of the two-point code approach is that a large proportion of the profiles encountered in most settings can be classified into a reasonably small number of two-point codes. Marks et al.

(1974), in their recent revision and extension of the earlier work by Marks and Seeman (1963), acknowledge that no appreciable loss in accuracy of extra-test descriptions resulted when they used two-point codes instead of their more complex rules for classifying MMPI profiles.

This chapter presents interpretive data for some MMPI two-point code types. As in the earlier chapters, the approach has been to examine existing literature concerning extra-test behavioral correlates of two-point codes,* to augment these data from the author's research and clinical experience, and to present a meaningful synthesis of all data. Although references are not cited for each descriptor presented, the sources consulted in preparing this chapter are listed at the end of the chapter. In general, in this chapter two-point codes are used interchangeably (e.g., the 12 and 21 codes are considered as the same type); absolute elevations of the two scales entering into the two-point code are not considered; and the relative elevations of the two scales are not taken into account. A careful examination of the existing literature suggests that in most cases the same basic extra-test behavioral correlates emerge for two-point codes irrespective of the order of the two scales and their absolute and relative elevations. When these features make a difference in interpretation, specific mention to that effect is made in the descriptive data for those particular codes in this chapter.

If two-point codes are used interchangeably, there are 40 possible two-point combinations of the 10 clinical scales. The two-point codes included in this chapter are those that occur reasonably frequently in a variety of settings† and for which an adequate amount of interpretive information is available in the literature. The reader will note that few codes including scales 5 and 0 are presented in this chapter. The reason is that in many research studies with two-point codes, scales 5 and 0 have been excluded because these two scales were added after the original publication of the MMPI and thus were not available for some subjects in some of the early studies. The descriptions provided below represent *modal* patterns and obviously do not describe unfailingly each and every such person. For profiles that do not fit any of the two-point codes presented here, the clinician will have to rely on interpretation of high and low scores on individual scales (see Chapter 4).

12/21‡

The most prominent features of the 12/21 code are somatic discomfort and pain. Individuals with this code present themselves as physically ill, although there may be no clinical evidence of an organic basis for their symptoms. They are very concerned about health and bodily functions, and

---

*Although useful interpretive data concerning two-point codes for adolescents have been published by Marks et al. (1974), their data are not included in this chapter because their classification of profiles is not based on K-corrected scores and utilizes specialized adolescent norms. The reader who is interested in interpretive information for two-point codes for adolescents should consult their book.

† A summary of the frequencies of occurrence of various two-point codes in a variety of settings is presented in Appendix M of *An MMPI Handbook,* Vol. 1 (Dahlstrom et al., 1972).

‡ Read this as "one-two/two-one."

they are likely to overreact to minor physical dysfunction. They may present multiple somatic complaints, or the symptoms may be restricted to one particular system. Although headaches and cardiac complaints may occur, the digestive system is more likely to be involved. Ulcers, particularly of the upper gastrointestinal tract, are common, and anorexia, nausea, and vomiting may be present. Individuals with the 12/21 code also may complain of dizziness, insomnia, weakness, fatigue, and tiredness. They tend to react to stress, including responsibility, with physical symptoms, and they resist attempts to explain their symptoms in terms of emotional or psychological factors.

12/21 individuals are generally anxious, tense, and nervous. Also, they are high-strung and tend to worry about many things, and they tend to be restless and irritable. Although pronounced clinical depression is not common for persons with the 12/21 code, they do report feelings of unhappiness or dysphoria, brooding, and loss of initiative.

Persons with the 12/21 code report feeling very self-conscious. They are introverted and shy in social situations, particularly with members of the opposite sex, and they tend to be somewhat withdrawn and seclusive. They harbor many doubts about their own abilities, and they show vacillation and indecision about even minor, everyday matters. They are hypersensitive concerning what other people think about them, and they may be somewhat suspicious and untrusting in interpersonal relations. They also tend to be passive-dependent in their relationships, and they may harbor hostility toward people who are perceived as not offering enough attention and support.

Excessive use of alcohol may be a problem for 12/21 individuals, especially among psychiatric patients. Their histories may include blackouts, job loss, arrests, and family problems associated with drinking. Persons with the 12/21 code most often are found to have been given a neurotic diagnosis (hypochondriacal, anxiety, or depressive), although a small proportion of individuals with this code may be diagnosed as having personality disorders or as schizophrenic. In this latter group (schizophrenia), scale 8 usually also is elevated along with scales 1 and 2.

Individuals with the 12/21 code are not seen as good risks for traditional psychotherapy. They can tolerate high levels of discomfort before becoming motivated to change. They utilize repression and somatization excessively, and they lack insight and self-understanding. In addition, their passive-dependent life styles make it difficult for them to accept responsibility for their own behavior. Although long term change after psychotherapy is not very likely, short-lived symptomatic changes often occur.

13/31

The 13/31 code is more common among women and older persons than among men and younger persons. Psychiatric patients with the 13/31 code almost always receive a psychophysiological or neurotic (hysterical, hypochondriacal) diagnosis. Classical conversion symptoms may be present, particularly if scale 2 is considerably lower than scales 1 and 3 (i.e., the so-called "conversion V" pattern). Whereas some tension may be reported by

13/31 persons, severe anxiety and depression usually are absent, as are clearly psychotic symptoms. Rather than being grossly incapacitated in functioning, the 13/31 individual is likely to continue functioning but at a reduced level of efficiency.

The somatic complaints presented by 13/31 persons include headaches, chest pain, back pain, and numbness or tremors of the extremities. Eating problems, including anorexia, nausea, vomiting, and obesity, are common. Other physical complaints include weakness, fatigue, dizziness, and sleep disturbance. The physical symptoms increase in times of stress, and often there is clear secondary gain associated with the symptoms.

Individuals with the 13/31 code present themselves as normal, responsible, and without fault. They make excessive use of denial, projection, and rationalization, and they blame others for their difficulties. They prefer medical explanations for their symptoms, and they lack insight into psychological factors underlying their symptoms. They manifest an overly optimistic and Pollyanish view of their situations and of the world in general, and they do not show appropriate concern about their symptoms and problems.

13/31 persons tend to be rather immature, egocentric, and selfish. They are insecure and have a strong need for attention, affection, and sympathy. They are very dependent, but they are uncomfortable with the dependency and experience conflict because of it. Although they are outgoing and socially extroverted, their social relationships tend to be shallow and superficial, and they lack genuine emotional involvement with other people. They tend to exploit social relationships in an attempt to fulfill their own needs. They lack skills in dealing with the opposite sex, and they may be deficient in heterosexual drive.

13/31 individuals harbor resentment and hostility toward other people, particularly those who are perceived as not fulfilling their needs for attention. Most of the time they are overcontrolled and likely to express their negative feelings in indirect, passive ways, but they occasionally lose their tempers and express themselves in angry, but not violent, ways. Behaving in a socially acceptable manner is important to 13/31 persons. They need to convince other people that they are logical and reasonable, and they are conventional and conforming in their attitudes and values.

Because of their unwillingness to acknowledge psychological factors underlying their symptoms, 13/31 persons are difficult to motivate in traditional psychotherapy. They expect the psychotherapist to provide definite answers and solutions to their problems, and they may terminate psychotherapy prematurely when the therapist fails to respond to their demands.

14/41

The 14/41 code is not encountered frequently in clinical practice and is much more likely to be found for males than for females. Persons with the 14/41 code frequently report severe hypochondriacal symptoms, particularly nonspecific headaches. They also may appear to be indecisive and anxious. Although they are socially extroverted, they lack skills with members of the opposite sex. They may feel rebellious toward home and parents, but direct expression of these feelings is not likely. Excessive use of alcohol may be a problem, and 14/41 persons may have a history of alcoholic benders, job loss, and family problems associated with their drinking behavior. In school or on the job the 14/41 persons lack drive and do not have well defined goals. They are dissatisfied and pessimistic in their outlook toward life, and they are demanding, grouchy, and referred to as bitchy in interpersonal relationships. Because they are likely to deny psychological problems, they tend to be resistant to traditional psychotherapy.

18/81

Persons with the 18/81 code harbor many feelings of hostility and aggression, and they are not able to express these feelings in a modulated, adaptive manner. They either inhibit expression almost completely, which results in the feeling of being "bottled up," or they are overly belligerent and abrasive.

18/81 persons feel socially inadequate, especially around members of the opposite sex. They lack trust in other people, keep other people at a distance, and feel generally isolated and alienated. A nomadic life style and a poor work history are common.

Psychiatric patients with the 18/81 code most often are diagnosed on strictly clinical criteria as schizophrenic, although diagnoses of anxiety neurosis and schizoid personality are sometimes given to them. 18/81 individuals tend to be unhappy and depressed, and they may display flat affect. They present somatic concerns (including headaches and insomnia) which at times are so intense that they border on being delusional. 18/81 individuals also may be confused in their thinking, and they are very distractible.

19/91

Persons with the 19/91 code are likely to be experiencing a great deal of distress and turmoil. They tend to be very anxious, tense, and restless. Somatic complaints, including gastrointestinal problems, headaches, and exhaustion, are common, and these people are reluctant to accept psychological explanations of their symptoms. Although on the surface 19/91 individuals appear to be verbal, socially extroverted, aggressive, and belligerent, they are basically passive-dependent persons who are trying to deny this aspect of their personalities.

19/91 persons have a great deal of ambition. They expect a high level of achievement from themselves, but they lack clear and definite goals. They are frustrated by their inability to achieve at a high level. The 19/91 code is sometimes found for brain-damaged individuals who are experiencing difficulty in coping with their limitations and deficits.

23/32

Although persons with the 23/32 code typically do not experience disabling anxiety, they do report feeling nervous, agitated, tense, and worried.

They also report feeling sad, unhappy, and depressed, and fatigue, exhaustion, and weakness are common. They lack interest and involvement in their life situations, and they have difficulty in getting started on things. Decreased physical activity is likely, and somatic complaints, usually gastrointestinal in nature, may occur.

23/32 individuals are rather passive, docile, and dependent. They are plagued by self-doubts, and they harbor feelings of inadequacy, insecurity, and helplessness. They tend to elicit nurturant and helpful attitudes from other people. Persons with the 23/32 code are very interested in achievement, status, and power. They may appear to be competitive, industrious, and driven, but they do not really place themselves in directly competitive situations where they might experience failure. They seek increased responsibility, but they dread the stress and pressure associated with it. They often feel that they do not get adequate recognition for their accomplishments, and they are easily hurt by even mild criticism.

23/32 persons are extremely overcontrolled. They have difficulty expressing their feelings, and they may feel bottled up much of the time. They tend to deny unacceptable impulses, and when denial fails they feel anxious and guilty. Persons with the 23/32 code feel socially inadequate, and they tend to avoid social involvement. They are especially uncomfortable with members of the opposite sex, and sexual maladjustment, including frigidity and impotence, is common.

The 23/32 code is much more common for women than for men. Rather than indicating incapacitating symptoms, it suggests a lowered level of efficiency for prolonged periods. Problems are long-standing, and the 23/32 persons have learned to tolerate a great deal of unhappiness. Among psychiatric patients, depressive neurosis is the most common diagnostic label assigned to persons with the 23/32 code, but the diagnosis of psychotic depression sometimes occurs. Psychopathic diagnoses are extremely rare for 23/32 persons.

Response to traditional psychotherapy is likely to be poor for the 23/32 persons. They are not introspective; they lack insight into their own behavior; they resist psychological formulations of their problems; and they tolerate a great deal of unhappiness before becoming motivated to change.

24/42

When persons with the 24/42 code come to the attention of professionals, it usually is after they have been in trouble with the law or with their families. 24/42 individuals are impulsive and unable to delay gratification of their impulses. They have little respect for social standards and often find themselves in direct conflict with societal values. Their acting out behavior is likely to involve excessive use of alcohol, and their histories include alcoholic benders, arrests, job loss, and family discord associated with drinking.

24/42 persons feel frustrated by their own lack of accomplishment and are resentful of demands placed on them by other people. They may react to stress by drinking excessively or by using addictive drugs. After periods of acting out, they express a great deal of remorse and guilt about their misdeeds. They may report feeling depressed, anxious, and worthless, but their expressions do not seem to be sincere. In spite of their resolutions to turn over a new leaf, they are likely to act out again in the future. It has been noted in the literature that when both scales 2 and 4 are grossly elevated, suicidal ideation and attempts are quite possible. Often the suicide attempts are directed at making other people feel guilty.

When they are not in trouble, 24/42 individuals tend to be energetic, sociable, and outgoing. They create favorable first impressions, but their tendencies to manipulate others produce feelings of resentment in long term relationships. Beneath the outer facade of competent, comfortable persons, 24/42 individuals tend to be introverted, self-conscious, and passive-dependent. They harbor feelings of inadequacy and self-dissatisfaction, and they are uncomfortable in social interactions, particularly ones involving members of the opposite sex.

Although persons with the 24/42 code may express the need for help and the desire to change, the prognosis for traditional psychotherapy is not good. They are likely to terminate psychotherapy prematurely when the situational stress subsides or when they have extracted themselves from their legal difficulties.

27/72

27/72 individuals tend to be anxious, nervous, tense, high-strung, and jumpy. They worry excessively, and they are vulnerable to real and imagined threat. They tend to anticipate problems before they occur and to overreact to minor stress. Somatic symptoms are common among 27/72 individuals. They usually involve rather vague complaints of fatigue, tiredness, and exhaustion, but insomnia, anorexia, and cardiac pain may be reported. Depression also is an important feature of the 27/72 code. Although 27/72 persons may not report feeling especially sad or unhappy, they show symptoms of clinical depression, including weight loss, slow personal tempo, slowed speech, and retarded thought processes. They are extremely pessimistic about the world in general and more specifically about the likelihood of overcoming their problems, and they brood and ruminate about their problems much of the time.

Individuals with the 27/72 code have a strong need for achievement and for recognition for their accomplishments. They have high expectations for themselves, and they feel guilty when they fall short of their goals. They tend to be rather indecisive, and they harbor feelings of inadequacy, insecurity, and inferiority. They are intropunitive, blaming themselves for all problems in their life situations. 27/72 individuals are rigid in their thinking and problem solving, and they are meticulous and perfectionistic in daily activities. They also may be excessively religious and extremely moralistic.

Persons with the 27/72 code tend to be rather docile and passive-dependent in their relationships with other people. In fact, they often find it difficult to be even appropriately assertive. They have the capacity for forming deep, emotional ties, and in times of stress they become overly clinging and dependent. They are not aggressive or belligerent, and they tend to elicit nurturance and helping behavior from other people. Because of the intense discomfort they experience, they are motivated for psychotherapy. They tend to remain in psychotherapy longer than many patients, and considerable improvement is likely.

Psychiatric patients with the 27/72 code are likely to receive a neurotic diagnosis (depressive, anxiety, obsessive-compulsive), but occasionally they are diagnosed as involutional melancholia or manic-depressive. Psychopathic diagnoses are very rare among persons with the 27/72 code.

28/82

Persons with the 28/82 code report feeling anxious, agitated, tense, and jumpy. Sleep disturbance, inability to concentrate, confused thinking, and forgetfulness also are characteristic of 28/82 people. Such persons are quite inefficient in carrying out their responsibilities, and they tend to be unoriginal in their thinking and stereotyped in problem solving. They are likely to present themselves as physically ill, and somatic complaints include dizziness, blackout spells, nausea, and vomiting. They resist psychological interpretations of their problems, and they are resistant to change. They underestimate the seriousness of their problems, and they tend to be unrealistic about their own capabilities.

28/82 individuals are basically dependent and ineffective, and they have problems in being assertive. They are irritable and resentful much of the time; they fear loss of control and do not express themselves directly. They attempt to deny undesirable impulses, and cognitive dissociative periods during which they act out may occur. Such periods are followed by guilt and depression. 28/82 persons are rather sensitive to the reactions of others, and they are quite suspicious of the motivations of others. They may have a history of being hurt emotionally, and they fear being hurt more. They avoid close interpersonal relationships, and they keep people at a distance emotionally. This lack of meaningful involvement with other people increases their feelings of despair and worthlessness.

If both scales 2 and 8 are very elevated, the 28/82 code is suggestive of serious psychopathology. The most common diagnoses given to psychiatric patients with this code are manic-depressive psychosis, involutional melancholia, and schizophrenia, schizoaffective type. 28/82 individuals have chronic, incapacitating symptomatology. They are guilt-ridden and appear to be clinically depressed. Withdrawal, soft and reduced speech, retarded stream of thought, and tearfulness are characteristic of 28/82 persons. Apathy, indifference, and feelings of worthlessness also are common. Psychiatric patients with the 28/82 code may be preoccupied with suicidal thoughts, and they are likely to have a specific plan for doing away with themselves.

29/92

29/92 persons tend to be self-centered and narcissistic, and they ruminate excessively about self-worth. Although they may express concern about achieving at a high level, it often appears that they set themselves up for failure. In younger persons, the 29/92 code may be suggestive of an identity crisis characterized by lack of personal and vocational direction.

29/92 persons report feeling tense and anxious, and somatic complaints, often centering in the upper gastrointestinal tract, are common. Although they may not appear to be clinically depressed at the time that they are examined, their histories typically suggest periods of serious depression. Excessive use of alcohol may be employed as an escape from stress and pressure.

The 29/92 code is found primarily among individuals who are denying underlying feelings of inadequacy and worthlessness and defending against depression through excessive activity. Alternating periods of increased activity and fatigue may occur. Whereas the most common diagnosis for psychiatric patients with the 29/92 code is manic-depressive psychosis, it sometimes is found for patients with brain damage who have lost control or who are trying to cope with deficits through excessive activity.

34/43

The most salient characteristic of 34/43 persons is chronic, intense anger. They harbor hostile and aggressive impulses, but they are unable to express their negative feelings appropriately. If scale 3 is higher than scale 4, passive, indirect expression of anger is likely. Persons with scale 4 higher than scale 3 appear to be overcontrolled most of the time, but brief episodes of aggressive, violent acting out may occur. Prisoners with the 43 code have histories of assaultive, violent crimes. In some rare instances, individuals with the 34/43 code successfully dissociate themselves from their aggressive acting out behavior. 34/43 individuals lack insight into the origins and consequences of their behavior. They tend to be extrapunitive and to blame other people for their difficulties. Other people may define the 34/43 person's behavior as problematic, but he or she is not likely to view it in the same way.

Persons with the 34/43 code are reasonably free of disabling anxiety and depression, but complaints of headaches, upper gastrointestinal discomfort, blackout spells, and eye problems may occur. Although these people may feel upset at times, the upset does not seem to be related directly to external stress.

Most of the 34/43 person's difficulties stem from deep, chronic feelings of hostility toward family members. They demand attention and approval from others. They are very sensitive to rejection, and they become hostile when criticized. Although they appear outwardly to be socially conforming, inwardly they are quite rebellious. They may be sexually maladjusted, and marital instability and sexual promiscuity are common. Suicidal thoughts and attempts are characteristic of 34/43 individuals; these are most likely to follow episodes of excessive drinking and acting out behavior. Personality disorder diagnoses are most commonly associated with the 34/43 code, with passive-aggressive personality and emotionally unstable personality being most common.

36/63

Individuals with the 36/63 code may report moderate tension and anxiety and may have physical complaints, including headaches and gastrointestinal discomfort, but their problems do not seem to be acute or incapacitating. Most of their difficulties stem from deep, chronic feelings of hostility toward family members. They do not express these feelings directly, and much of the time they may not even recognize the hostile feelings within themselves. When they do become aware of their anger, they try to justify it in terms of the behavior of others. In general, 36/63 individuals are defiant, uncooperative, and hard to get along with. They may express mild suspiciousness and resentment about others, and they are very self-centered and narcissistic. They deny serious psychological problems and express a very naive, Pollyanish attitude toward the world.

38/83

Persons with the 38/83 code appear to be in a great deal of psychological turmoil. They report feeling anxious, tense, and nervous. Also, they are fearful and worried, and phobias may be present. Depression and feelings of hopelessness are common among 38/83 individuals, and they have difficulties in making even minor decisions. A wide variety of physical complaints (gastrointestinal and musculoskeletal discomfort, dizziness, blurred vision, chest pain, genital pain, headaches, insomnia) may be presented. 38/83 persons tend to be quite vague and evasive when talking about their complaints and difficulties.

38/83 persons are rather immature and dependent, and they have strong needs for attention and affection. They display intropunitive reactions to frustration. They are not involved actively in their life situations, and they are apathetic and pessimistic. They approach problems in an unoriginal, stereotyped manner. Although response to insight-oriented psychotherapy is not likely to be good for 38/83 persons, they often benefit from a supportive psychotherapeutic relationship.

The 38/83 code suggests the presence of disturbed thinking. Individuals with this code complain of not being able to think clearly, of problems in concentration, and of lapses of memory. They express unusual, unconventional ideas, and their ideational associations may be rather loose. Obsessive ruminations, blatant delusions and/or hallucinations, and irrelevant, incoherent speech may be present. The most common diagnosis for psychiatric patients with the 38/83 code is schizophrenia, but they are sometimes diagnosed as suffering from hysterical neurosis.

45/54

Persons with the 45/54 code tend to be rather immature and narcissistic. They are emotionally passive, and they harbor very strong unrecognized dependency needs. They have difficulty in incorporating societal values into their own personalities. They are nonconforming, and they seem to be defying convention through their dress, speech, and behavior. In the 45/54 configuration, scale 5 indicates that these individuals have adequate control and are not likely to act out in obviously delinquent ways. However, a low frustration tolerance, coupled with intense feelings of anger and resentment, can lead to brief periods of aggressive acting out. Temporary remorse and guilt may follow the acting out behavior, but 45/54 persons are not likely to be able to inhibit similar episodes in the future. The modal diagnosis for psychiatric patients with the 45/54 code is passive-aggressive personality.

45/54 persons are likely to be experiencing great difficulty with sex role identity. They are rebelling against stereotyped sex roles, and overt homosexuality is a definite possibility, particularly if both scales 4 and 5 are markedly elevated. Males with the 45/54 code fear being dominated by females, and they are extremely sensitive to the demands of females.

46/64

Persons with the 46/64 code are immature, narcissistic, and self-indulgent. They are passive-dependent individuals who make excessive demands on others for attention and sympathy, but they are resentful of even the most mild demands made on them by others. Females with the 46/64 code seem overly identified with the traditional female role and are very dependent on males. Both 46/64 males and females do not get along well with others in social situations, and they are especially uncomfortable around members of the opposite sex. They are suspicious of the motivations of others and avoid deep emotional involvement. They generally have poor work histories, and marital problems are quite common. Repressed hostility and anger are characteristic of 46/64 persons. They appear to be irritable, sullen, argumentative, and generally obnoxious. They seem to be especially resentful of authority and may derogate authority figures.

Individuals with the 46/64 code tend to deny serious psychological problems. They rationalize and transfer blame to others, and they accept no responsibility for their own behavior. They are somewhat unrealistic and grandiose in their self-appraisals. Because they deny serious emotional problems, they generally are not receptive to traditional counseling or psychotherapy.

Among psychiatric patients, diagnoses associated with the 46/64 code are about equally divided between passive-aggressive personality and schizophrenia, paranoid type. In general, as the elevation of scales 4 and 6 increases and as scale 6 becomes higher than scale 4, a prepsychotic or psychotic disorder becomes more likely. 46/64 individuals present vague emotional and physical complaints. They report feeling moderately nervous and depressed, and they are indecisive and insecure. Physical symptoms may include asthma, hay fever, hypertension, headaches, blackout spells, and cardiac complaints.

47/74

Persons with the 47/74 code may alternate between periods of gross insensitivity to the consequences of their actions and excessive concern about the effects of their behavior. Episodes of acting out, which may include excessive drinking and sexual promiscuity, may be followed by temporary expressions of guilt and self-condemnation. However, the remorse does not inhibit further episodes of acting out. 47/74 individuals may present vague somatic complaints, including headaches and stomach pain. They also may report feeling tense, fatigued, and exhausted. They are rather dependent, insecure individuals who require almost constant reassurance of their self-worth. In psychotherapy they tend to respond symptomatically to support and reassurance, but long term changes in personality are unlikely.

48/84

48/84 individuals do not seem to fit into their environments. They are seen by others as odd, peculiar, and queer. They are nonconforming and resentful of authority, and they often espouse radical religious or political views. Their behavior is erratic and unpredictable, and they have marked problems with impulse control. They tend to be angry, irritable, and resentful, and they act out in asocial ways. When crimes are committed by 48/84 persons they tend to be vicious and assaultive, and they often appear to be senseless, poorly planned, and poorly executed. Prostitution, promiscuity, and sexual deviation are fairly common among 48/84 individuals. Excessive drinking and drug abuse (particularly involving hallucinogens) may also occur. Histories of 48/84 individuals usually indicate underachievement, uneven performance, and marginal adjustment.

Persons with the 48/84 code harbor deep feelings of insecurity, and they have exaggerated needs for attention and affection. They have poor self-concepts, and it seems as if they set themselves up for rejection and failure. They may have periods during which they become obsessed with suicidal ideation. 48/84 persons are quite distrustful of other people, and they avoid close relationships. When they are involved interpersonally, they have impaired empathy and try to manipulate others into satisfying their needs. They lack basic social skills and tend to be socially withdrawn and isolated. The world is seen as a threatening and rejecting place, and their response is to withdraw or to strike out in anger as a defense against being hurt. They accept little responsibility for their own behavior, and they rationalize excessively, blaming their difficulties on other people. 48/84 persons tend to harbor serious concerns about their masculinity or femininity. They may be obsessed with sexual thoughts, but they are afraid that they cannot perform adequately in sexual situations. They may indulge in antisocial sexual acts in an attempt to demonstrate sexual adequacy.

Psychiatric patients with the 48/84 code tend to be diagnosed as schizophrenia (paranoid type), asocial personality, schizoid personality, or paranoid personality. If both scales 4 and 8 are very elevated, and particularly if scale 8 is much higher than scale 4, the likelihood of psychosis and bizarre symptomatology, including unusual thinking and paranoid suspiciousness, increases.

49/94

The most salient characteristic of 49/94 individuals is a marked disregard for social standards and values. They frequently get into trouble with the environment because of antisocial behavior. They have poorly developed consciences, easy morals, and fluctuating ethical values. Alcoholism, fighting, marital problems, sexual acting out, and a wide array of delinquent acts are among the difficulties in which they may be involved.

49/94 individuals are narcissistic, selfish, and self-indulgent. They are quite impulsive and are unable to delay gratification of their impulses. They show poor judgment, often acting without considering the consequences of their acts, and they fail to learn from experience. They are not willing to accept responsibility for their own behavior, rationalizing shortcomings and failures and blaming difficulties on other people. They have a low tolerance for frustration, and they often appear to be moody, irritable, and caustic. They harbor intense feelings of anger and hostility, and these feelings get expressed in occasional emotional outbursts.

49/94 persons tend to be ambitious and energetic, and they are restless and overactive. They are likely to seek out emotional stimulation and excitement. In social situations they tend to be uninhibited, extroverted, and talkative, and they create a good first impression. However, because of their self-centeredness and distrust of people, their relationships are likely to be superficial and not particularly rewarding. They seem to be incapable of deep emotional ties, and they keep others at an emotional distance. Beneath the facade of self-confidence and security, the 49/94 individuals are immature, insecure, and dependent persons who are trying to deny these feelings. A diagnosis of antisocial personality or emotionally unstable personality is usually associated with the 49/94 code, although patients with the code occasionally are diagnosed as having manic-depressive psychosis.

68/86

Persons with the 68/86 code harbor intense feelings of inferiority and insecurity. They lack self-confidence and self-esteem, and they feel guilty about perceived failures. Withdrawal from everyday activities and emotional apathy are common, and suicidal ideation may be present. 68/86 persons are not emotionally involved with other people. They are suspicious and distrustful of others, and they avoid deep emotional ties. They are seriously deficient in social skills, and they are most comfortable when alone. They are quite resentful of demands placed on them, and other people see them as moody, irritable, unfriendly, and negativistic. In general, their life styles can be characterized as schizoid.

Although some persons with the 68/86 code are diagnosed as paranoid personality or schizoid personality, among psychiatric patients this configuration usually is associated with a diagnosis of schizophrenia, paranoid type, particularly if scales 6 and 8 are very elevated and both are considerably higher than scale 7. 68/86 individuals are likely to manifest clearly psychotic behavior. Thinking is described as autistic, fragmented, tangential, and circumstantial, and thought content is likely to be bizarre. Difficulties in concentrating and attending, deficits in memory, and poor judgment are common. Delusions of persecution and/or grandeur and hallucinations may be present, and feelings of unreality may be reported. Persons with the 68/86 code often are preoccupied with abstract or theoretical matters to the exclusion of specific, concrete aspects of their life situations. Affect may be blunted, and speech may be rapid and at times incoherent. Effective defenses seem to be lacking, and these persons respond to stress and pressure by withdrawing into fantasy and daydreaming. Often it is difficult for the 68/86 person to differentiate between fantasy and reality.

69/96

69/96 individuals are rather dependent and have strong needs for affection. They are vulnerable to real or imagined threat, and they feel anxious and tense much of the time. In addition, they may appear to be tearful and trembling. A marked overreaction to minor stress also is characteristic of persons with the 69/96 code. A typical response to severe stress is withdrawal into fantasy. 69/96 individuals are unable to express emotions in an adaptive, modulated way, and they may alternate between overcontrol and direct, uncontrolled emotional outbursts.

Psychiatric patients with the 69/96 code almost always receive a diagnosis of schizophrenia, paranoid type, and they are likely to show signs of a thought disorder. They complain of difficulties in thinking and concentrating, and their stream of thought is retarded. They are ruminative, overideational, and obsessional. They may have delusions and hallucinations, and their speech seems to be irrelevant and incoherent. They appear to be disoriented and perplexed, and they may show poor judgment.

78/87

78/87 individuals typically are in a great deal of turmoil. They are not hesitant to admit to psychological problems, and they seem to lack adequate defenses to keep them reasonably comfortable. They report feeling depressed, worried, tense, and nervous. When first seen professionally they may appear to be confused and in a state of panic. They show poor judgment and do not seem to profit from experience. They are introspective and they are characterized as ruminative and overideational.

Persons with the 78/87 code harbor chronic feelings of insecurity, inadequacy, and inferiority, and they tend to be quite indecisive. They lack even an average number of socialization experiences, and they are not socially poised or confident. As a result, they withdraw from social interactions. They are passive-dependent individuals who are unable to take a dominant role in interpersonal relationships. Mature heterosexual relationships are especially difficult for the 78/87 persons. They feel quite inadequate in the traditional sex role, and sexual performance may be poor. In an apparent attempt to compensate for these deficits, they engage in rich sexual fantasies.

Neurotic, psychotic, and personality disorder diagnoses all are represented among individuals with the 78/87 code. The most common neurotic diagnoses are obsessive-compulsive and depressive. Many different psychotic labels may be applied to 78/87 individuals, but manic-depressive disorders rarely occur. Schizoid is the personality disorder diagnosis most often found. The relative elevations of scales 7 and 8 are important in differentiating neurotics from psychotics or schizoid personality disorders. As scale 8 becomes greater than scale 7, the likelihood of a neurotic diagnosis decreases, and if scale 8 is extremely higher than scale 7 a psychotic diagnosis is likely. Even when a psychotic label is applied, blatant psychotic symptoms may not be present.

89/98

Persons with the 89/98 code tend to be rather self-centered and infantile in their expectations of other people. They demand a great deal of attention and may become resentful and hostile when their demands are not met. Because they fear emotional involvement, they avoid close relationships and tend to be socially withdrawn and isolated. They seem especially uncomfortable in heterosexual relationships, and poor sexual adjustment is common.

89/98 persons also are characterized as hyperactive and emotionally labile. They appear to be agitated and excited, and they may talk excessively in a loud voice. They are unrealistic in self-appraisal, and they impress others as grandiose, boastful, and fickle. They are vague, evasive, and denying in talking about their difficulties, and they may state that they do not need professional help.

Although 89/98 persons have a high need to achieve and may feel pressured to do so, their actual performance tends to be mediocre. Their feelings of inferiority and inadequacy and their low self-esteem limit the extent to which they involve themselves in competitive or achievement-oriented situations.

The 89/98 code is suggestive of serious psychological disturbance, particularly if scales 8 and 9 are grossly elevated. The modal diagnosis for 89/98 persons is schizophrenia, with catatonic, schizoaffective, and paranoid types being represented. Severe disturbance in thinking is likely. 89/98 individuals are confused, perplexed, and disoriented, and they report feelings of unreality. They have difficulty concentrating and thinking, and they are unable to focalize on issues. Thinking also may appear to be odd, unusual, autistic, and circumstantial. Speech may be bizarre and may include clang associations, neologisms, and echolalia. Delusions and hallucinations may be present. The 89/98 code frequently is found among adolescents who are using drugs.

SOURCES CONSULTED IN PREPARING CHAPTER 5

Carson, R. C., Interpretive manual to the MMPI. In J. N. Butcher (Ed.), *MMPI: Research developments and clinical applications*. New York: McGraw-Hill, 1969.

Dahlstrom, W. G., Welsh, G. S., & Dahlstrom, L. E. *An MMPI Handbook: Volume I. Clinical Interpretation*. Minneapolis: University of Minnesota Press, 1972.

Davis, K. R., & Sines, J. O. An antisocial behavior pattern associated with a specific MMPI profile. *Journal of Consulting and Clinical Psychology, 1971, 36,* 229–234.

Drake, L. E., & Oetting, E. R. *An MMPI Codebook for Counselors*. Minneapolis: University of Minnesota Press, 1959.

Duckworth, J. C., & Duckworth, E. *MMPI Interpretive Manual for Clinicians and Counselors*. Muncie, Ind.: Accelerated Development, Inc., 1975.

Gilberstadt, H., & Duker, J. *A Handbook for Clinical and Actuarial MMPI Interpretation*. Philadelphia: Saunders, 1965.

Good, P. K. E., & Brantner, J. P. *The Physician's Guide to the MMPI*. Minneapolis: University of Minnesota Press, 1961.

Gynther, M. D., Altman, H., & Sletten, I. W. Replicated correlates of MMPI two-point types: the Missouri Actuarial System. *Journal of Clinical Psychology, 1973,* Monograph Supplement No. 39.

Hovey, H. B., & Lewis, E. G. Semiautomatic interpretation of the MMPI. *Journal of Clinical Psychology, 1967,* Monograph Supplement no. 22.

Lachar, D. *The MMPI: Clinical Assessment and Automated Interpretation*. Los Angeles: Western Psychological Services, 1974.

Lewandowski, D., & Graham, J. R. Empirical correlates of frequently occurring two-point code types: a replicated study. *Journal of Consulting and Clinical Psychology*, 1972, *39*, 467–472.

Marks, P. A., Seeman, W., & Haller, D. L. *The Actuarial Use of the MMPI with Adolescents and Adults*. Baltimore: Williams & Wilkins, 1974.

Persons, R. W., & Marks, P. A. The violent 4-3 MMPI personality type. *Journal of Consulting and Clinical Psychology*, 1971, *36*, 189–196.

Schubert, H. J. P. *A Wide-Range MMPI Manual*. Unpublished manuscript, 1971.

6

Frequently Scored Research Scales

In addition to its utilization in the construction of the standard validity and clinical scales, the MMPI item pool has been used to develop numerous other scales by variously recombining the 566 items using item analytic, factor analytic, or intuitive procedures. Dahlstrom, Welsh, and Dahlstrom (1975) presented more than 450 additional scales. These scales have quite diverse labels, ranging from more traditional ones, such as Dominance and Suspiciousness, to more unusual ones, such as Success in Baseball and Yeshiva College Subcultural Scale. The scales also differ greatly in the care with which they were constructed and the extent to which they have been cross-validated. Most of the additional scales have not been cross-validated adequately and thus are not suitable for routine clinical use.

The following 12 of these additional scales have become more familiar to the clinician because they are reported routinely by some of the MMPI scoring and interpretation services:

A	– Anxiety	Dy – Dependency	
R	– Repression	Do – Dominance	
Es	– Ego Strength	Re – Social Responsibility	
MAS	– Manifest Anxiety	Pr – Prejudice	
Lb	– Low Back Pain	St – Social Status	
Ca	– Caudality	Cn – Control	

A major reason for selecting these scales for computer scoring was that normative data have been published for them (Hathaway & Briggs, 1957; Taylor, 1953). Although a review of the existing literature for the present chapter did not yield much information for most of the scales, they are discussed here in the hope that clinicians will be stimulated to use the scales in order that more information about them will become available.

The format for discussing each scale is the same. Scale development information is presented, and, to the extent that they are available, reliability and validity data are reported. Interpretive information for high and low scores on each scale also is summarized. As with the clinical and validity scales, no absolute cutoffs for high and low scores can be determined. In general, T-scores greater than 70 should be considered as high scores, and T-scores below 40 should be considered as low scores. Whenever information about specific cutoff scores for a scale is available, such information is presented. The higher the scores are, the more likely it is that the interpretive information for high scores will apply. Similarly, the lower the scores are, the more likely it is that interpretive information for low scores will apply. Although an attempt was made to rely on research studies for interpretive information, in some cases so little research data are available that more subjective information, including analysis of item content and clinical impressions, is included.

The composition and scoring of each scale are presented in Appendix B. It should be noted that the research scales can be scored only if the entire 566-item MMPI is administered. A table for converting raw scores on the scales to T-scores is presented in Appendix C. For all scales except the Manifest Anxiety scale the values in this table were calculated by Dahlstrom et al. (1960) from data presented by Hathaway and Briggs (1957). The norm group included 226 males and 315 females selected from the original general Minnesota normal sample utilized in computing T-score values for the standard validity and clinical scales of the MMPI. For the Manifest Anxiety scale, the values were calculated from data on 1971 normal college males and females reported by Taylor (1953).* Although no scoring keys or profile sheets are available commercially for use with the research scales, they easily can be constructed from the data in Appendices B and C.

ANXIETY (A) AND REPRESSION (R) SCALES

Scale Development

Whenever the basic validity and clinical scales of the MMPI have been statistically factor-analyzed to reduce them to their most common denominators, two basic dimensions have emerged consistently (e.g., Block, 1965; Eichman, 1961, 1962; Welsh, 1956). Welsh (1956) developed the Anxiety (A) and Repression (R) scales to assess these two basic dimensions.

By factor-analyzing MMPI scores for male Veterans Administration patients, Welsh identified a factor which he originally labeled "general maladjustment." A scale was developed to assess this factor by identifying items that were most highly associated with the factor. This original scale was administered to new groups of psychiatric patients, and it was refined by utilizing internal consistency procedures. The 39 items which ultimately were statistically identified in this manner constitute the final A scale. Welsh suggested from an examination of these 39 items that the content of the A scale items falls into four categories: thinking and thought processes; negative emotional tone and dysphoria; lack of energy and pessimism; and malignant mentation. The items are keyed in such a way that high scores on the A scale are associated with more psychopathology.

---

* Because Taylor did not report a standard deviation for the norm group, the T-score calculations had to be based on a frequency polygon and therefore the values are approximate rather than precise.

The R scale was constructed by Welsh (1956) to measure the second major dimension emerging from factor analyses of the basic validity and clinical scales of the MMPI. A procedure similar to that used in developing the A scale also was employed with the R scale, and it resulted in a final scale that contained 40 items. Welsh suggested the following clusters based on the content of the R scale items: health and physical symptoms; emotionality, violence, and activity; reactions to other people in social situations; social dominance, feelings of personal adequacy, and personal appearance; and personal and vocational interests.

Reliability and Validity

Welsh (1956) reported reliability data for the A and R scales based on research by Kooser and Stevens. For 108 college undergraduates the split-half reliability coefficients for A and R were .88 and .48, respectively. When 60 college sophomores were given the A and R scales on two occasions, separated by 4 months, test-retest reliability coefficients for A and R were .70 and .74, respectively. Gocka (1965) reported Kuder-Richardson 21 (internal consistency) values of .94 and .72 for the A and R scales, respectively, for 220 male Veterans Administration psychiatric patients.

It has been suggested by some writers that the major sources of variance in MMPI responses are associated with *response sets*. A response set exists when the individual taking the test answers the items from a particular perspective or attitude about how he would like to have the items show him to be. Edwards (1964) has argued that the first factor of the MMPI, the one assessed by the A scale, simply assesses the examinee's willingness while describing himself on the test to endorse socially undesirable items. Messick and Jackson (1961) have suggested that R scores simply indicate the extent to which examinees are willing to admit (acquiesce) on the test to all kinds of emotional difficulties. This interpretation appears to be supported by the fact that all of the items in the R scale are keyed in the false direction. Block (1965) has refuted the response set or bias arguments by demonstrating that the same two major factor dimensions emerge even when the MMPI scales are altered to control for social desirability and acquiescence effects using techniques developed by Edwards (1964) and others. Block also was able to identify through his research reliable extra-test correlates for the two factor dimensions.

Welsh (1956) reported some unpublished data supplied by Gough for a group of normal subjects. Gough found that A scale scores correlated negatively with the K and L scales and with scale 1 of the MMPI, and correlated positively with the F scale and with scales 9 and 0. Gough also reported that high A scorers showed slowness of personal tempo, pessimism, vascillation, hesitancy, and inhibitedness. Sheriffs and Boomer (1954) found that high A scorers showed more self-doubt in examination situations. Welsh (1956) reported a study by Welsh and Roseman that indicated that patients who showed the most positive change during insulin shock therapy also showed marked decreases in A scale scores after such therapy. There also is evidence that A scores tend to decrease during psychiatric hospitalization (Lewinsohn, 1965). Duckworth and Duckworth

(1975) suggested that a high A score indicates that a person is experiencing enough discomfort that he/she is likely to be motivated to change in psychotherapy. Block and Bailey (1955) reported reliable extra-test correlates for high and low scores on the A scale. These correlates are presented below in the discussion of the interpretation of high and low A scores.

Welsh (1956) also reported that in the study by Welsh and Roseman the patients who were judged as most improved during their course of insulin shock therapy also showed some decreases in R scores in addition to the decrease in A scores. Lewinsohn (1965) found that only small changes were found in R scores during psychiatric hospitalization. Welsh (1956) reported data provided by Gough indicating that in a sample of normal subjects, R scale scores were positively correlated with the L and K scales and with scales 1 and 2 of the MMPI and negatively correlated with scale 9. Duckworth and Duckworth (1975) described high R scorers as denying, rationalizing, and lacking self-insight. Block and Bailey (1955) identified extra-test correlates of high and low R scores. These correlates are included below in connection with the interpretation of high and low scores on the R scale. Below is summarized what these various studies on the A and R scales seem to have revealed.

Interpretation of High A Scores

A high score on the A scale is indicative of an individual who (is):
1. anxious, uncomfortable
2. has slow personal tempo
3. pessimistic
4. apathetic, unemotional, unexcitable
5. shy, retiring
6. lacks confidence in own abilities
7. hesitant, vascilating
8. inhibited, overcontrolled
9. influenced by diffuse personal feelings
10. defensive
11. rationalizes; blames others for difficulties
12. lacks poise in social situations
13. overly accepting of authority, conforming
14. submissive, compliant, suggestible
15. cautious
16. fussy
17. if male, has behavior which tends to be effeminate
18. cool, distant, uninvolved
19. becomes confused, disorganized, and maladaptive under stress
20. uncomfortable enough to be motivated to change in psychotherapy

In summary, a high scoring A scale individual, if from a normal population, is a rather miserable and unhappy person. If the high scoring A scale individual is in a psychiatric setting, he/she fits such summarizing rubrics as neurotic, maladjusted, submissive, and overcontrolled. Because of his/her discomfort, the high A scorer usually is highly motivated for psychotherapy or counseling.

Interpretation of Low A Scores

A low score on the A scale is indicative of an individual who (is):
1. does not feel anxious or uncomfortable
2. active, vigorous
3. expressive, colorful, verbally fluent
4. frank, outspoken
5. outgoing, sociable, friendly, informal
6. assumes ascendant role in relation to others
7. persuasive
8. ostentatious, exhibitionistic
9. efficient, capable, clear thinking
10. versatile, resourceful
11. self-confident
12. competitive; values success and achievement
13. interested in power, status, recognition
14. manipulates other people
15. unable to delay gratification of impulses
16. prefers action to thought; acts without considering consequences of actions

In summary, the low A scoring individual is characterized as extroverted, competent, confident, and somewhat impulsive. Although such an individual is not likely to be experiencing serious psychological turmoil, he/she may or may not have adjustment problems.

Interpretation of High R Scores

A high score on the R scale is indicative of an individual who (is):
1. submissive
2. unexcitable
3. conventional, formal
4. clear thinking
5. slow; painstaking

In summary, a high R scorer is an internalizing individual who has adopted a rather careful and cautious life style.

Interpretation of Low R Scores

A low score on the R scale is indicative of an individual who (is):
1. outgoing, outspoken, talkative
2. excitable, emotional
3. enthusiastic
4. spunky, daring
5. informal
6. robust, jolly
7. courageous
8. generous
9. dominant
10. impulsive
11. aggressive, bossy
12. sarcastic, argumentative

13. self-seeking, self-indulgent
14. shrewd, wary, guileful, deceitful

In summary, the low R scorer tends to be rather outgoing, emotional, and spontaneous in his/her life style, and such an individual takes an ascendant role in interpersonal relationships.

Conjoint Interpretation of A and R Scales

Welsh (1956, 1965) has suggested that a more complete understanding of an examinee is possible if the A and R scores are considered conjointly. Welsh (1956) reported some preliminary work carried out by Welsh and Pearson in which protocols of Veterans Administration psychiatric inpatients were categorized as high A-low R, high A-high R, low A-low R, and low A-high R. Different psychiatric diagnostic labels were associated with cases in the four quadrants (e.g., depressive diagnoses most often occurring in the high A-high R quadrant and character disorder diagnoses most often occurring in the low A-low R quadrant). Gynther and Brillant (1968) reported that Welsh's results were not replicated when the quadrant approach was utilized by them with their own sample of psychiatric outpatients.

More recently, Welsh (1965) has suggested dividing each scale (A and R) into high, medium, and low categories to form nine categories or novants. Using male Veterans Administration patients, Welsh identified protocols that fit each of his novants. He then determined the typical profiles for the novants and inferred personality descriptions from the profile configurations (See Table 6.1). Welsh noted that the descriptions are biased toward patient groups rather than normal individuals, and that the descriptions are intended to lead to hypotheses for further investigation and should not be taken literally and should *not* be used for "cook-book" interpretation of profiles. Duckworth and Duckworth (1975) reported that they have not found Welsh's descriptions of the novants to be very accurate for college counselees, except for the high A- high R interpretation.

MANIFEST ANXIETY SCALE (MAS)

Scale Development

The Manifest Anxiety scale (MAS) was developed originally by Taylor (1951, 1953) to select experimental subjects with high and low drive (anxiety) levels in order to study the effects of drive level on performance in a number of experimental situations. The scale was rationally constructed. Five clinicians were given a definition of manifest anxiety and were asked to designate items from the original MMPI item pool that were indicative of manifest anxiety. Sixty-five items on which there was 80% agreement among the judges and 135 additional buffer items constituted the original scale which was called the Biographical Inventory to disguise its intended purpose from examinees. After several subsequent revisions, a 225-item scale was developed. In addition to 50 of the original 65 items that showed the highest correlations with total anxiety scores, items from the MMPI L, F, and K scales and from a rigidity scale were included as buffer items.

Table 6.1. Summary of clinical descriptors for each novant in Welsh's A and R Scale Schema[a]

Novant	Descriptors
High A-low R	Subjects falling into this novant may be expected to be introspective, ruminative and overideational, with complaints of worrying and nervousness. There may be chronic feelings of inadequacy, inferiority, and insecurity which are often accompanied by rich fantasies with sexual content. Emotional difficulties may interfere with judgment, so that they are seen as lacking common sense. Patients in this novant do not use somatic defenses, and although they seem able to admit problems readily, the prognosis is poor.
High A-medium R	Severe personality difficulties may be expected, with loss of efficiency in carrying out duties. There may be periods of confusion, inability to concentrate, and other evidence of psychological deficit. Symptoms of depression, anxiety, and agitation predominate, although hysterical disorders sometimes appear. Subjects are often described as unsociable.
High A-high R	Depression is often encountered, with accompanying tenseness and nervousness as well as complaints of anxiety, insomnia, and undue sensitivity. Generalized neurasthenic features of fatigue, chronic tiredness, or exhaustion may be seen. These subjects are seen as rigid and worrying in a psychasthenic way, and suffer from feelings of inadequacy and a brooding preoccupation with their personal difficulties.
Medium A-low R	This novant profile represents a heterogeneous group of subjects, but often there are headaches and upper gastrointestinal tract symptoms after periods of tension and restlessness. Symptoms are often noted in response to frustration and situational difficulties, although subjects are reluctant to accept the psychogenic nature of their complaints. Patients tend to drop out of treatment quickly, so that a superficial approach is frequently all that is possible. Ambition is often noted, but the level of adjustment may be poor with excessive use of alcohol.
Medium A-medium R	Somatic symptomatology in this group tends to be specific rather than generalized, with epigastric and upper gastrointestinal pain predominating. In some cases there may be an active ulcer. Patients not showing somatic symptoms may complain of tension and depression. Frequently noted is the ability of these patients to tolerate discomfort rather than acting out.

Table 6.1—*Continued*

Novant	Descriptors
Medium A-high R	Subjects are often described as inadequate or immature and tend to use illness as an excuse for not accomplishing more. Lack of insight is often noted, with mechanisms of repression and denial prominent in adjustment attempts. Patients give a chronic hypochondriacal history with somatic overconcern, particularly in the alimentary system; abdominal pain is common. Response to treatment is not often favorable, because they seem to have learned to use somatic complaints to solve emotional problems.
Low A-low R	Aggression and hostility may be noted in many subjects, and they are often described as arrogant, boastful, and self-centered; some are seen as dishonest and suspicious. Patients may show episodic attacks of acute distress in various organ systems, but these physical problems are not severe and generally yield to superficial treatment.
Low A-medium R	Although subjects in this novant are characterized by attempts at self-enhancement they are not viewed favorably by others; they tend to be seen as irritable, immature, and insecure. Under stress they are prone to develop symptoms which are usually localized rather than diffuse. Patients suffer from complaints arrived at after protracted periods of mild tension; these are rarely incapacitating, although there is an indifferent response to treatment, and marginal adjustment is often noted.
Low A-high R	Lack of self-criticism with impunitive behavior may be found in subjects in this novant, and they are often self-centered, with many physical complaints. Occasionally there is mild anxiety and tension, but little depression occurs. Patients more often have pain in the extremities and the head rather than the trunk, but precordial and chest pain may be noted. They profit from reassurance, although insight is lacking into the nature of their symptoms.

a Welsh indicated that he viewed these descriptions as providing the basis for hypotheses for further investigation, and he warned against their literal interpretation or use for cook-book interpretation of profiles. (From W. G. Dahlstrom, G. S. Welsh, & L. E. Dahlstrom, *An MMPI Handbook, Vol. I.* The University of Minnesota Press, Minneapolis. Copyright 1960, 1972 by the University of Minnesota. Reproduced with permission.)

Although subsequent revisions in the MAS have taken place, including attempts to simplify the vocabulary and sentence structure of items, the 50 anxiety items from the 225-item scale constitute the MAS that can be scored from the standard MMPI protocol. Although Taylor (1953) cautioned against scoring the MAS from a standard MMPI administration because of differences in buffer items, the scale typically is scored in this manner.

The 50 items in the MAS cover a rather wide variety of behaviors. Whereas many of the items clearly deal with overt signs of anxiety (e.g., sweating, blushing, shakiness, etc.), other items contain subjective reports of feeling nervous, tense, anxious, upset, etc. There also are many items that involve somatic complaints (e.g., nausea, headaches, diarrhea, stomach trouble, etc.). Difficulties in concentration and feelings of excitement and/or restlessness also are suggested by some of the items. Some items suggest lack of self-confidence, extreme sensitivity to the reactions of other people, and feelings of unhappiness and uselessness. The items are keyed in such a way that higher scores are indicative of greater anxiety.

Reliability and Validity

Hilgard, Jones, and Kaplan (1951) reported a split-half reliability coefficient of .92 for the MAS, and Gocka (1965) obtained a Kuder-Richardson 21 (internal consistency) value of .92 for 220 male Veterans Administration psychiatric patients. Taylor (1953), using a sample of college students, obtained test-retest reliability coefficients of .89, .82, and .81 over periods of 3 weeks, 5 months, and 7 to 19 months, respectively.

The MAS originally was developed to measure drive level in studies seeking to test Hullian predictions concerning the relationship between drive level and learning. Spence and Spence (1966) summarized these predictions and reviewed empirical evidence relevant to them. It was predicted that on simple learning tasks high scorers on the MAS would perform better than low scorers, whereas on more complex tasks high MAS scorers would perform worse than low scorers. Although the data relevant to these predictions are not completely consistent, in general they seem to support the predictions. However, it has become obvious that the relationship between anxiety and learning is not a simple one, and additional variables such as task difficulty, degree of perceived stress, etc., must be taken into account.

Byrne (1974) and Speilberger (1966ab) have reviewed numerous studies conducted to clarify the relationship between anxiety, as assessed by the MAS, and many other extra-test characteristics. They concluded that the relationship between anxiety and intelligence is not as strong as has been inferred from simple observation. Whereas most studies have reported small and often nonsignificant correlations between MAS scores and intelligence test scores, Spielberger (1966a) indicated that higher negative correlations are obtained with samples that include larger proportions of subjects of lower intellectual levels. The relationship between anxiety and academic achievement is generally insignificant across all ability levels. However, for subjects of middle level ability, higher MAS scores are negatively correlated with grades obtained and positively related to academic problems.

Byrne (1974) concluded from his literature review that MAS scores are positively correlated with other anxiety scale scores (e.g., separation anxiety, test anxiety) and to physiological measures of anxiety such as palmar sweating. Likewise, high MAS scorers tend to be rated high on manifest anxiety by observers. That MAS scores are related to general psychological maladjustment is suggested by data indicating that psychiatric patients achieve higher MAS scores than do medical patients or college students. In addition, high MAS scorers admit to more medical and psychiatric symptoms than low MAS scorers. MAS scores after psychotherapy tend to be lower than pretherapy scores. There also are data that suggest that high MAS scorers tend to perceive the environment as threatening and uncontrollable and that they are less able than low MAS scorers to control autonomic reactions to stress situations. High MAS scorers tend to focus on the present rather than the future and to rely on very recent past experiences in developing expectancies.

Spielberger (1966b) has differentiated between trait and state anxiety. Trait anxiety refers to relatively stable, acquired tendencies to respond in an anxious manner in a stressful situation. State anxiety refers to temporary feelings of tension and apprehension and activation of the autonomic nervous system that fluctuate in response to situational changes. The MAS clearly assesses trait rather than state anxiety. MAS scores do not change in response to situational changes such as relaxation training or a stressful interview.

Interpretation of High MAS Scores

A high score on the MAS indicates that the person is predisposed to experience great emotional discomfort in stressful situations. In such situations, he/she feels anxious, tense, and jumpy and is likely to experience some physiological changes such as excessive perspiration, increased pulse rate, etc. He/she perceives the environment as threatening and feels that he/she is at the mercy of forces beyond his/her control. He/she emphasizes the present more than the future and develops expectancies on the basis of immediate past experiences. Whereas a high MAS scorer may do well on simple performance tasks, performance on more complex tasks, such as work or school performance, is likely to be impaired. In addition, a high MAS score is indicative of an individual who (is):
1. reports numerous physical or somatic complaints
2. feels excited or restless much of the time
3. has difficulties in concentrating
4. lacks self-confidence
5. overly sensitive to the reactions of others
6. feels unhappy and useless

Interpretation of Low MAS Scores

A low MAS score indicates that the person is not predisposed to experience extreme emotional discomfort in stressful situations. He/she remains calm and unruffled in such situations and feels as if he/she is in control of the situation. In complex learning situations the low MAS scorer is expected to perform better than the high MAS scorer. In addition, a low MAS score indicates that an individual is self-confident and relatively free of physical or somatic complaints.

EGO STRENGTH (Es) SCALE

Scale Development

The Ego Strength (Es) scale was developed by Barron (1953) specifically to predict the response of neurotic patients to individual psychotherapy. The 68 Es scale items were identified empirically from the 566 MMPI item pool by comparing item response frequencies of 17 patients who were judged independently as clearly improved after 6 months of psychotherapy with response frequencies of 16 patients who were judged as unimproved after 6 months of psychotherapy. The Es scale items deal with physical functioning, seclusiveness, attitudes toward religion, moral posture, personal adequacy and ability to cope, phobias, and anxieties.

Reliability and Validity

The Es scale was cross-validated by Barron (1953) using three different samples of neurotic patients for whom ratings of improvement during brief, psychoanalytically oriented psychotherapy were available. Because pretherapy Es scores were positively related to rated improvement for all three samples, Barron concluded that the Es scale is useful in predicting personality change during psychotherapy. Barron also reported that the odd-even reliability of the Es scale for a sample of 126 patients was .76 and that the test-retest reliability, using a 3-month interval between testings, was .72 for a sample of 30 cases. Gocka (1965) reported a Kuder-Richardson 21 (internal consistency) value of .78 for the Es scale for 220 male Veterans Administration psychiatric patients.

Unfortunately, subsequent attempts by others to cross-validate the Es scale as a predictor of response to psychotherapy or other treatment approaches have yielded inconsistent findings. Some data indicate that psychiatric patients who change most during treatment have higher pretreatment Es scores than patients who show less change (e.g., Wirt, 1955, 1956), whereas other data suggest that change in treatment is unrelated to pretreatment Es scores (e.g. Ends & Page, 1957; Fowler, Teel, & Coyle, 1967; Getter & Sundland, 1962; Sullivan, Miller, & Smelser, 1958). Distler, May, and Tuma (1964) found that pretreatment Es scores were positively related to hospitalization outcome for male psychiatric patients and negatively related to hospitalization outcome for female psychiatric patients. Simmett (1962) reported that Veterans Administration psychiatric patients with higher pretreatment Es scores showed more personality growth during treatment, which included psychotherapy, than did patients with lower scores, but pretreatment Es scores were unrelated to rated symptomatic change for these same patients. It should be noted that many of the failures to replicate Barron's finding that Es scores were related to change after *psychotherapy* utilized change after *hospitalization* and therefore did not represent a true replication of his study.

Dahlstrom et al. (1975) have tried to explain the inconsistent findings concerning the relationship between Es scores and treatment outcome.

They suggest that when high Es scores occur for persons who obviously are having difficulties but who are denying them, the high Es scores may not be predictive of a favorable treatment outcome. However, high Es scores for persons who are admitting to emotional problems may suggest a favorable response to treatment. It is clear from the existing literature that the relationship between Es scores and treatment outcome is not a simple one and that factors such as kind of patients, type of treatment, and nature of the outcome measures must be taken into account. In general, however, high Es scores are predictive of positive personality change for neurotic patients who receive traditional, individual psychotherapy.

There also are research data indicating that the Es scale can be viewed as an indication of overall psychological adjustment. Higher scores on the Es scale are associated with more favorable adjustments levels as assessed by other MMPI indices and extra-test criteria. Es scores tend to be lower for psychiatric patients than for nonpatients and for people receiving psychiatric or psychological treatment than for people who are not involved in such treatment (Gottesman, 1959; Himelstein, 1964; Kleinmuntz, 1960; Quay, 1955; Spiegel, 1969; Taft, 1957). However, it has been reported that the Es scale fails to differentiate between delinquent and nondelinquent adolescents (Gottesman, 1959). Whereas Es scores tend to be higher for neurotic patients than for psychotic patients, the scale fails to discriminate among more specific diagnostic categories (Hawkinson, 1962; Rosen, 1963; Tamkin, 1957; Tamkin & Klett, 1957).

There are some data that indicate that Es scores tend to go up as a result of psychotherapy or other treatment procedures. Lewinsohn (1965) has reported that psychiatric patients showed an increase in level of Es scores from hospital admission to discharge. However, Barron and Leary (1955) found that Es scores did not change more for patients who received individual or group psychotherapy than for patients who remained on a waiting list for a similar period of time. It also has been reported that psychotherapy patients who were self-referred scored higher on the Es scale than those who were referred by someone else (Himelstein, 1964), suggesting that high Es scorers are more aware of internal conflicts than are low Es scorers.

Scores on the Es scale are related positively to intelligence (Tamkin & Klett, 1967; Wirt, 1955) and to formal education (Tamkin & Klett, 1967). The relationship between Es scores and age is less clear. Tamkin and Klett (1967) found no relationship between Es scores and age, but Getter and Sundland (1962) reported that older persons tended to score lower on the Es scale. Consistent sex differences in Es scores have been reported, with males obtaining higher scores than females (Distler et al., 1964; Getter & Sundland, 1962; Taft, 1957). This sex difference originally was interpreted as reflecting the greater willingness of females to admit to problems and complaints (Getter & Sundland, 1962). However, a more reasonable explanation of the sex difference on the Es scale is that males score higher than females because the scale contains a number of items dealing with masculine role identification (Holmes, 1967).

Interpretation of High Es Scores

From the above discussion, it may be concluded that high scorers on the Es scale generally tend to show more positive personality change during treatment than do low scorers. However, the relationship between Es scores and treatment prognosis is not a simple one, and patient and treatment variables must be taken into account. Also, high Es scorers tend to be better adjusted psychologically, and they are more able than low scorers to cope with problems and stresses in their life situations. Among psychiatric patients, high Es scores are likely to be associated with neurotic diagnoses and low Es scores are more likely to be found for psychotic patients.

In addition, published studies (e.g., Barron, 1953, 1956; Dahlstrom et al., 1975; Duckworth & Duckworth, 1975; Good & Brantner, 1961; Quay, 1955) reveal that a high Es score is indicative of an individual who (is):

1. lacks chronic psychopathology
2. stable, reliable, responsible
3. tolerant; lacks prejudice
4. alert, adventuresome
5. determined, persistent
6. self-confident, outspoken, sociable
7. intelligent, resourceful, independent
8. has a secure sense of reality
9. deals effectively with others
10. creates favorable first impressions
11. gains acceptance of others
12. opportunistic, manipulative
13. has strongly developed interests
14. if male, has appropriately masculine style of behavior
15. hostile, rebellious toward authority
16. competitive
17. sarcastic, cynical
18. seeks help because of situational problems
19. can tolerate confrontations in psychotherapy

In summary, a person with a high Es score appears to be one who is fairly well put together. In nonpsychiatric settings, such a person is not likely to have serious emotional problems. Among persons with emotional problems, a high Es score suggests that problems are likely to be situational rather than chronic, that the person has psychological resources that can be drawn upon in helping him/her to solve the problems, and that the prognosis for positive change in psychotherapy or counseling is good.

Interpretation of Low Es Scores

In general, low Es scorers tend to be less well adjusted psychologically than high Es scorers, and they are not well equipped to deal with problems and stresses. In general, low scorers are likely to show less positive personality change during treatment. Among psychiatric patients, low Es scorers are more likely to be diagnosed as psychotic than as neurotic or personality disorder. In addition, Barron (1953, 1956), Dahlstrom and Welsh (1960), Dahlstrom et al. (1975), Duckworth and Duckworth (1975), and Good and Brantner (1961) have suggested that a low score on the Es scale is indicative of an individual who (is):

1. has poor self-concept; feels worthless; broods
2. feels helpless
3. confused
4. has chronic physical complaints
5. has chronic fatigue
6. has fears, phobias
7. withdrawn, seclusive
8. inhibited, unadaptive
9. shows stereotyped, unoriginal approach to problems
10. mannerly, mild
11. has fundamental religious beliefs
12. rigid, moralistic
13. if male, has effeminate style of behavior
14. exaggerates problems as "cry for help"
15. has a poor work history
16. has problems that are characterological rather than situational in nature
17. expresses good intentions to change in psychotherapy but does not act on them

In sumary, a person with a low Es score does not seem to be very well put together. Such a person is likely to be seriously maladjusted psychologically. Problems are likely to be long-standing in nature; personal resources for coping with problems are extremely limited; and the prognosis for positive change in psychotherapy is poor.

LOW BACK PAIN (Lb) SCALE

Scale Development

The Low Back Pain (Lb) scale was developed empirically by Hanvik (1949, 1951) to help with an important clinical challenge, namely, to differentiate between patients with chronic low back pain but with no evidence of organic disease and patients with similar pain but with clear evidence of organic disease. The 25 items in the Lb scale were identified from the total MMPI item pool by comparing the response frequencies of two groups of patients with low back pain (Dahlstrom & Welsh, 1960). One group consisted of 30 patients whose pain was diagnosed independently by other clinical criteria as due to protruding intervertebral disc, and the other group included 30 patients for whom comparable pain was diagnosed as quite likely not resulting from organic disease. The 25 items are keyed in such a way that high Lb scores are suggestive of functional pain (i.e., pain in which psychological factors are believed to be preeminent) and low Lb scores are suggestive of pain resulting from organic disease. The content of the Lb items includes multiple physical complaints, denial of social anxiety and negative feelings about people, lack of some traditional religious beliefs, restlessness, dysphoria, and failure to express one's attitudes and beliefs to others. Hanvik recommended that a raw score cutoff of 11 be used to discriminate between patients with functional versus organic pain.

Reliability and Validity

Gocka (1965) reported a Kuder-Richardson 21 (internal consistency) value of .22 for the Lb scale for 220 male Veterans Administration psychiatric patients. Dahlstrom (1954) reported that the Lb scale was useful in identifying patients with chronic low back pain for which no physical explanation could be found. He also indicated that recovery after surgery for known physical defects was poorer for patients with higher Lb scores. Lewinsohn (1965) found that Lb scores of psychiatric patients were lower at the time of hospital discharge than at admission.

Interpretation of High Lb Scores

In persons who are reporting chronic low back pain, high scores, on the Lb scale indicate that the pain may be functional in nature, particularly if no medical evidence of an organic defect can be found. Whereas Hanvik (1949, 1951) found that a raw score cutoff of 11 yielded the best discrimination between functional and organic patient groups, Good and Brantner (1961) suggested using a T-score cut-off of 70. Although an optimal cutoff score quite likely should be established separately in each clinical setting where the scale is used, the higher Lb the scores are, the more likely it is that chronic low back pain is functional in nature. Although no other research data are available concerning other extra-test correlates of high Lb scores, an examination of the content of the Lb scale items suggests that a high Lb score may turn out to be indicative of an individual who (is):
1. experiences physical discomfort in addition to the back pain (headaches, heart pounding, shortness of breath)
2. restless
3. denies getting angry or irritated with other people
4. somewhat dysphoric
5. does not express his/her opinions or beliefs to others
6. comfortable in interacting in social situations
7. does not have traditional religious beliefs
8. tries to cover up inadequacies and insecurities

In summary, when used along with other appropriate clinical criteria, a high Lb score suggests that psychological factors may be preeminent in reported low back pain. A person with a high Lb score tends to direct feelings and problems inwardly, where they may find expression in somatic symptoms.

Interpretation of Low Lb Scores

Among persons who report chronic low back pain, low scores on the Lb scale may be contraindicative of a functional disorder. Some medical evidence of an organic cause for their discomfort usually is available. As with high scores, no additional research data other than those cited above are available concerning other extra-test correlates of low Lb scores.

However, a reading of the content of the Lb scale items indicates that a low Lb score may be indicative of an individual who (is):

1. does not report physical or somatic discomfort other than the low back pain
2. happy and contented
3. admits getting angry and irritated with other people
4. expresses his/her opinions or beliefs to others
5. uncomfortable and shy in social situations
6. has traditional religious beliefs
7. rather open about his/her inadequacies and insecurities.

In summary, when used along with other appropriate clinical criteria, a low Lb score suggests that organic rather than psychological factors may be preeminent in reported low back pain. A person with a low Lb score tends to be rather open and honest about his feelings and insecurities.

CAUDALITY (Ca) SCALE

Scale Development

Although the differential diagnosis of frontal versus parietal lobe damage has been and should continue to be made primarily on the basis of neurological and other medical evidence, there have been several efforts to develop MMPI scales to help in this important clinical problem. Although no responsible clinician would use a paper-and-pencil test for making a clinical diagnosis as important as frontal versus nonfrontal cortical damage, such scales may offer an additional item of information if and when they are adequately validated.

The present Caudality (Ca) scale is a revision and extension of an earlier scale developed by Friedman (1950) in an attempt to discriminate between patients with frontal lobe and parietal lobe brain damage. In developing the present Ca scale, Williams (1952) cross-validated Friedman's scale on new samples of frontal and parietal lobe cases, identified new items from the MMPI item pool that differentiated patients with frontal lobe damage from patients with parietal lobe damage, and combined some of the new items with some items from the Friedman scale to form the 36-item Ca scale. The items are keyed in such a way that high Ca scores are believed to be predictive of nonfrontal damage, and low Ca scores are alleged to be indicative of frontal damage. The 36 Ca scale items deal with anxiety, depression, somatic complaints, social introversion, problems in emotional control, and fear of loss of control of thought processes.

Reliability and Validity

Gocka (1965) reported a Kuder-Richardson 21 (internal consistency) value of .86 for the Ca scale for 220 male Veterans Administration psychiatric patients. Williams (1952) reported that when a raw score of 11 on the Ca scale was used as a cutoff, 78% accuracy was achieved in separating patients with frontal lobe damage from those with parietal lobe damage (as compared with a 50% base rate in the samples utilized). Williams' data also indicated that scores on the Ca scale are positively related to scores on scale 7 of the MMPI and negatively related to the MMPI K scale.

Meier and French (1964) found that a T-score cutoff of 50 led to accurate identification of patients with temporal lobe abnormalities. One year after surgery to remove the tissue generating the electrographic focus, Ca scores were lower than the presurgery scores, and the T-score cutoff of 50 no longer accurately identified the patients who previously had manifested temporal lobe abnormalities. Meier and French concluded that when used along with other appropriate clinical evidence the Ca scale may be effective in helping to localize temporal lobe abnormalities, and that the higher Ca scores among patients with temporal lobe involvement may turn out to be the result of personality changes (anxiety, guilt, feelings of inadequacy, etc.) associated with the temporal lobe damage.

Interpretation of High Ca Scores

When dealing with patients with focalized organic brain pathology as determined by standard neurological and related indices, high Ca scores may be suggestive of posterior localization of damage. Although the Ca scale should not be used alone in localizing brain damage, it can be a useful addition to other data. Whereas no research data are available concerning other extra-test correlates of high Ca scores, study of the content of the Ca scale items suggests that a high Ca score is indicative of an individual who (is):

1. feels anxious, guilty, depressed
2. reports multiple physical complaints
3. feels inadequately equipped to handle stresses in his/her life situation
4. worries excessively
5. socially extroverted
6. has problems in controlling emotional expression
7. fears losing control of his/her thought processes

In summary, although the Ca scale should be viewed primarily as a research tool which is not yet adequately validated, when it is used in conjunction with other appropriate clinical evidence, high Ca scores may be suggestive of parietal localization of cortical damage. High Ca scorers tend to have problems in emotional and cognitive control, which is consistent with clinical observations of patients with parietal damage.

Interpretation of Low Ca Scores

When dealing with patients with focalized brain damage as identified by the usual neurological criteria, low Ca scores may be indicative of frontal lobe involvement. Whereas research data are not available concerning the other extra-test correlates of low Ca scores, the content of the Ca scale items suggests that a low Ca score describes an individual who (is):

1. denying anxiety, complaints and discomfort
2. free of somatic complaints and discomfort
3. presents self as comfortable and confident in social situations
4. feels in control of emotions and thought processes

In summary, although the Ca scale should be viewed primarily as a research tool which as yet has not been adequately validated, when it is used in conjunction with other appropriate clinical evidence, low Ca scores may be suggestive of frontal localization of cortical damage. Low Ca scorers appear to be in control of emotions and cognitive processes.

DEPENDENCY (Dy) SCALE

Scale Development

The Dependency (Dy) scale was derived rationally by Navran (1954) to assess the strength of dependency needs. After an unsuccessful attempt to develop the scale empirically, Navran asked 16 judges independently to identify those MMPI items that, based on their own clinical experience, they felt were related to dependency. The initial 157 items identified by these 16 judges were administered to two samples of 50 psychiatric patients each, and internal consistency procedures were employed to identify further the items that had the most discriminability for both samples. The 57 items which resulted constitute the Dy scale. The items are keyed in such a way that higher scores are indicative of more dependency. The Dy scale items deal with problems such as feeling misunderstood, indecision, lack of self-confidence, excessive sensitivity to the reactions of others, somatic complaints, shyness in social situations, and religious concerns.

Reliability and Validity

Navran (1954) reported that the reliability (internal consistency) of the 57-item Dy scale for the 100 patients in the derivation samples was .91, and Gocka (1965) reported an identical Kuder-Richardson 21 (internal consistency) value based on 220 male Veterans Administration psychiatric patients. Button (1956), using a 1-week interval between two testings, found a test-retest reliability coefficient of .85 for the Dy scale for a sample of 64 alcoholic patients in a state mental hospital.

In his original article on the development of the Dy scale, Navran (1954) reported that psychiatric patients scored significantly higher on Dy than did normals from the original MMPI standardization group utilized by Hathaway and McKinley, that the standardization group normals scored significantly higher than a group of graduate students, and that within the psychiatric patient samples nonparanoid schizophrenics scored significantly higher than paranoid schizophrenics. In another study Button (1956) found that alcoholic patients did not score significantly differently on the Dy scale than did normal subjects, but both alcoholic and normal samples scored lower than psychiatric patient samples. Dahlstrom and Welsh (1960) reported a study by Warn which found that tuberculosis patients and epileptics scored higher than controls on the Dy scale, but paraplegics did not score differently from controls on the Dy scale. Zuckerman, Levitt, and Lubin (1961) combined items from the Dy scale with items from Gough's Dominance scale and found that a total score based on these two scales showed significant, but modest, relationships with peer ratings and self-ratings of dependency. Pruitt and Van deCastle (1962) found that higher Dy scores were associated with greater chronicity among welfare recipients. Pruitt and Van deCastle also reported the results of a study by Nelson (1959) which indicated that Dy scores were not predictive of length of therapy but that high Dy scorers were more likely to continue in therapy for at least one session after an initial intake interview. Button (1956) cited a personal communication in which Navran indicated that he viewed the Dy scale as a self-report of degree of dependency and not necessarily as an accurate measure of dependency. Conflict, in the sense of ambivalence, about dependency needs is suggested if scores on the Dy scale are not consistent with behavior or other evidence of dependency.

Interpretation of High Dy Scores

High scores on the Dy scale tend to be associated with general psychological maladjustment. A conflict about dependency needs is suggested when an individual has a high Dy score but his behavior and other test data are not indicative of strong dependency needs. An examination of the content of the Dy scale items suggests that a high Dy score also is indicative of an individual who (is):
1. admits to strong dependency needs
2. feels misunderstood
3. feels dysphoric, unhappy
4. experiences somatic discomfort
5. lacks self-confidence
6. feels shy and embarassed in social situations
7. excessively sensitive to the reactions of others
8. has traditional religious beliefs and may be worried about religious matters

In summary, a person with a high Dy score is likely to have very strong dependency needs that are not being fulfilled adequately. Such a person also may have serious emotional problems that lead to feelings of dysphoria and unhappiness.

Interpretation of Low Dy Scores

In general, low Dy scores are associated with satisfactory psychological adjustment. A conflict about dependency needs is suggested if a person has a low Dy score but behaves in a dependent manner. Examination of the content of the Dy scale items indicates that a low Dy score is indicative of an individual who (is):
1. does not admit to strong dependency needs
2. feels that other people understand him/her
3. feels happy
4. free of somatic discomfort
5. feels self-confident
6. comfortable and confident in social situations
7. not excessively sensitive to reactions of others
8. does not hold traditional religious beliefs and is not worried about religious matters

In summary, a person with a low Dy score is denying strong dependency needs and is not excessively sensitive to the reactions of others. Such a person is likely to be rather well adjusted psychologically and to feel happy and confident.

DOMINANCE (Do) SCALE

Scale Development

The Dominance (Do) scale was developed by Gough, McClosky, and Meehl (1951) as part of a larger project concerned with political participation. The 60-item scale includes a subscale of 28 MMPI items that can be scored separately from the total 60-item scale and for which normative data are available. The remaining 32 items are not MMPI items. High school and college students were given a definition of dominance ("strength" in face-to-face personal situations; ability to influence others; not readily intimidated or defeated; feeling safe, secure, and confident in face-to-face situations) and were asked to nominate peers who were most dominant and least dominant. High and low dominance criterion groups were defined on the basis of these peer nominations, and both groups were given a 150-item questionnaire, which included some MMPI items. Item analyses of the responses identified 60 items, including 28 MMPI items, that differentiated between the high and low dominance criterion groups. The items are keyed in such a way that a high score on the Do scale is suggestive of high dominance. The 28 MMPI items included in the Do scale deal with a number of different content areas, including concentration, obsessive-compulsive behaviors, self-confidence, discomfort in social situations, concern about physical appearance, perseverance, and political opinions.

Reliability and Validity

Gough et al. (1951) reported a reliability coefficient (Kuder-Richardson 21) of .79 for the 60-item Do scale, and Gocka (1965) reported a Kuder-Richardson value of .60 for the 28-item Do scale for 220 male Veterans Administration psychiatric patients. A test-retest reliability coefficient of .86 for Marine Corps officers was reported by Knapp (1960). Knapp also reported correlations of .75 and .79 between Do scores based on the 28 MMPI items and Do scores on the total 60-item scale.

Gough et al. (1951) found that a raw score cutoff of 36 on the 60-item Do scale identified 94% of their high and low dominance high school subjects, whereas a raw score cutoff of 39 on the 60-item scale correctly identified 92% of high and low dominance college students. Correlations between Do scores based on the 28 MMPI items and peer ratings and self-ratings of dominance were .52 and .65, respectively, for college students and .60 and .41, respectively, for high school students.

Knapp (1960) found that Marine Corps officer pilots scored significantly higher on the 28-item Do scale than did enlisted men. The mean scores for the officers and enlisted men were quite similar to mean scores reported for high and low dominance high school and college students. Knapp interpreted his data as supporting the use of the Do scale as a screening device in selecting officers. However, Olmstead and Monachesi (1965) reported that the MMPI Do scale was not able to differentiate between firemen and fire captains. Eschenback and Dupree (1959) found that Do scores did not change as a result of situational stress (a realistic survival test). It would be interesting to know whether Do scores change as individuals change their dominance roles (e.g., when an enlisted man becomes an officer). Unfortunately, no data of this kind are available at this time.

Interpretation of High Do Scores

High scorers on the Do scale see themselves and are seen by others as stronger in face-to-face personal situations, as not readily intimidated, and as feeling safe, secure, and self-confident. Although there is some limited evidence that high scores on the Do scale are more common among persons holding positions of greater responsibility and leadership, no data are available concerning the adequacy of performance in such positions as a function of Do scores. Also, a high Do score is indicative of an individual who (is):

1. appears poised and self-assured
2. self-confident
3. appears free to behave in straightforward manner
4. optimistic
5. resourceful, efficient
6. realistic, task-oriented
7. feels adequate to handle problems
8. perseverant
9. has a dutiful sense of morality
10. has a strong need to face reality

In summary, the high Do scorer is a person who is confident of his/her abilities in coping with problems and stresses in his/her life situation.

Interpretation of Low Do Scores

Low scorers on the Do scale see themselves and are seen by others as submissive, weaker in face-to-face contacts, unassertive, unable to stand up for their own rights and opinions, and easily influenced by other people. Low Do scorers are less likely than high Do scorers to be in positions of responsibility and leadership. Based on an examination of the content of the Do scale items, it appears that a low Do score is indicative of an individual who (is):

1. lacks self-confidence
2. pessimistic
3. inefficient, stereotyped in approach to problems
4. feels inadequate to handle problems
5. gives up easily
6. does not feel sense of duty to others
7. does not face up to the realities of his/her own life situation

In summary, a low Do scorer tends to be an individual who has problems in asserting himself/herself. In addition, he/she is not very effective in handling problems and stresses in his/her life situation.

SOCIAL RESPONSIBILITY (Re) SCALE

Scale Development

The Social Responsibility (Re) scale was developed by Gough, McClosky, and Meehl (1952) as part of a larger project concerning political participation. The original Re scale contained 56 items, with 32 items coming from the MMPI item pool. A score based on the 32 MMPI items can be obtained in addition to a score based on all 56 items, and normative data are available for the 32 MMPI item Re scale.

The four samples used in constructing the Re scale were 50 college fraternity men, 50 college sorority women, 123 social science students from a high school, and 221 ninth grade students. In each sample, the most and least responsible individuals were identified empirically. The definition of responsibility utilized emphasized willingness to accept the consequences of one's own behavior, dependability, trustworthiness, integrity, and sense of obligation to the group. For the high school and college samples, high and low criterion ratings were based on peer nominations. Teachers provided ratings of responsibility for students in the ninth grade sample. The responses of the most responsible and least responsible subjects so identified in each sample to the items in the MMPI item pool and to a questionnaire containing rationally generated items were examined. Items that revealed the best discrimination between most and least responsible subjects in all samples became the Re scale. The 32 MMPI items constituting the Re scale deal with concern for social and moral issues, disapproval of privilege and favor, emphasis on duties and self-discipline, conventionality versus rebelliousness, trust and confidence in the world in general, and poise, assurance, and personal security (Gough et al., 1952).

Reliability and Validity

Gough et al. (1952) reported an uncorrected split-half coefficient of .73 for the 56-item scale for a sample of ninth grade students. Gocka (1965) reported a Kuder-Richardson 21 (internal consistency) value of .63 for the 32-item Re scale for 220 male Veterans Administration psychiatric patients. Gough and his colleagues also reported correlations of .84 and .88 between Re scores based on all 56 items and scores based on the 32 MMPI items in the Re scale for their college and high school samples.

Correlations between MMPI Re scale scores and criterion ratings of responsibility in the derivation samples were .47 for college students and .53 for high school students. For college students the correlation between MMPI Re scores and self-ratings of responsibility was .20, and the correlation between these two variables for the high school students was .23. Optimal cutting scores for the MMPI Re scale yielded correct classification of 78% to 87% of the most and least responsible individuals in the various derivation samples. Gough et al. (1952) reported some limited cross-validational data for the total (56-item) Re scale. They obtained a correlation of .22 between Re scores and ratings of responsibility for a sample of medical students. A correlation of .33 between Re scores and ratings of positive character integration was reported for a sample of 4th year graduate students.

In two studies, persons with higher Re scores tended to have positions of leadership and responsibility. Knapp (1960) found that Marine Corps officers scored significantly higher on the MMPI Re scale than did enlisted men. Olmstead and Monachesi (1956) reported that fire captains scored higher on the MMPI Re scale than firemen, but the difference was not statistically significant.

Duckworth and Duckworth (1975) suggested that the Re scale measures acceptance (high score) or rejection (low score) of a previously held value system, usually that of one's parents. For persons above the age of 25, high Re scorers tend to accept their present value system and intend to continue using it, and low scorers may be questioning their current value system or rejecting their most recently held value system. For younger persons, high Re scores indicate that they accept the value system of their parents, whereas low Re scores indicate questioning or rejection of parental value systems. Duckworth and Duckworth also suggest that high Re scorers, regardless of age, are more rigid in acceptance of values and are less willing to explore other values. They also indicated that older persons tend to score higher than younger persons on the Re scale and that college students who are questioning parental values often receive quite low Re scores.

Interpretation of High Re Scores

High Re scorers tend to see themselves and are seen by others as willing to accept the consequences of their own behavior, as dependable and trustworthy, and as having integrity and a sense of responsibility to the group. They also are more likely than low Re scorers to be in positions of leadership and responsibility. High Re scorers are rigid in acceptance of values and are unwilling to explore other values. Younger persons with high Re scores tend to accept the values of their parents. Also, a high Re score is indicative of an individual who (is):

1. has deep concern over ethical and moral problems
2. has a strong sense of justice
3. sets high standards for self
4. rejects privilege and favor
5. has excessive emphasis on carrying his/her own share of burdens and duties
6. self-confident
7. has trust and confidence in the world in general

In summary, a high Re scorer is a person who has incorporated societal and cultural values and is committed to behaving in a manner consistent with those values. In addition, he/she places high value on honesty and justice.

Interpretation of Low Re Scores

Low Re scorers do not see themselves and are not seen by others as willing to accept responsibility for their own behaviors. They are lacking or deficient in dependability, trustworthiness, integrity, and sense of responsibility to the group. They are less likely than high Re scorers to be in positions of leadership and responsibility. Low Re scorers also are less rigid than high Re scorers in acceptance of values and are more willing to explore other values. Younger persons with low Re scores tend to deny the value system of their parents and to substitute another value system for the parental one. Older persons with low Re scores question or deny their most recently held value system and may have adopted new religious or political outlooks.

PREJUDICE (Pr) SCALE

Scale Development

The Prejudice (Pr) scale was developed by Gough (1951a) to identify persons with anti-Semitic prejudices. The Levinsohn-Sanford Anti-Semitism Scale was administered to 271 high school seniors in a midwestern community, and the 40 highest scoring students (high prejudice) and the 40 lowest scoring students (low prejudice) were identified. The MMPI was administered to the students and item analyses were conducted to compare the responses of high and low prejudiced students to the MMPI items. The 47 items that discriminated significantly between the high and low prejudice groups were included in the Pr scale. The items in the Pr scale deal with such diverse things as intellectual interests, optimism versus pessimism, interpersonal trust, hostility and aggression, personal discontentment, self-assurance, inflexible thinking, and feelings of isolation and estrangement.

Reliability and Validity

Gocka (1965) reported a Kuder-Richardson 21 (internal consistency) value of .82 for the Pr scale for 220 male Veterans Administration psychiatric patients. Split-half reliability coefficients of .79 and .81 for college students have been reported for the Pr scale (Gough, 1951a; Jensen, 1957). Jensen also reported a test-retest reliability coefficient of .56 for the Pr scale for a sample of college freshmen.

After the scale was developed on a high school sample, correlations of .45 and .49 were reported between the Pr scale and the Levinsohn-Sanford Anti-Semitism Scale for college students (Gough, 1951ab). When Pr scores and scores on the California Ethnocentrism-Fascism Scale were correlated for high school and college students, coefficients ranging from .30 to .62 were obtained (Altus & Tafejian, 1953; Gough, 1951ab; Jensen, 1957; Sundberg & Bachelis, 1956; Tafejian, 1951). Pr scores also have been found to correlate positively with Tafejian's 40-item prejudice scale (Stricker, 1961) and negatively with the Purdue Attitude Scale toward Jews (Gough, 1951a; high scores on the Purdue scale indicate favorable attitudes).

Pr scores do not seem to be related to the sex of the respondent (Jensen, 1957). However, there is evidence that high Pr scorers are more likely to come from lower social classes (Gough, 1951b), to have lower IQ scores (Gough, 1951b; Jensen, 1957), and to show poor academic achievement (Jensen, 1957). College students are more likely to score lower on Pr than high school students (Duckworth & Duckworth, 1975; Jensen, 1957). Also, students with different college majors differ in terms of Pr scores (Jensen, 1957). There also are data indicating that high Pr scorers are less well adjusted psychologically, as indicated by other MMPI indices of adjustment and faculty evaluations of student adjustment (Gough, 1951b; Jensen, 1957). Sundberg & Bachelis (1956) demonstrated that subjects can produce higher Pr scores when asked to respond as someone who was prejudiced and intolerant would respond and lower Pr scores when asked to respond as someone who was tolerant and unprejudiced would respond.

Interpretation of High Pr Scores

Persons with high Pr scores are intolerant and prejudiced in their opinions and beliefs. They are extremely rigid in their beliefs, and they often will not even consider points of view different from their own. High Pr scorers are more common among persons of lower socioeconomic status, less intelligent persons, and persons with less formal education. High Pr scorers show poor academic performance and are less well adjusted psychologically than are low Pr scorers. In addition, a high Pr score is indicative of an individual who (is):

1. anti-intellectual
2. pessimistic; lacks hope and confidence in the future
3. cynical, distrustful, doubtful, suspicious
4. feels other cannot be trusted
5. fears exploitation by others
6. lacks self-regard, self-integrity
7. resentful of others; discredits achievements and abilities of others
8. hostile, bitter
9. discontented with current status
10. has a dogmatic style of thinking
11. lacks poise, self-assurance
12. feels isolated, estranged

In summary, a high Pr scorer is a person who is very rigid and intolerant in his/her beliefs. Also, such a person has a generally cynical, distrustful attitude toward other people and the world in general.

Interpretation of Low Pr Scores

Low Pr scorers tend to be tolerant and unprejudiced. They are flexible in their thinking and are open-minded and able to consider points of view that differ from their own. Low Pr scores are more common among persons from higher social classes, with higher IQ scores, and with more formal education. College students often score very low on the Pr scale. Low Pr scorers tend to show high academic achievement, and they are well adjusted psychologically. In addition, a low Pr score is indicative of an individual who (is):

1. has intellectual interests
2. optimistic
3. can place trust in other people
4. self-confident, self-assured, poised
5. free of excessive hostility and bitterness
6. satisfied with current status

In summary, a low Pr scorer tends to be open-minded and tolerant of attitudes and beliefs that differ from his/her own. He/she has a generally positive perception of the world and is effective in coping with his/her life situation.

SOCIAL STATUS (St) SCALE

Scale Development

The Social Status (St) scale was developed by Gough (1948a) by comparing MMPI item responses of high socioeconomic status and low socioeconomic status high school seniors. Status was assessed by an objective scale, and the 38 highest scoring and 38 lowest scoring students from a group of 223 high school seniors were designated as high status and low status groups, respectively. Item analyses identified 34 items that differentiated the two criterion groups. Gough (1948a) suggested that the items of the St scale can be grouped into five general categories: literary-esthetic attitudes; social poise, security, confidence in self and others; denial of fears and anxieties; broad minded attitudes toward moral, religious, and sexual matters; and positive, dogmatic, self-righteous opinions.

Reliability and Validity

Gough (1948a) reported a corrected split-half reliability coefficient of .74 for the St scale for the 223 students in the original derivation sample. A test-retest reliability coefficient of .87 for a smaller sample of 101 students also was reported by Gough. Gocka (1965) reported a Kuder-Richardson 21 (internal consistency) value of .55 for the St scale for 220 male Veterans Adminstration psychiatric patients.

Gough (1949) reported a correlation of .67 between St scores and the objective status measure used in the derivation sample. In a separate cross-validational sample, he found a correlation of .50 between St scores of high school students and socioeconomic status as measured by an objective scale different from the one used in the original derivation of the St scale.

Among high school students, high scorers on the St scale have been reported to be less insecure, to have higher intelligence test and college aptitude test scores, and to show superior academic achievement (Gough, 1948b). High scorers also have been described by Gough as socially extroverted, defensive and reserved in regard to personal problems, and conventional. They tend to have fewer somatic complaints and to be generally better adjusted psychologically.

Gough (1949) and Duckworth and Duckworth (1975) suggested that for some individuals the St scale measures desired social status more than actual status. This is particularly likely when objective evidence of status (income, education, etc.) is not consistent with St scores. Gough described persons with congruent objective status and St scores and those with discrepancies between objective status and St scores. Individuals with objective indices of high status and high St scores come from good families, are ambitious and dependable, and have the potential for high levels of achievement. When both objective indices and St scores indicate low status, persons are seen as obedient and compliant and as lacking drive and confidence. When St scores suggest a higher status than is indicated by objective indices, persons tend to be upwardly mobile and not as submissive and acquiescent. Individuals with low St scores and objective indices of high status are submissive and acquiescent.

Duckworth and Duckworth (1975) characterized high St scorers as desiring some of the nicer things in life, such as good books or nice homes, and as complaining of job dissatisfaction if their status needs are not met on their jobs. If a person seeking help with serious emotional problems has a high St score, good motivation for counseling or psychotherapy is suggested. Low scores on St may indicate poor self-esteem and lack of self-confidence. Low scorers may feel that they deserve a better life but they do not seem to be willing to work to better themselves.

Interpretation of High St Scores

A high score on the St scale is indicative of an individual who (is):
1. from a higher social class or has status desires similar to someone from a higher social class
2. intelligent
3. has a history of superior academic achievement
4. secure, socially extroverted
5. desires some of the nicer things in life (good books, nice home, etc.)
6. complains of job dissatisfaction if status needs are not met on the job
7. defensive and reserved in regard to personal problems
8. conventional
9. generally well adjusted psychologically
10. ambitious, dependable
11. motivated to change in counseling or psychotherapy

In summary, a high scorer on the St scale is a person who has needs and desires generally characteristic of higher socioeconomic subjects (phsycial luxuries, power, etc.). In lower socioeconomic subjects, a high St score suggests a desire to better one's social position in life. A high St scorer generally achieves at high levels and makes satisfactory adjustments to problems and stresses.

Interpretation of Low St Scores

A low score on the St scale is indicative of an individual who (is):
1. from a lower social class or has status desires similar to someone from a lower social class
2. feels that he/she deserves a better life but is not willing to work to improve himself/herself
3. lacks drive
4. lacks self-confidence
5. obedient, submissive, compliant

In summary, a low St scorer is a person who has values and desires similar to lower socioeconomic subjects. Although the low scorer may feel that he/she deserves a better life, he/she does not seem willing to work to attain it.

CONTROL (Cn) SCALE

Scale Development

Cuadra (1953) reasoned that the essential difference between persons with equal psychopathology who are hospitalized and those who are treated as outpatients is that the latter have more control over the expression of their pathology. The Cn scale was developed to assess this control dimension. Cuadra collected 30 pairs of MMPI profiles in which the members of a pair were similar in terms of age, sex, and profile elevation and configuration. However, in each pair one profile was of a person who was hospitalized for psychiatric treatment, and the other profile was of a person who was receiving outpatient psychiatric treatment. By comparing the MMPI item responses of the two groups of patients, 50 items were identified that were answered differently by the two groups of patients. The items were keyed in such a way that high Cn scores indicate responses similar to those of the nonhospitalized patients. The content of the Cn scale items included awareness of one's own weaknesses, sensitivity to social criticism, religious beliefs, and involvement in exciting or risky activities.

Cuadra (1953) reported that scores on the Cn scale were significantly different for his two criterion groups, with nonhospitalized patients scoring higher, but he did not report any cross-validational data. Negative correlations between the Cn scale and the L and K scales of the MMPI and a positive correlation between Cn scores and F scale scores led Cuadra to conclude that one important dimension being tapped by the Cn scale is realistic self-appraisal.

Reliability and Validity

Gocka (1965) reported a Kuder-Richardson 21 (internal consistency) value of .58 for the Cn scale for 220 male Veterans Administration psychiatric patients. No additional validity studies of the Cn scale have been reported.

Interpretation of High Cn Scores

High Cn scorers who have serious psychological problems are not likely to exhibit problem behaviors to others and are more likely than low scorers to be able to handle their problems without being hospitalized. Duckworth and Duckworth (1975) indicated that the Cn scale must be interpreted in relation to the MMPI clinical scales. For persons with very elevated clinical scales, a high Cn score indicates an ability to control problems and to show only what they wish others to observe. Such control can be an asset, but it also can be a liability if the person chooses to hide problems from the psychotherapist and others who are involved in the treatment process. When a high Cn score occurs in the absence of marked elevations in the clinical scales, it is suggestive of an individual who is reserved and unemotional. Such persons may express a desire to be able to be more expressive of their emotions. In addition, a high Cn score is indicative of an individual who (is):

1. described by others as sophisticated and realistic
2. impatient with naive, moralistic, and opinionated people
3. aware of his/her own weaknesses
4. inwardly sensitive to social criticism
5. not accepting of traditional religious beliefs
6. rebellious toward authority
7. explores and experiments with the environment even though it may involve risk of social disapproval

In summary, a high scoring subject on the Cn scale who has serious psychological problems tends to keep the problems to himself/herself rather than revealing them to others. Although this tendency allows such a person to avoid hospitalization, it also may prevent him/her from admitting the need for help.

Interpretation of Low Cn Scores

When low Cn scores are found for persons with serious emotional problems, they indicate an inability to control problem behaviors and suggest that hospitalization may be required. Duckworth and Duckworth (1975) suggested that when low Cn scores are found in persons who do not have marked elevations on the clinical scales of the MMPI they suggest the absence of serious psychological problems. In addition, a low Cn score is indicative of an individual who (is):

1. conventional
2. moralistic
3. not likely to experiment with or explore the environment
4. has traditional religious beliefs
5. has unrealistic self-appraisal

In summary, a low Cn score for a person with serious psychological problems suggests that such a person cannot control his/her problem behaviors and may require hospitalization. Interestingly, low Cn scores also are found among persons who are free of serious psychological problems.

A FINAL CAUTION

The reader is again reminded that the scales discussed in this chapter are research scales. The reliability and validity of many of them have not yet been demonstrated. They have been presented here in the hope of stimulating additional research that will lead to a better understanding of what the scales are measuring. If they are used in clinical interpretation of the MMPI, any inferences derived from the scales should be viewed as very tentative and should be validated against other clinical and test data.

7

Other MMPI Scales

As pointed out in the introductory chapters, empirical keying procedures were employed by Hathaway and McKinley in the construction of
the original MMPI scales. Items were included in a scale if they empirically differentiated between external criterion groups. No emphasis was
placed on the content of the items identified in this manner, and no
attempt was made to ensure that the resulting scales were homogeneous
or internally consistent. However, two other major strategies for scale
construction have been used in subsequent efforts to develop additional
scales for the MMPI from the original item pool. These are the *logical* and
the *homogeneous* keying approaches. The logical keying procedure involves grouping together items that are judged, on the basis of an examination of their content, to assess the trait or characteristic under investigation. Although empirical validity studies may be conducted later to
determine the relationships between scores on such logically derived
scales and external criterion measures, logically constructed scales typically simply are assumed to be measuring the characteristics suggested by
the scale names and are used accordingly without further empirical
validation.

Another alternative to the empirical keying procedure is the homogeneous keying approach to scale construction. In this technique the test
constructor has no a priori notions about what scales are to be developed.
A large pool of heterogeneous items is assembled and administered to a
group of subjects. The resulting item responses are intercorrelated, and
the intercorrelation matrix is factor-analyzed. The factors that emerge are
considered to be the relevant dimensions being tapped by the inventory,
and scales are constructed to assess them by choosing individual MMPI
items that have high loadings on each such factor. The resulting scales
tend to be quite consistent internally. Names or labels are assigned to the
scales by examining the content of items in each scale. As with the scales
constructed by the logical keying approach, the factor scales often are
assumed to be measuring the characteristic suggested by the scale name,

and empirical studies typically are not conducted. In the case of the MMPI, the homogeneous keying procedure also has been used in a somewhat modified manner. Instead of intercorrelating item responses, a task which until recently has exceeded the capacity of most computers, the original MMPI scales are administered to subjects and the resulting scores are intercorrelated and factor-analyzed. The Anxiety (A) and Repression (R) scales discussed in Chapter 6 were constructed using this modified homogeneous keying procedure.

The purpose of this chapter is to discuss some MMPI scales that were constructed utilizing the logical and homogeneous keying approaches. Because several hundred such scales have been developed using these approaches, only selected scales can be considered here. The scales discussed in this chapter were chosen for inclusion because they emerged from comprehensive research efforts, as opposed to the one-shot construction of a single scale, and/or because they have gained some popularity among clinicians who use the MMPI routinely. It should be emphasized that these scales should be viewed as *supplementary* to the standard MMPI scales and should not be used instead of these standard scales.

THE HARRIS SUBSCALES FOR THE MMPI

Subscale Development

As mentioned above, the standard MMPI clinical scales were constructed by empirical keying procedures. Because no attention was given by Hathaway and McKinley to scale homogeneity, the standard clinical scales are quite heterogeneous in terms of item content. The same total raw score on a clinical scale can be achieved by individuals endorsing any combinations of quite different kinds of items. A number of investigators have suggested that systematic analysis of these subgroups of items within the standard clinical scales can add significantly to the interpretation of MMPI protocols (e.g., Comrey, 1957abc, 1958bcde; Comrey & Marggraff, 1958; Graham, Schroeder, & Lilly, 1971; Harris & Lingoes, 1955, 1968; Pepper & Strong, 1958). The subscales developed by Harris represent the most comprehensive effort of this kind. His scales have come to be widely used clinically and are routinely scored and reported by some of the automated MMPI scoring and interpretation services.

Harris and Lingoes (1955, 1968) reported the construction of subscales for 6 of the 10 standard clinical scales (scales 2, 3, 4, 6, 8, 9). They did not develop subscales for scales 1, 5, 7, and 0. Each subscale was constructed logically by examining the content of items within a standard clinical scale and grouping together items that seemed similar in content or were judged to reflect a single attitude or trait. A new label was assigned to each subscale on the basis of Harris and Lingoes' clinical judgment of the content of items in that subscale. Although it was assumed that the resulting subscales would be more homogeneous than their parent scales, no statistical estimates of subscale homogeneity were provided by Harris and Lingoes. Although 31 subscales were developed, three subscales that are obtained by summing scores on other subscale generally are not used in clinical interpretation. The other 28 Harris subscales are listed in Table 7.1, and the numbers of the items included in each subscale, along with the scored response for each item, are presented in Appendix D of this *Guide*.* No scoring keys or profile sheets are available commercially for use with the Harris subscales. However, scoring templates can be constructed using the information in Appendix D. If a profile sheet for plotting the Harris subscales is desired, one can be constructed from the data in Appendix E.

No attempt was made by Harris to avoid placing an item in more than one subscale. Thus, item overlap among the subscales is considerable and may account for the high correlations among subscale scores. Table 7.2 summarizes these intercorrelations as presented by Harris and Lingoes (1968).

Subscale Norms

Harris and Lingoes (1955) presented no normative data for their subscales when they were first described, but a later paper (Harris & Lingoes, 1968) reported means and standard deviations for psychiatric patients at the Langley Porter Clinic. Gocka and Holloway (1963) presented means and standard deviations for 68 male Veterans Administration psychiatric patients. Dahlstrom et al. (1972) developed tables for converting raw scores on the Harris subscales to T-scores based on the scores of normal adult male and female subjects who were used in the original MMPI derivational work. These Dahlstrom et al. norms for normal subjects, which are the ones that should be used for general clinical interpretation of the Harris subscales, are reproduced in Appendix E of this *Guide*.

Subscale Reliability

Gocka (1965) presented reliability data for the Harris subscales. He calculated Kuder-Richardson 21 values (internal consistency) for the subscales based on 220 male admissions to a Veterans Administration Hospital. These values are reported in Table 7.1. Although several of the Harris subscales have rather low coefficients, most of the subscales have a high degree of internal consistency.

Subscale Validity

Although the Harris subscales have been in existence for about 30 years and have come to gain fairly wide usage among clinicians (partly because they are scored routinely by some automated scoring and interpretation services), disappointingly little empirical research concerning the subscales has been published. The factor analytic work of Comrey (1957abc, 1958bcde; Comrey & Marggraff, 1958) indirectly offers some support for the construct validity of the Harris subscales. Comrey reported factor analyses of the intercorrelations of items *within* each scale, separately for each of the clinical scales of the MMPI (excluding scales 5 and 0). Al-

---

* In their 1968 paper Harris and Lingoes presented corrections to their earlier paper in terms of items included in some of the subscales. These corrected scale compositions are the ones presented in Appendix D and throughout the discussion of the Harris subscales.

Table 7.1. Internal consistency values (Kuder-Richardson 21) for the Harris subscales of the MMPI[a]

Scale		Subscale	Kuder-Richardson relia-bility
1—Hypochondriasis		None	
2—Depression	D1	Subjective Depression	.82
	D2	Psychomotor Retardation	.11
	D3	Physical Malfunctioning	.24
	D4	Mental Dullness	.80
	D5	Brooding	.73
3—Hysteria	Hy1	Denial of Social Anxiety	.72
	Hy2	Need for Affection	.65
	Hy3	Lassitude-Malaise	.85
	Hy4	Somatic Complaints	.84
	Hy5	Inhibition of Aggression	.31
4—Psychopathic Deviate	Pd1	Familial Discord	.67
	Pd2	Authority Problems	.04
	Pd3	Social Imperturbability	.67
	Pd4A	Social Alienation	.71
	Pd4B	Self-alienation	.78
5—Masculinity-Femininity		None	
6—Paranoia	Pa1	Persecutory Ideas	.85
	Pa2	Poignancy	.48
	Pa3	Naivete	.70
7—Psychasthenia		None	
8—Schizophrenia	Sc1A	Social Alienation	.71
	Sc1B	Emotional Alienation	.37
	Sc2A	Lack of Ego Mastery, Cognitive	.82
	Sc2B	Lack of Ego Mastery, Conative	.76
	Sc2C	Lack of Ego Mastery, Defective Inhibition	.74
	Sc3	Bizarre Sensory Experiences	.80
9—Hypomania	Ma1	Amorality	.46
	Ma2	Psychomotor Acceleration	.19
	Ma3	Imperturbability	.51
	Ma4	Ego Inflation	.50
0—Social Introversion		None	

[a] Source: Gocka (1965).

though there are some significant differences between the logically derived Harris subscales and the corresponding factor-analytically derived Comrey factors, in general the Comrey studies revealed factors within each clinical scale that are similar to the Harris subscales and supported Harris' notion that the clinical scales are not homogeneous and unidimensional. The reader who is interested in a detailed comparison of the Harris subscales and the Comrey factors is referred to Appendix F of this *Guide,* where item overlap for the subscales and the factors is presented.

Table 7.2.   Intercorrelations for Harris subscales[a]

	D	D1	D2	D3	D4	
D1	.92					
D2	.70	.65				
D3	.64	.60	.18			
D4	.86	.91	.63	.50		
D5	.70	.85	.45	.42	.83	
	Hy	Hy1	Hy2	Hy3	Hy4	
Hy1	.25					
Hy2	.31	.28				
Hy3	.67	−.26	−.19			
Hy4	.71	−.13	−.15	.55		
Hy5	.38	.25	.36	−.06	−.01	
	Pd	Pd1	Pd2	Pd3	Pd4A	
Pd1	.58					
Pd2	.48	.12				
Pd3	−.33	−.39	−.03			
Pd4A	.72	.44	.25	−.53		
Pd4B	.77	.37	.29	−.56	.74	
	Pa	Pa1	Pa2			
Pa1	.68					
Pa2	.67	.53				
Pa3	.31	−.29	−.24			
	Sc	Sc1A	Sc1B	Sc2A	Sc2B	Sc2C
Sc1A	.87					
Sc1B	.78	.63				
Sc2A	.74	.52	.58			
Sc2B	.80	.63	.85	.76		
Sc2C	.79	.87	.53	.45	.55	
Sc3	.72	.47	.40	.44	.44	.68
	Ma	Ma1	Ma2	Ma3		
Ma1	.66					
Ma2	.75	.40				
Ma3	−.14	−.14	−.46			
Ma4	.77	.40	.56	−.30		

[a] Source: Harris and Lingoes (1968).

Lingoes (1960) factor-analyzed scores on the Harris subscales and on the Wiener subtle-obvious subscales of the MMPI (Wiener, 1948) in an attempt to determine the statistical factor structure of the MMPI. He concluded that the dimensionality of the MMPI is more complex than the 6 standard scales from which the various subscales were derived, but simpler than the 36 subscales (Harris, Wiener) included in his own factor analysis. Harris (1955) reasoned intuitively that his subscales should be more homogeneous than the parent scales from which they were drawn, but he did not offer any evidence in this regard. Calvin (1974) statistically examined the homogeneity of the 5 Harris subscales for scale 2 (Depression). He separately factor-analyzed inter-item correlations for each of the five subscales, and he concluded that four of the subscales appeared to be unidimensional, whereas one subscale (Psychomotor Retardation) was two-dimensional (loss of interest in life activities and inhibition of hostility).

Harris and Christiansen (1946) studied pretherapy MMPI differences between neurotic patients who were judged to have been successful in psychotherapy and similar patients who were judged to have been unsuccessful in psychotherapy. They found that the successful patients scored lower on scales 4, 6, 8, and 9 of the MMPI, suggesting that they had more ego strength. Significant differences between successful and unsuccessful patients also were identified for eight Harris subscales. Successful patients scored lower on the Pd1 (Familial Discord), Pd2 (Authority Problems), and Pd4A (Social Alienation) subscales, on the Pa1 (Persecutory Ideas) subscale, on the Sc2C (Defective Inhibition) and Sc3 (Bizarre Sensory Experiences) subscales. Harris and Christiansen did not address themselves to the question of whether greater accuracy of prediction of psychotherapy outcome was possible with the subscales than with only the standard clinical scales. They felt, however, that the subscale information could lead to a better understanding of how the successful therapy patient views himself and the environment in which he lives.

Gocka and Holloway (1965) correlated scores of psychiatric patients on the Harris subscales with other MMPI scales assessing social desirability, introversion-extroversion, and dissimulation, with a number of demographic variables (intelligence, occupational level, marital status), with legal competency status at the time of hospital admission, and with number of days of hospitalization. Most Harris subscales were related to the social desirability scale, and some Harris subscales were related to the introversion-extroversion and dissimulation scales. Few significant correlations were found between Harris subscale scores and demographic variables. Two Harris subscale scores correlated significantly with competency status, and no Harris subscale correlated significantly with length of hospitalization.

Panton (1959) compared the Harris subscale scores of black and white prison inmates. He found that whites scored higher on Pd2 (Authority Problems), suggesting that whites had more authority problems and aggressive tendencies than blacks. Blacks scored higher on Pa1 (Persecutory Ideas), Sc1A (Social Alienation), and Ma4 (Ego Inflation), suggesting more psychotic trends for blacks than for whites. Panton also compared the Harris subscale scores of prison inmates with the psychiatric norms presented by Harris and Lingoes (1968). He found that prison inmates were higher than the psychiatric patients on Pd4A (Social Alienation), Pd4B (Self-Alienation), and Ma1 (Amorality). Prisoners were lower than the psychiatric patients on D1 (Subjective Depression), D2 (Psychomotor Retardation), D4 (Mental Dullness), Hy2 (Need for Affection), Hy3 (Lassitude-Malaise), Hy5 (Inhibition of Aggression), Sc2A (Lack of Cognitive Ego Mastery), Sc2B (Lack of Conative Ego Mastery), and Ma2 (Psychomotor Acceleration).

Calvin (1975) attempted to identify empirical behavioral correlates for the Harris subscales for a sample of hospitalized psychiatric patients. He compared high scorers on each Harris subscale with other scorers on that subscale on a number of extra-test variables, including psychiatric diagnosis, reasons for hospitalization, nurses' ratings, and psychiatrists' ratings. Although 10 of the 28 Harris subscales were determined to have reliable behavioral correlates, Calvin concluded that in most cases the Harris subscales are not likely to add significantly to protocol analysis based on the standard clinical scales for psychiatric patients. The results of Calvin's study are included in the interpretive descriptions that are presented in the following section.

Interpretation of Subscales

As with the other scales previously discussed, it is not possible to establish absolutely firm cutoff scores to define high and low scorers on the subscales. As the clinician gains experience with the subscales, he/she will come to establish specific cutoff scores for the settings in which the MMPI is used. The individual who is just beginning to use the subscales for MMPI interpretation should find it useful to consider T-scores greater than 70 as high scores and T-scores less than 40 as low scores.

The descriptions that follow for high and low scorers on each of the subscales are based on the descriptions provided by Harris and Lingoes (1955, 1968), on the validity studies reviewed in the previous section, on the author's own clinical experience, and on examination of the content of the items in each subscale. The resulting descriptions should be viewed as preliminary. As the subscales are used more frequently and as more empirical research is conducted to determine extra-test correlates for the subscales, more comprehensive, and perhaps more accurate, descriptions can be developed. The descriptions presented are *modal* ones, and as such they will not apply completely to every examinee who achieves high or low scores on the subscales. It should be emphasized again that the Harris subscales should be used to *supplement* the standard validity and clinical scales and should not replace them.

Subjective Depression (D1)

A high score on the D1 subscale is indicative of an individual who (is):
1. feels unhappy, blue, or depressed much of the time
2. lacks energy for coping with problems of his/her everyday life
3. not interested in what goes on around him/her
4. feels nervous or tense much of the time
5. have difficulties in concentrating and attending
6. has a poor appetite and trouble sleeping
7. broods and cries frequently
8. lacks self-confidence
9. feels inferior and useless
10. easily hurt by criticism
11. feels uneasy, shy, and embarrassed in social situations
12. tends to avoid interactions with other people, except for relatives and close friends
13. if a hospitalized psychiatric patient, likely to receive a clinical diagnosis of depressive neurosis

A low score on the D1 subscale is indicative of an individual who (is):
1. feels happy and satisfied
2. interested in and stimulated by his/her environment
3. denies tension, difficulties in concentration and attendance, poor appetite, sleep disturbances, and frequent brooding or crying
4. self-confident
5. socially extroverted
6. likes to be around other people
7. at ease in social situations

Psychomotor retardation (D2)

A high score on the D2 subscale is indicative of an individual who (is):
1. characterized as immobilized and withdrawn
2. lacks energy to cope with everyday activities
3. avoids other people
4. denies hostile or aggressive impulses or actions
A low score on the D2 subscale is indicative of an individual who (is):
1. describes himself/herself as active and involved
2. has no difficulty getting started on things
3. views everyday life as interesting and rewarding
4. admits to having hostile and aggressive impulses at times

Physical malfunctioning (D3)

A high score on the D3 subscale is indicative of an individual who (is):
1. preoccupied with his/her own physical functioning
2. denies good health
3. reports a wide variety of specific somatic symptoms that may include weakness, hay fever or asthma, poor appetite, constipation, nausea or vomiting, and convulsions
A low score on the D3 subscale is indicative of an individual who (is):
1. presents himself/herself as being in good physical health
2. does not report the wide variety of specific somatic symptoms characteristic of high scorers on this subscale

Mental Dullness (D4)

A high score on the D4 subscale is indicative of an individual who (is):
1. lacks energy to cope with the problems of everyday life
2. feels tense
3. complains of difficulties in concentrating
4. complains of poor memory and judgment
5. lacks self-confidence
6. feels inferior to others
7. gets little enjoyment out of life
8. appears to have concluded that life is no longer worthwhile
A low score on the D4 subscale is indicative of an individual who (is):
1. views life as interesting and worthwhile
2. feels capable of coping with everyday problems
3. denies tension

4. denies difficulties in concentrating
5. claims that memory and judgment are satisfactory
6. self-confident
7. compares himself/herself favorably with other people

Brooding (D5)

A high score on the D5 subscale is indicative of an individual who (is):
1. broods, ruminates, and cries much of the time
2. lacks energy to cope with problems
3. seems to have concluded that life is no longer worthwhile
4. feels inferior, unhappy, and useless
5. easily hurt by criticism
6. feels that he/she is losing control of his/her thought processes
   A low score on the D5 subscale is indicative of an individual who (is):
1. feels happy most of the time
2. feels that life is worthwhile
3. denies lack of energy, brooding, and frequent crying
4. self-confident
5. not excessively sensitive to criticism

Denial of Social Anxiety (Hy1)

A high score on the Hy1 subscale is indicative of an individual who (is):
1. socially extroverted
2. feels quite comfortable in interacting with other people
3. finds it easy to talk with other people
4. not easily influenced by social standards and customs
   A low score on the Hy1 subscale is indicative of an individual who (is):
1. socially introverted
2. shy and bashful in social situations
3. finds it difficult to talk with other people
4. greatly influenced by social standards and customs

Need for Affection (Hy2)

A high score on the Hy2 subscale is indicative of an individual who (is):
1. expresses naively optimistic and trusting attitudes toward other people
2. sees others as honest, sensitive, and reasonable
3. denies having negative feelings about other people
4. tries to avoid unpleasant confrontations whenever possible
5. has strong needs for attention and affection from others and fears that these needs will not be met if he/she is more honest about his/her feelings and attitudes
   A low score on the Hy2 subscale is indicative of an individual who (is):
1. has very negative, critical, and suspicious attitudes toward other people
2. sees others as dishonest, selfish, and unreasonable
3. admits to negative feelings toward other people who are perceived as treating him/her badly

Lassitude-Malaise (Hy3)

A high score on the Hy3 subscale is indicative of an individual who (is):
1. generally uncomfortable and not in good health
2. feels weak, fatigued, or tired
3. does not present specific somatic complaints
4. reports difficulties in concentrating, poor appetite, and sleep disturbance
5. feels unhappy and blue
6. describes home environment as unpleasant and uninteresting.
A low score on the Hy3 subscale is indicative of an individual who (is):
1. comfortable and in good health
2. does not have difficulties in concentrating, poor appetite, or disturbed sleep
3. feels happy and satisfied with his/her life situation
A low score on the Hy3 subscale is indicative of an individual who (is):
1. comfortable and in good health
2. does not have difficulties in concentrating, poor appetite, or disturbed sleep
3. feels happy and satisfied with his/her life situation

Somatic Complaints (Hy4)

A high score on the Hy4 subscale is indicative of an individual who (is):
1. presents multiple somatic complaints
2. complains of pain in head and/or chest
3. complains of fainting spells, dizziness, or balance problems
4. complains of nausea and vomiting, poor vision, shakiness, and feeling too hot or too cold
5. utilizes repression and conversion of affect
6. expresses little or no hostility toward other people
A low score on the Hy4 subscale is indicative of an individual who (is):
1. does not report the multiple somatic symptoms characteristic of high scorers on this subscale

Inhibition of Aggression (Hy5)

A high score on the Hy5 subscale is indicative of an individual who (is):
1. denies hostile and aggressive impulses
2. says he/she is not interested in reading about crime and violence
3. sensitive about how others respond to him/her
4. says he/she is decisive
A low score on the Hy5 subscale is indicative of an individual who (is):
1. admits to hostile and aggressive impulses
2. expresses an interest in reading about crime and violence
3. sees himself/herelf as indecisive
4. says he/she is not very concerned about how other people view him/her

Familial Discord (Pd1)

A high score on the Pd1 subscale is indicative of an individual who (is):
1. describes his/her home and family situation as quite unpleasant

2. has felt like leaving the home situation
3. describes his/her home as lacking in love, understanding, and support
4. describes his/her family as critical, quarrelsome, and refusing to permit adequate freedom and independence

A low score on the Pd1 subscale is indicative of an individual who (is):
1. describes his/her home and family situation in very positive terms
2. sees his/her family as offering love, understanding, and support
3. describes his/her family as not being overly controlling or domineering

Authority Problems (Pd2)

A high score on the Pd2 subscale is indicative of an individual who (is):
1. resentful of societal and parental standards and customs
2. admits to having been in trouble in school or with the law
3. has definite opinions about what is right and wrong
4. stands up for what he/she believes
5. not greatly influenced by the values and standards of others

A low score on the Pd2 subscale is indicative of an individual who (is):
1. tends to be very socially conforming and accepting of authority
2. does not express personal opinions or beliefs openly
3. easily influenced by other people
4. denies having been in trouble in school or with the law

Social Imperturbability (Pd3)

A high score on the Pd3 subscale is indicative of an individual who (is):
1. presents himself/herself as comfortable and confident in social situations
2. likes to interact with other people
3. experiences no difficulty in talking with other people
4. tends to be somewhat exhibitionistic and "show-offish"
5. has strong opinions about many things and is not reluctant to defend his/her opinions vigorously

A low score on the Pd3 subscale is indicative of an individual who (is):
1. experiences a great deal of discomfort and anxiety in social situations
2. does not like to meet new people
3. finds it difficult to talk in interpersonal situations
4. is socially conforming
5. does not express personal opinions or attitudes

Social Alienation (Pd4A)

A high score on the Pd4A subscale is indicative of an individual who (is):
1. feels alienated, isolated, and estranged
2. believes that other people do not understand him/her
3. feels lonely, unhappy, and unloved
4. feels that he/she gets a raw deal from life
5. blames other people for his/her problems and shortcomings
6. concerned about how other people react to him/her
7. self-centered and insensitive to the needs and feelings of others
8. acts in inconsiderate ways toward other people

9. verbalizes regret and remorse for his/her actions
   A low score on the Pd4A subscale is indicative of an individual who (is):
1. feels that he/she belongs in his/her social environment
2. sees other people as loving, understanding, and supportive
3. finds interpersonal relationships gratifying
4. not overly influenced by the values and attitudes of others
5. willing to settle down; finds security in routine

Self-Alienation (Pd4B)

A high score on the Pd4B subscale is indicative of an individual who (is):
1. describes himself/herself as uncomfortable and unhappy
2. has problems in concentrating
3. does not find daily life interesting or rewarding
4. verbalizes regret, guilt, and remorse for past deeds but is vague about the nature of this misbehavior
5. finds it hard to settle down
6. may use alcohol excessively
   A low score on the Pd4B subscale is indicative of an individual who (is):
1. presents himself/herself as comfortable and happy
2. finds daily life stimulating and rewarding
3. willing to settle down
4. denies excessive use of alcohol
5. does not express regret, remorse, or guilt about past misdeeds

Persecutory Ideas (Pa1)

A high score on the Pa1 subscale is indicative of an individual who (is):
1. views the world as a threatening place
2. feels that he/she is getting a raw deal from life
3. feels misunderstood
4. feels that others have unfairly blamed or punished him/her
5. suspicious and untrusting of other people
6. blames others for his/her problems and shortcomings
7. in extreme cases may have delusions of persecution
   A low score on the Pa1 subscale is indicative of an individual who (is):
1. feels that he/she is understood and fairly treated
2. able to trust other people
3. does not project blame for problems and shortcomings
4. denies the persecutory ideas expressed by high scorers on this subscale

Poignancy (Pa2)

A high score on the Pa2 subscale is indicative of an individual who (is):
1. sees himself/herself as more high-strung and more sensitive than other people
2. says that he/she feels more intensely than others
3. feels lonely and misunderstood
4. looks for risky or exciting activities to make him/her feel better
   A low score on the Pa2 subscale is indicative of an individual who (is):
1. feels understood and accepted

2. does not present himself/herself as more sensitive than others
3. avoids risky or dangerous activities

Naivete (Pa3)

A high score on the Pa3 subscale is indicative of an individual who (is):
1. expresses extremely naive and optimistic attitudes about other people
2. sees others as honest, unselfish, generous, and altruistic
3. presents himself/herself as trusting
4. says he/she has high moral standards
5. denies hostility and negative impulses

A low score on the Pa3 subscale is indicative of an individual who (is):
1. has rather negative and suspicious attitudes toward other people
2. sees others as dishonest, selfish, and untrustworthy
3. admits to some hostility and resentment toward people who make demands on or take advantage of him/her

Social Alienation (Sc1A)

A high score on the Sc1A subscale is indicative of an individual who (is):
1. feels that he/she is getting a raw deal from life
2. feels that other people do not understand him/her
3. feels that other people have it in for him/her
4. feels that other people are trying to harm him/her
5. describes family situation as lacking in love and support
6. feels that family treats him/her more as a child than an adult
7. feels lonely and empty
8. admits that he/she has never had a love relationship with anyone
9. reports hostility and hatred toward family members
10. avoids social situations and interpersonal relationships whenever possible

A low score on the Sc1A subscale is indicative of an individual who (is):
1. feels understood and loved
2. reports having rewarding emotional involvements with other people
3. describes his/her family situation in positive terms
4. denies feelings of hatred and resentment toward family members

Emotional Alienation (Sc1B)

A high score on the Sc1B subscale is indicative of an individual who (is):
1. reports feelings of depression and despair; wishes he/she were dead
2. is apathetic and frightened
3. may exhibit sadistic and/or masochistic needs

A low score on the Sc1B subscale is indicative of an individual who (is):
1. denies feelings of depression and despair
2. not apathetic and frightened
3. feels that life is worth living
4. denies sadistic or masochistic needs

Lack of Ego Mastery, Cognitive (Sc2A)

A high score on the Sc2A subscale is indicative of an individual who (is):
1. feels that he/she might be losing his/her mind
2. reports strange thought processes and/or feelings of unreality
3. reports difficulties in concentration and memory

A low score on the Sc2A subscale is indicative of an individual who (is):
1. denies concern about loss of control of thought processes
2. does not admit to strange or unusual thought processes
3. does not admit to feelings of unreality
4. does not admit difficulties in concentration and memory

Lack of Ego Mastery, Conative (Sc2B)

A high score on the Sc2B subscale is indicative of an individual who (is):
1. feels that life is a strain; admits feelings of depression and despair
2. has difficulty in coping with everyday problems; worries excessively
3. responds to stress by withdrawing into fantasy and daydreaming
4. does not find his/her daily activities interesting and rewarding
5. has given up hope of things getting better
6. may wish that he/she were dead

A low score on the Sc2B subscale is indicative of an individual who (is):
1. feels that life is interesting and very much worthwhile
2. has the energy to cope with everyday problems
3. denies feelings of depression, excessive worry, suicidal ideation

Lack of Ego Mastery, Defective Inhibition (Sc2C)

A high score on the Sc2C subscale is indicative of an individual who (is):
1. feels that he/she is not in control of his/her emotions and impulses and is frightened by this perceived loss of control
2. tends to be restless, hyperactive, and irritable
3. may have periods of laughing and crying that he/she cannot control
4. may report episodes during which he/she did not know what was being done and later could not remember what had been done

A low score on the Sc2C subscale is indicative of an individual who (is):
1. denies concern about loss of control of impulses and emotions
2. does not admit to restlessness, hyperactivity, or irritability
3. does not admit to periods of activity that he/she could not control or could not later remember

Bizarre Sensory Experiences (Sc3)

A high score on the Sc3 subscale is indicative of an individual who (is):
1. experiences feeling that his/her body is changing in strange or unusual ways
2. reports skin sensitivity, feeling hot or cold, voice changes, muscle twitching, clumsiness, problems in balance, ringing or buzzing in the ears, paralysis, weakness
3. admits to hallucinations, unusual thought content, ideas of external influence

A low score on the Sc3 subscale is indicative of an individual who (is):

1. denies bodily changes, feelings of depersonalization, and other strange experiences characteristic of high scorers on this scale

Amorality (Ma1)

A high score on the Ma1 subscale is indicative of an individual who (is):
1. perceives other people as selfish, dishonest, and opportunistic, and because of these perceptions feels justified in behaving in similar ways
2. seems to derive vicarious satisfaction from the manipulative exploits of others

A low score on the Ma1 subscale is indicative of an individual who (is):
1. denies that other people are selfish, dishonest, or opportunistic and finds such behaviors unacceptable in himself/herself
2. denies receiving vicarious gratification from the manipulative exploits of others

Psychomotor Acceleration (Ma2)

A high score on the Ma2 subscale is indicative of an individual who (is):
1. experiences acceleration of speech, thought processes, and motor activity
2. feels tense and restless
3. feels excited or elated without cause
4. becomes bored easily and seeks out risk, excitement, or danger as a way of overcoming the boredom
5. admits to impulses to do something harmful or shocking

A low score on the Ma2 subscale is indicative of an individual who (is):
1. calm and placid
2. denies hyperactivity, restlessness, or tension
3. satisfied with a life situation that many other people might judge to be dull or boring
4. avoids situations or activities involving risk or danger

Imperturbability (Ma3)

A high score on the Ma3 subscale is indicative of an individual who (is):
1. denies social anxiety
2. feels comfortable around other people
3. has no problem in talking with others
4. professes little concern about or sensitivity to the opinions, values, and attitudes of other people
5. feels impatient and irritable toward others

A low score on the Ma3 subscale is indicative of an individual who (is):
1. quite uncomfortable around other people
2. has problem in talking with others
3. easily influenced by the opinions, values, and attitudes of those around him/her
4. denies resentment, impatience, irritability toward others

Ego Inflation (Ma4)

A high score on the Ma4 subscale is indicative of an individual who (is):

1. has an unrealistic evaluation of his/her own abilities and self-worth
2. resentful and opportunistic when others make demands on him/her, particularly if the persons making those demands are perceived as less capable

A low score on the Ma4 subscale is indicative of an individual who (is):

1. has a realistic notion of his/her own self worth or may even be extremely self-critical
2. denies resentment toward others who make demands on him/her

SUBSCALES FOR SCALES 5 AND 0

Development of the Subscales

As stated in the previous section, Harris and Lingoes (1955, 1968) did not develop subscales for scales 5 (Masculinity-Femininity) and 0 (Social Introversion) of the MMPI. Their omission of these scales was consistent with other early research efforts that did not consider scales 5 and 0 as standard clinical scales. In recent years there has been an increasing awareness of the importance of scales 5 and 0 in the clinical interpretation of MMPI protocols.

An early effort by Pepper and Strong (1958), who used clinical judgment in forming subgroups of items for scale 5, has received little attention among MMPI users. No published studies are available concerning subscales for scale 0. More recently, factor analyses of scales 5 and 0 (Graham et al., 1971) have provided the basis for the construction of subscales for these two scales. The factor analyses were conducted on scale 5 and 0 item responses of psychiatric inpatients, psychiatric outpatients, and normal subjects. For each of the two scales seven factors emerged, one of which represented demographic variables included in the analysis.

Serkownek (1975) utilized the data from Graham et al.'s factor analyses to develop subscales for scales 5 and 0. Items that loaded higher than .30 on a factor were selected for the scale to assess that factor dimension. Labels were assigned to the subscales on the basis of an examination of the content of the items included in the scale. Whereas most of the items in the subscales are scored in the same direction as for the parent scales, 14 items from the scale 5 subscales and 7 items from the scale 0 subscales are scored in the opposite direction from the parent scales, to be consistent with their factor loadings. The scale 5 and scale 0 subscales are listed in Table 7.3. Item composition and scoring directions for each subscale are presented in Appendix G of this *Guide*. Although scoring keys for the scale 5 and scale 0 subscales are not available commercially, they can be constructed from the data presented in Appendix G.

Subscale Norms

Serkownek (1975) provided norms for the scale 5 and scale 0 subscales for a group of normal subjects. T-score conversion tables for males and females separately are reproduced in Appendix H of this *Guide*. If a profile sheet for plotting the subscales is desired, one can be constructed from the data in Appendix H.

Table 7.3. Subscales for scales 5 and 0 of the MMPI[a]

Scale		Subscale
5 – Masculinity-Femininity	Mf1	Narcissism-Hypersensitivity
	Mf2	Stereotypic Feminine Interests
	Mf3	Denial of Stereotypic Masculine Interests
	Mf4	Heterosexual Discomfort-Passivity
	Mf5	Introspective-Critical
	Mf6	Socially Retiring
0 – Social Introversion	Si1	Inferiority-Personal Discomfort
	Si2	Discomfort with Others
	Si3	Staid-Personal Rigidity
	Si4	Hypersensitivity
	Si5	Distrust
	Si6	Physical-Somatic Concerns

[a] Source: Serkownek (1975).

Subscale Reliability and Validity

Although no reliability data are available for the scale 5 and scale 0 subscales, because of the factor analytic basis for scale construction, one can assume that the subscales possess a high level of internal consistency. No validity data are available for the subscales.

Interpretation of Scores on the Subscales

Because the scale 5 and scale 0 subscales only recently have been made available for general clinical use, no tradition exists concerning cutoffs for high and low scores on the subscales. Until additional data become available, the best procedure is to use the same cutoff scores as for the Harris subscales. Subscale T-scores greater than 70 should be considered as high scores, and subscale T-scores less than 40 should be considered as low scores. Because no validity data and only limited clinical experience are available for the subscales, the interpretive descriptions that follow are based on an examination of the content of items included in each subscale. The descriptions should be considered as preliminary, and should be expanded and/or modified on the basis of future research data and clinical experience with the subscales.

Narcissism-Hypersensitivity (Mf1)

A high score on the Mf1 subscale is indicative of an individual who (is):
1. self-centered, narcissistic
2. concerned about his/her physical appearance
3. sees himself/herself as extremely sensitive and easily hurt
4. lacks self-confidence
5. preoccupied with sexual matters
6. expresses resentment and hostility toward his/her family
7. characterizes other people as insensitive, unreasonable, and dishonest
   A low score on the Mf1 subscale is indicative of an individual who (is):
1. self-confident
2. free of worry

3. denies concern about sexual matters
4. not very sensitive to the reactions of others
5. denies negative feelings about his/her family
6. characterizes other people as sensitive, reasonable, and honest

Stereotypic Feminine Interests (Mf2)*

A high score on the Mf2 subscale is indicative of an individual who (is):
1. expresses interest in culturally feminine occupations (e.g., nurse, librarian, etc.)
2. enjoys culturally feminine activities and pastimes (e.g., reading poetry or love stories, growing plants, cooking, etc.)
3. as a child liked culturally feminine play activities (e.g., dolls, hopscotch, etc.)

Denial of Stereotypic Masculine Interests (Mf3)

A high score on the Mf3 subscale is indicative of an individual who (is):
1. not interested in culturally masculine occupations (e.g., forest ranger, soldier, building contractor, etc.)
2. does not enjoy culturally masculine activities or interests (e.g., science, hunting, reading mechanics magazines, etc.)
A low score on the Mf3 subscale is indicative of an individual who (is):
1. interested in culturally masculine occupations (e.g., forest ranger, soldier, building contractor, etc.)
2. enjoys culturally masculine activities and interests (e.g., science, hunting, reading mechanics magazines, etc.)

Heterosexual Discomfort — Passivity (Mf4)

A high score on the Mf4 subscale is indicative of an individual who (is):
1. attracted by members of his/her own sex
2. uncomfortable talking about sex
3. passive
4. unaspiring
A low score on the Mf4 subscale is indicative of an individual who (is):
1. denies being attracted by members of his/her own sex
2. comfortable talking about sex
3. assertive
4. aspiring

Introspective-Critical (Mf5)

A high score on the Mf5 subscale is indicative of an individual who (is):
1. introverted
2. dislikes crowds

---

* Empirical data (Graham et al., 1971) suggest that scores on the Mf2 subscale (Stereotypic Feminine Interests) and the Mf3 subscale (Denial of Stereotypic Masculine Interests) are relatively independent of each other. Thus, an individual can score high on both, low on both, or high on one and low on the other. For example, although a high score on Mf2 indicates interest in feminine activities, it does not necessarily indicate a lack of interest in masculine activities.

3. lacks self-confidence
4. does not subscribe to some fundamentalist religious beliefs (e.g., devil, hell, afterlife)

A low score on the Mf5 subscale is indicative of an individual who (is):

1. extroverted
2. enjoys and feels comfortable in loud, active social gatherings
3. self-confident
4. subscribes to some fundamentalist religious beliefs (e.g., devil, hell, afterlife)

Socially Retiring (Mf6)

A high score on the Mf6 subscale is indicative of an individual who (is):

1. socially introverted
2. tries to avoid being the center of attention
3. does not stand up for his/her own rights or argue in support of his/her opinions
4. does not seek out excitement, danger, or risk

A low score on the Mf6 subscale is indicative of an individual who (is):

1. socially extroverted
2. exhibitionistic; enjoys being the center of attention
3. stands up for his/her rights; argues in support of his/her opinions
4. seeks out excitement, risk, or danger

Inferiority—Personal Discomfort (Si1)

A high score on the Si1 subscale is indicative of an individual who (is):

1. lacks social skills
2. shy, easily embarrassed in social situations
3. finds it difficult to talk in social situations
4. does not make friends easily
5. avoids social interactions whenever possible
6. sensitive to criticism
7. socially suggestible
8. feels unhappy; views himself/herself as failure
9. indecisive; obsessive
10. impatient
11. has problems in concentrating
12. does not face up to problems

A low score on the Si1 subscale is indicative of an individual who (is):

1. socially extroverted; comfortable in social situations
2. makes friends easily
3. finds it easy to talk in social situations
4. not overly sensitive to criticism
5. feels happy and successful
6. patient, decisive
7. faces up to problems
8. denies problems in concentrating

Discomfort with Others (Si2)

A high score on the Si2 subscale is indicative of an individual who (is):

1. uncomfortable around most other people
2. dislikes crowds and large social gatherings
3. withdraws from social interactions whenever possible
4. lacks self-confidence; gives up easily
    A low score on the Si2 subscale is indicative of an individual who (is):
1. enjoys being around other people
2. feels comfortable around most other people
3. seeks out excitement
4. self-confident; does not give up easily

Staid — Personal Rigidity (Si3)

A high score on the Si3 subscale is indicative of an individual who (is):
1. dislikes social groups (clubs, etc.) and parties
2. does not seek out excitement
3. avoids placing himself/herself in risky or competitive situations
4. has no desire to assume leadership role
    A low score on the Si3 subscale is indicative of an individual who (is):
1. enjoys social groups (clubs, etc.) and parties
2. seeks out excitement, risk, and competition
3. has periods of hyperactivity
4. blames others for his/her failure to accomplish great things

Hypersensitivity (Si4)

A high score on the Si4 subscale is indicative of an individual who (is):
1. overly sensitive to reactions of others; easily hurt
2. enjoys being the center of attention
3. broods; has problems in concentrating
4. does not face up to problems; gives up easily
    A low score on the Si4 subscale is indicative of an individual who (is):
1. avoids being the center of attention
2. not especially sensitive to reactions of others
3. denies problems in concentrating
4. faces up to problems; does not give up easily

Distrust (Si5)

A high score on the Si5 subscale is indicative of an individual who (is):
1. has generally negative perception of other people
2. sees others as selfish, dishonest, insensitive, and untrustworthy
3. feels overwhelmed by problems and responsibilities
4. indecisive; obsessive
5. lacks self-confidence
    A low score on the Si5 subscale is indicative of an individual who (is):
1. has naively optimistic perception of other people
2. sees others as trustworthy, honest, unselfish, and sensitive
3. faces up to problems; responsible
4. self-confident

Physical-Somatic Concerns (Si6)

A high score on the Si6 subscale is indicative of an individual who (is):

1. reports somatic symptoms including changes in speech and hearing, hay fever, or asthma
2. concerned about his/her physical appearance
3. broods; worries
4. socially introverted

A low score on the Si6 subscale is indicative of an individual who (is):

1. denies somatic symptoms such as changes in speech or hearing and hay fever or asthma
2. not especially concerned about physical appearance
3. does not brood or worry excessively
4. socially extroverted

WIGGINS CONTENT SCALES

Wiggins Content Scale Development

Although Hathaway and McKinley (1940) presented 26 categories for classifying the content of the MMPI item pool, they did so only to demonstrate that the items sampled a wide array of behaviors. The empirical keying procedure used in developing the original MMPI scales did not necessitate consideration of the content of individual items. Items were selected for inclusion in the original scales because they *empirically* differentiated criterion groups, and the content of the items was of no concern. With the exceptions discussed earlier in this chapter, among many MMPI users a tradition has developed that consideration of the *content* of an examinee's individual item responses might interfere with the empirical nature of the test.

Recently, some investigators have suggested that the content of responses to items on the MMPI and other structured personality assessment techniques can add significantly to the understanding of an examinee's personality and behavior (e.g., Goldberg, 1972; Hase & Goldberg, 1967; Jackson, 1971; Koss & Butcher, 1973). Whereas a number of efforts have been made to construct MMPI scales on the basis of item content, Wiggins and his associates have accomplished the most complete investigation of the content dimensions of the MMPI and have developed psychometrically sound scales for assessing the content dimensions (Wiggins, 1966, 1969; Wiggins, Goldberg, & Applebaum, 1971; Wiggins & Vollmar, 1959).

Wiggins (1969) has pointed out that two examinees with exactly the same profile based on the standard 4 validity and 10 clinical scales can have quite different patterns of scores on his content scales, which are listed in Table 7.4. He has argued that consideration of the content scales in addition to the standard profile can add significantly to the understanding of the examinee. In common with what was stated above, he does not suggest that the content scales be used instead of the standard scales, but in addition to them.

Wiggins (1969) has discussed in some detail the procedures utilized in developing the content scales. Hathaway and McKinley (1940) suggested that the original MMPI item pool could be clustered on the basis of content into 26 categories. Initially, Wiggins treated each of these 26 categories as

Table 7.4. Wiggins' content scales[a]

Scale symbol	Scale name
SOC	Social Maladjustment
DEP	Depression
FEM	Feminine Interests
MOR	Poor Morale
REL	Religious Fundamentalism
AUT	Authority Conflict
PSY	Psychoticism
ORG	Organic Symptoms
FAM	Family Problems
HOS	Manifest Hostility
PHO	Phobias
HYP	Hypomania
HEA	Poor Health

[a] Source: Wiggins (1969).

a scale, and a score was obtained for each scale by keying items in the scale in the deviant direction (i.e., the infrequent response of the Minnesota normal group). The internal consistency of these 26 scales was determined by analyzing the scores of 500 college students. Because the internal consistency of some of these 26 scales left much to be desired, Wiggins revised the scales based on the 26 categories suggested by Hathaway and McKinley by collapsing several categories into a single one, by reassigning items from one category to another, by eliminating some original categories, and by adding new categories. The internal consistencies of the revised content scales were determined for a number of different samples, and several more scales were eliminated because of lack of homogeneity. This series of revisions yielded a final set of 13 content scales (see Table 7.4) that are mutually exclusive, internally consistent, moderately independent, and representative of the major content dimensions of the MMPI. Cohler, Weiss, and Grunebaum (1974) demonstrated that the content scales can be scored from a shortened (400-item) version of the MMPI. The abbreviated content scales are internally consistent and show high correspondence with the longer scales.

The item composition and scoring directions for the content scales are presented in Appendix I of this *Guide*. Although scoring keys for the content scales are not available commercially, they can be constructed from the data in Appendix I.

Norms for Wiggins Content Scales

Normative data for the Wiggins content scales have been reported for a number of different samples. Gilberstadt (1970), in the automated scoring and interpretation service that he developed in the Veterans Administration, uses T-score values for the Wiggins content scales based on a sample of Air Force enlisted men. Fowler and Coyle (1970) have reported normative data for students at a southern university. Wiggins et al. (1971) have presented normative data for the Wiggins content scales separately for a university sample (from three different schools) and for a Minnesota normative group. This latter sample is the same one utilized by Hathaway and Briggs (1957) in presenting norms for the research scales of the MMPI (see Chapter 6). Because the Minnesota sample is the same one used for the frequently scored research scales and is quite similar to the sample used in determining norms for the standard validity and clinical scales of the MMPI, it is the most appropriate group to be used in converting raw scores on the Wiggins content scales to T-scores for general clinical use. Wiggins (1971) constructed tables for converting raw scores on his content scales to T-scores based on the Minnesota normal sample, and these tables are reproduced in Appendix J of this *Guide*.

Wiggins Content Scale Reliability

The only published reliability data for the Wiggins content scales have been reported by Wiggins (1969). Internal consistency estimates (Cronbach's coefficient α) for the content scales in seven samples are presented in Table 7.5. An examination of these values indicates that most of the content scales have a high degree of internal consistency.

Wiggins Content Scale Validity

Some evidence concerning concurrent validity of the content scales is available from studies that have related scores on the content scales to other measures of the same or similar characteristics. Wiggins et al. (1971) correlated scores on the Wiggins content scales with a variety of other MMPI scales, with scales from the Edwards Personal Preference Schedule, the California Psychological Inventory, and the Adjective Check List, and with scales assessing masculinity and femininity from the Strong Vocational Interest Blank. They obtained numerous significant correlations and concluded that their data offered evidence for the concurrent validity

Table 7.5. Coefficient α internal consistency estimates for MMPI content scales in seven normal samples[a]

Content scale	Air Force enlisted men	University of Minnesota Men (n = 96)	University of Minnesota Women (n = 125)	University of Oregon Men (n = 95)	University of Oregon Women (n = 108)	University of Illinois Men (n = 100)	University of Illinois Women (n = 83)
SOC	.829	.856	.835	.830	.862	.856	.843
DEP	.872	.860	.831	.821	.756	.842	.854
FEM	.585	.523	.505	.594	.566	.650	.542
MOR	.857	.866	.825	.804	.753	.867	.804
REL	.674	.892	.861	.842	.756	.817	.793
AUT	.681	.794	.772	.743	.669	.766	.698
PSY	.877	.794	.687	.738	.662	.763	.806
ORG	.863	.772	.645	.662	.695	.749	.731
FAM	.707	.712	.789	.712	.694	.806	.643
HOS	.764	.819	.794	.788	.651	.776	.765
PHO	.765	.663	.721	.568	.701	.705	.770
HYP	.671	.701	.715	.682	.632	.679	.667
HEA	.743	.557	.713	.555	.537	.673	.651

[a] Reproduced with permission from J. S. Wiggins, Content dimensions in the MMPI. In J. N. Butcher (Ed.), *MMPI: Research Developments and Clinical Applications.* New York: McGraw-Hill, 1969. Copyright 1969 by McGraw-Hill Book Company.

of the Wiggins content scales. Of special interest in the Wiggins et al. study are correlations between the content scales and the standard MMPI scales (see Table 7.6). Some of the content scales correlate so highly with corresponding standard scales that they can be interpreted in similar ways. The Social Maladjustment and Social Introversion scales seem to be measuring very similar characteristics, as are the Poor Health and Hypochondriasis scales. Other scales have high correlations with corresponding standard scales (e.g., Depression and Depression, Feminine Interests and Masculinity-Femininity, Psychoticism and Schizophrenia, Organic Symptoms and Hypochondriasis, Hypomania and Hypomania), but the correlations are low enough that one suspects that each scale is assessing some unique characteristics as well as some common ones. Other content scales have only moderate correlations with the standard MMPI scales and seem to be measuring unique characteristics.

Taylor, Ptacek, Carithers, Griffin, and Coyne (1972) compared scores of psychiatric patients on the Wiggins content scales with other scales and self-ratings judged to be assessing the same or similar characteristics. They found generally good agreement between content scale scores and the other measures of the corresponding characteristics.

Boerger (1975) was able to identify empirical extra-test correlates for some of the Wiggins content scales. In general, the correlates reflected closely the content of the Wiggins scales. Although many fewer extra-test correlates were identified for the Wiggins content scales than for the standard clinical scales, as many correlates were identified for the content scales as for two different sets of factor analytically derived MMPI scales.

Payne and Wiggins (1972) examined the self-report of psychiatric patients whose profiles had been classified according to scores and configurations of scores on the standard MMPI validity and clinical scales. They found that when more complex rules were utilized for classification, the self-report of patients within a given profile type was more homogeneous. In addition, descriptions of the profile types based on self-report (the Wiggins content scales) were similar to descriptions based on empirical extra-test correlates for the same types.

A number of studies have demonstrated that scores on the Wiggins content scales differ for various kinds of criterion groups. Wiggins (1969) compared his content scale scores of seven groups: normal Air Force males, male psychiatric inpatients, female psychiatric inpatients, male psychiatric outpatients, female psychiatric outpatients, college males, and college females. He found differences among the groups on many of his content scales. The largest differences were between college students and psychiatric patients, but substantial differences also were found between college males and Air Force males and between male and female psychiatric outpatients. Wiggins (1969) also has reported data concerning the ordering of means on his content scales for groups differing in degree of psychopathology. He concluded that his content scales do not provide measures of pathology that are consistent with the conventional meaning of the term.

Wiggins (1969) used his 13 content scales as predictors of diagnostic classification for 6 categories of psychiatric patients. The diagnostic groups used were brain disorders, personality disorders, sociopathic disorders,

Table 7.6.   Correlations between Wiggins content scales and standard MMPI validity and clinical scales[a]

Content scale	Standard MMPI scales												
	L	F	K	1	2	3	4	5	6	7	8	9	0
males													
SOC	-001	325	-472	335	481	-180	083	305	132	598	488	-192	899
DEP	-282	561	-708	618	557	-027	438	444	315	877	788	257	685
FEM	013	203	-158	275	206	131	144	684	237	317	295	079	231
MOR	-256	460	-711	524	479	-136	314	384	197	847	700	200	725
REL	036	-264	055	-009	-165	-089	-139	-137	084	019	-073	-152	037
AUT	-349	388	-632	294	038	-385	301	-049	-273	422	440	531	243
PSY	-193	535	-577	449	223	-148	344	345	359	694	725	499	367
ORG	-153	520	-442	772	399	247	408	345	328	599	665	360	386
FAM	-139	449	-432	412	328	062	584	295	129	427	517	399	362
HOS	-375	408	-719	388	092	-348	277	143	-001	571	592	548	321
PHO	-236	283	-466	418	311	-092	169	270	176	561	471	115	491
HYP	-368	313	-601	323	021	-150	175	169	030	535	515	617	145
HEA	-207	457	-413	800	437	176	379	371	247	597	561	252	417
females													
SOC	013	336	-356	177	485	-249	-021	188	171	456	352	-260	894
DEP	-267	501	-642	530	611	077	476	241	363	879	774	305	570
FEM	-141	-140	058	105	051	123	-055	587	131	073	-065	-079	-033
MOR	-307	460	-686	467	550	-063	336	237	267	851	689	232	663
REL	120	-265	142	-059	-212	023	-093	-062	020	-050	-088	-067	-055
AUT	-381	364	-597	214	021	-319	222	-268	-302	350	466	490	126
PSY	-245	566	-590	441	217	-023	363	112	361	694	765	530	301
ORG	-186	451	-403	738	328	339	312	120	244	560	643	379	233
FAM	-099	360	-462	274	225	028	551	151	143	446	534	404	190
HOS	-385	458	-698	292	045	-253	277	-098	038	560	645	585	215
PHO	-182	180	-385	321	273	043	072	181	123	487	354	040	385
HYP	-333	287	-563	334	019	-011	216	036	097	510	531	688	-060
HEA	-163	407	-305	835	408	394	311	285	188	527	484	280	248

[a] Source: unpublished materials provided by Lewis Goldberg, Oregon Research Institute.

affective psychoses, schizophrenic psychoses, and psychoneurotic disorders. His content scales were related significantly to diagnostic classification for both male and female patients. The Authority Conflict, Poor Morale, Hostility, Psychoticism, and Depression scales were the most important contributors to group discrimination, but the Family Problems, Organic Symptoms, and Hypomania scales also were related to diagnostic classification.

Cohler et al. (1974) compared women hospitalized for psychiatric treatment after childbirth with an appropriate control group and found that the two groups differed for 11 of the 13 Wiggins content scales. Mezzich, Damarin, and Erickson (1974) reported significant relationships between psychiatric diagnosis of depression and 8 of the 13 Wiggins content scales. Comprehensive study of the protocols of 25 males who were given the MMPI while in college and many years later were found to be alcoholics indicated that the prealcoholic males and a control group of male college students who did not become alcoholic differed significantly on 2 of the 13 Wiggins content scales (Loper, Kammeier, & Hoffman, 1973). In addition, the scores of the college males who later became alcoholics showed changes for 5 of the 13 Wiggins content scales when they were retested while in treatment for their alcoholism (Hoffman, Loper, & Kammeier, 1974; Kammeier, Hoffman, & Loper, 1973).

A factor analysis of scores on the 13 Wiggins content scales (Wiggins, 1969) has identified five important factor dimensions. Factor I, Anxiety Proneness versus Ego Resiliency, is similar to Welsh's first factor (Anxiety) and to Block's Ego Resiliency dimension (see Chapter 6). It has high loadings for the Poor Morale, Social Maladjustment, and Depression scales. Factor II, Impulsivity versus Control, is similar to Welsh's second factor (Repression) and to Block's Control dimension (see Chapter 6). It has high loadings for the Hypomania scale for males and for the Manifest Hostility and Authority Conflict scales for females. Factor III, Health Concern, is identified by the Organic Symptoms and Poor Health scales. Factor IV, Social Desirability Role Playing, is defined by a special social desirability scale included in the factor analysis and by the Religious Fundamentalism scale. Factor V, Feminine Interests, is virtually identical to the Feminine Interests scale.

It may be concluded that whereas validity studies of the Wiggins content scales currently available are limited, they do support the notion that scores on the content scales are related to important aspects of extra-test behavior for a variety of populations. More empirical research is needed to specify more clearly how the content scales can be used in understanding an examinee's behavior and personality.

Interpretation of Wiggins Content Scale Scores

Most suggestions for interpreting scores on the content scales have been based on examination of the content of items in each scale. Wiggins (1966, 1969) provided the most complete interpretive information for the content scales, and the descriptions that follow are based to a large extent on his information. Also, inferences based on the data from the validity studies described above are included in the descriptions that are presented below.

Although some limited information is available about low scores on the content scales, most interpretive efforts to date have dealt only with high scores. In the absence of descriptive information about low scores on a content scale, it may be inferred that low scorers are not reporting the behaviors, feelings, ideas, and so forth characteristic of high scorers on that scale. However, it should not be assumed that low scorers on a content scale necessarily are the opposite of high scorers.

Because the use of the Wiggins content scales as part of routine MMPI interpretation is relatively new and infrequent, no strong tradition exists concerning cutoff scores for considering scores on the content scales as high or low. Boerger (1975) defined high scores on the content scales as those falling within the top 25% of his sample of psychiatric patients and low scores as those falling within the bottom 25% for the same sample. Using Wiggins' norms, these cutoffs for the most part ranged from T-scores of 60 to 70 for high scores and from 40 to 50 for low scores. As with other scales discussed in earlier chapters of this *Guide*, the higher the scores are, the most likely it is that interpretive material presented for high scores will apply, and the lower the scores are, the more likely it is that interpretive information presented for low scores will apply. Although the practicing clinician will come to establish his/her own cutoff scores as he/she gains experience with the content scales, persons who are just beginning to use the content scales will find it useful to consider T-scores above 70 as high and T-scores below 40 as low. It should be understood that the descriptions that follow are based on limited empirical data and thus should be viewed as preliminary and tentative. The content scales are most useful for clinical assessment if used along with other MMPI scales and extra-test information.

Social Maladjustment (SOC)

A high score on the SOC scale is indicative of an individual who (is):
1. self-conscious and introverted
2. feels bashful, embarassed, and shy in social situations
3. tends to be reserved and reticent
4. if a psychiatric patient, reports feeling blue and depressed
5. if a psychiatric patient, is less grandiose than other patients

A low score on the SOC scale is indicative of an individual who (is):
1. outgoing and extroverted
2. gregarious and fun-loving
3. appears to be the "life of the party"
4. self-conscious
5. assertive
6. relates easily and quickly to other people
7. experiences no difficulty in speaking before groups

Depression (DEP)

A high score on the DEP scale is indicative of an individual who (is):
1. clinically depressed

2. experiences guilt, regret, worry, and unhappiness
3. feels that life has lost its zest
4. has little motivation to pursue things
5. has difficulty in concentrating
6. anxious and apprehensive about the future
7. feels misunderstood
8. convinced of his/her unworthiness and believes that he/she deserves to be punished
9. if a psychiatric patient, is more likely than other patients to show evidence of thinking disturbance, to talk or mutter to self, and to be slow moving and sluggish

A low score on the DEP scale is indicative of an individual who (is):
1. presents himself/herself as happy and satisfied with his/her life situation
2. stimulated by his/her everyday activities
3. optimistic about the future
4. denies anxiety, worry, and depression
5. has a high degree of self-esteem
6. if a psychiatric patient, is more likely than other patients to be irritable, impatient, and grouchy
7. if a psychiatric patient, is less likely than other patients to feel anxious, depressed, or guilty, or to show motor retardation

Feminine Interests (FEM)

A high score on the FEM scale is indicative of an individual who (is):
1. expresses more interest in activities, games, and occupations that are stereotypically feminine than most members of his/her sex
2. as children liked games such as drop-the-handkerchief and hopscotch
3. likes activities such as cooking and growing flowers
4. says he/she would like occupations such as florist, nurse, or dressmaker
5. has romantic outlook on life
6. identifies with females
7. denies liking sterotypically masculine activities such as hunting, fishing, or auto racing
8. says that he/she would not like occupations such as forest ranger or building contractor
9. has cultural and aesthetic interests such as poetry, literature, theatre, etc.
10. if male, is more likely to come from higher socioeconomic class

A low score on the FEM scale is indicative of an individual who (is):
1. denies liking for stereotypically feminine activities, games, and interests
2. professes interest in and liking of traditional masculine activities and occupations
3. not likely to have strong cultural or aesthetic interests
4. if male, has a strong traditional masculine identification
5. if female, is rejecting the traditional female role and sees herself as a "liberated woman"

Poor Morale (MOR)

A high score on the MOR scale is indicative of an individual who (is):
1. lacks self-confidence
2. feels like a failure in life
3. overwhelmed by feelings of uselessness and despair
4. pessimistic about the future; has given up hope
5. avoids facing up to difficulties and responsibilities
6. sensitive to the reactions of other people
7. socially suggestible
8. feels misunderstood but does not express these feelings for fear of offending others
9. if a psychiatric patient, more likely than other patients to express paranoid symptomatology including conceptual disorganization, suspiciousness, and hostility

A low score on the MOR scale is indicative of an individual who (is):
1. very self-confident
2. faces up to difficulties and responsibilities
3. not overly dependent on other people for reinforcements
4. at times may seem to be quite insensitive to feelings of others
5. appears to be inner-directed; not socially suggestible
6. feels successful in activities
7. optimistic about the future
8. if a psychiatric patient, less likely than other patients to manifest paranoid symptomatology

Religious Fundamentalism (REL)

A high score on the REL scale is indicative of an individual who (is):
1. presents himself/herself as a very religious person who attends church regularly
2. subscribes to a number of fundamentalist religious beliefs, including literal interpretation of the Bible, the second coming of Christ, and the existence of hell and the devil
3. believes his/her religion is the only true one; intolerant of persons whose religious beliefs are different
4. if a psychiatric patient, more likely than other patients to display conceptual disorganization, unusual thought content, and religious delusions

A low score on the REL scale is indicative of an individual who (is):
1. may have strong religious convictions but does not subscribe to the fundamentalist religious beliefs characteristic of high scorers on this scale
2. tolerant of religious beliefs and practices that differ from his/her own
3. if a psychiatric patient, less likely than other patients to have delusions

Authority Conflict (AUT)

A high score on the AUT scale is indicative of an individual who (is):
1. sees the world as a jungle in which everyone must fight to exist

2. characterizes other people as dishonest, untrustworthy, and motivated primarily by selfish needs
3. expresses little respect for laws or for authority figures
4. may have been in trouble with the law
5. feels that it is acceptable to lie to keep out of trouble
6. enjoys excitement and risk
7. obtains vicarious gratification from the activities of other people who engage in asocial or antisocial behavior
8. because of his/her negative perceptions of other people, feels justified in behaving in selfish, insensitive ways

A low score on the AUT scale is indicative of an individual who (is):
1. has a trusting attitude toward the world
2. sees other people as sensitive, honest, and law-abiding
3. respects the law, social standards, and authority figures
4. feels that it is best to be honest, even if honesty gets him/her into trouble
5. denies having been in trouble with the law
6. does not seek out excitement and risk
7. if a psychiatric patient, less likely than other patients to hallucinate, to talk or mutter to self, or to have conceptual disorganization

Psychoticism (PSY)

A high score on the PSY scale is indicative of an individual who (is):
1. admits to a wide variety of clearly psychotic symptoms, including:
   a. hallucinations
   b. confused thinking; unusual thought content
   c. mannerisms or posturing
   d. clearly paranoid orientation
   e. loss of control of thinking and behavior
2. feels misunderstood, mistreated, and persecuted
3. feels that other people are trying to influence his/her behavior
4. responds to a threatening and hostile world by withdrawing into fantasy and daydreaming
5. has unrealistic self-appraisal
6. sees self as important, sensitive, and dutiful person who could be of great benefit to the world if given a fair chance

A low score on the PSY scale is indicative of an individual who (is):
1. does not admit to the wide variety of psychotic symptoms characteristic of high scorers on this scale
2. does not have exaggerated appraisal of his/her own worth
3. does not tend to withdraw from people
4. does not engage in excessive fantasy or daydreaming

Organic Symptoms (ORG)

A high score on the ORG scale is indicative of an individual who (is):
1. reports symptoms that could be suggestive of a neurological disorder (e.g., fits or convulsions, paralysis, clumsiness, loss of balance, double vision, etc.)

2. reports many somatic symptoms that could be functional in origin:
   a. nausea, vomiting
   b. back pain, head pain
   c. skin sensitivity or numbness
   d. dizziness
   e. shaky hands; twitching muscles
   f. problems with speech, hearing, or vision
   g. weakness, fatigue
3. has difficulties in memory and concentration
4. unable to understand what is read
5. shows poor judgment
6. admits having had periods during which he/she carried out activities without awareness of what he/she was doing
7. if a psychiatric patient, more likely than other patients to be anxious and to experience conceptual disorganization

A low score on the ORG scale is indicative of an individual who (is):
1. presents few, if any, somatic complaints
2. denies difficulties in concentration, attention, or memory

Family Problems (FAM)*

A high score on the FAM scale is indicative of an individual who (is):
1. describes his/her home and family situation as unpleasant†
2. says his/her home situation is lacking in love and understanding
3. admits to having had the desire to run away from the home situation
4. sees his/her parents as nervous, critical, quick-tempered, and quarrelsome
5. feels that his/her parents object to his/her friends and acquaintances
6. reports that his/her family does frightening and irritating things
7. feels that his/her family treats him/her more like a child than like an adult
8. if a psychiatric patient, more likely than other patients to have been given clinical diagnosis of personality or transient disorder

Manifest Hostility (HOS)

A high score on the HOS scale is indicative of an individual who (is):
1. harbors intense hostile and aggressive impulses
2. usually expresses negative impulses in passive, indirect ways such as teasing animals, poking fun at people, being uncooperative, and being very critical of the shortcomings of others
3. resentful of demands placed on him/her by other people
4. resents being taken advantage of

---

* This scale seems to assess the same characteristics as the Pd1 Harris subscale (Familial Discord) discussed earlier in this chapter.

† Because some of the items in the FAM scale are phrased with specific reference to the parental home and other items are much more vague, high scorers may be describing their parental homes, their current homes, or both. The examiner may find it useful to examine responses to individual items on the FAM scale to try to differentiate between the two home situations.

5. retaliatory in interpersonal relationships
6. cross, grouchy, and argumentative
7. competitive; socially aggressive
   A low score on the HOS scale is indicative of an individual who (is):
1. does not admit to strong hostile or aggressive impulses
2. not critical and resentful in interpersonal relationships
3. seen by others as easygoing and somewhat passive

Phobias (PHO)

A high score on the PHO scale is indicative of an individual who (is):
1. admits to generalized fear, worry, or anxiety
2. admits to fear or anxiety associated with many different objects and/or situations including:
   a. animals (snakes, spiders, etc.)
   b. storms
   c. closed places
   d. open places
   e. heights
   f. darkness
   g. fire
   h. money
   i. blood
   j. disease
3. fearful of people, particularly groups or crowds
4. if T-score is greater than 70, experiences a generalized and incapacitating fear or anxiety that may be masking more serious psychopathology
   A low score on the PHO scale is indicative of an individual who (is):
1. does not admit to the multiple fears characteristic of high scorers on the scale (although some specific fear(s) may be reported)
2. comfortable around groups of people

Hypomania (HYP)

A high score on the HYP scale is indicative of an individual who (is):
1. characterized by periods of excitement, happiness, or cheerfulness that often are unexplainable
2. tense, restless, high-strung
3. becomes bored easily
4. seeks out excitement and change
5. has broad interests, often undertaking more than he can handle
6. dislikes details and routine; often does not see things through to completion
7. impulsive; makes quick decisions without carefully considering the consequences of the decisions
8. has poor tolerance for frustration; flies off the handle easily
9. does not harbor grudges; quick to forgive and forget
   A low score on the HYP scale is indicative of an individual who (is):
1. has limited drive and energy level
2. may have difficulty getting started on things

3. reliable, persistent; likely to see a job through to completion
4. does not anger easily
5. seems satisfied with a life style that others might judge to be boring and uneventful

Poor Health (HEA)

A high score on the HEA scale is indicative of an individual who (is):
1. expresses concern about health and physical functioning in general
2. admits to some physical preoccupation, often gastrointestinal in nature (eating, drinking, stomach discomfort, elimination, etc.)
3. presents other somatic complaints including:
    a. coughing
    b. pains in heart or chest
    c. hay fever; asthma
    d. breaking out of skin
    e. shortness of breath
    f. difficulties with sex organs
    g. tiredness, fatigue
4. does not complain of difficulties in motor activity or in cognitive functioning

A low score on the HEA scale is indicative of an individual who (is):
1. not preoccupied with health and physical functioning
2. does not admit to the somatic complaints characteristic of high scorers on the scale

TRYON, STEIN, AND CHU CLUSTER SCALES

Cluster Scale Development

Early factor analytic studies of the MMPI utilized scores on the 4 standard validity and 10 clinical scales as variables. One important reason for this approach was that early computers could not accommodate the 550 individual MMPI items as variables in a factor analysis. Tryon and his colleagues (Chu, 1966; Stein, 1968; Tryon, 1966; Tryon & Bailey, 1965) subsequently developed cluster analysis procedures and programs that can handle such large numbers of variables. When these cluster analytic procedures were applied to the MMPI item responses of 70 male Veterans Administration outpatient schizophrenics, 150 male Veterans Administration outpatients diagnosed as having anxiety reaction, and 90 normal military officers, seven clusters of items were identified that were judged to be homogeneous both statistically and in content meaning. Scales were developed to assess each cluster by selecting items with high loadings on the cluster. Lables were assigned logically to the scales by examining the content of items in each scale. Table 7.7 lists the seven Tryon, Stein, and Chu (TSC) cluster scales. The items and scoring directions for each of the cluster scales are presented in Appendix K of this *Guide*. Although scoring keys for the cluster scales are not available commercially, they can be constructed from the data presented in Appendix K.

Intercorrelations among the TSC scales for the psychiatric sample used in developing the scales are reported in Table 7.8. As Tryon (1966) pointed

Table 7.7.   Reliability coefficients for TSC cluster scales[a]

Cluster scale	Reliability (α coefficient)
I. Social Introversion versus Interpersonal Poise and Outgoingness	.93
II. Body Symptoms versus Lack of Physical Complaints	.92
III. Suspicion and Mistrust versus Absence of Suspicion	.85
IV. Depression and Apathy versus Positive and Optimistic Outlook	.94
V. Resentment and Aggression versus Lack of Resentment and Aggression	.87
VI. Autism and Disruptive Thoughts versus Absence of Such Disturbance	.86
VII. Tension, Worry, Fears versus Absence of Such Complaints	.92

[a] Adapted with permission from R. C. Tryon, Unrestricted cluster and factor analysis with applications to the MMPI and Holzinger-Harmon problems. *Multivariate Behavioral Research*, 1966, *1*, 229–244. Copyright 1966 by Society of Multivariate Experimental Psychology, Inc.

Table 7.8.   Intercorrelations among TSC cluster scales[a]

	I	II	III	IV	V	VI
I. Introversion						
II. Body Symptoms	.48					
III. Suspicion	.28	.32				
IV. Depression	.75	.60	.40			
V. Resentment	.61	.53	.63	.74		
VI. Autism	.48	.59	.60	.67	.71	
VII. Tension	.68	.76	.48	.85	.79	.75

[a] Adapted with permission from R. C. Tryon, Unrestricted cluster and factor analysis with applications to the MMPI and Holzinger-Harmon problems. *Multivariate Behavioral Research*, 1966, *1*, 229–244. Copyright 1966 by the Society of Multivariate Experimental Psychology, Inc.

out, the first three scales (Introversion, Body Symptoms, Suspicion) are the most independent ones. The remaining four scales are highly correlated with each other and with the first three scales.

Norms for the TSC Cluster Scales

Normative data for the TSC scales have been presented by Stein (1968) for 20 male and 13 female samples. The samples included normal subjects, medical patients, psychiatric inpatients, and psychiatric outpatients. Stein also reported normative data for composite samples of normal males and females. The male composite ($n = 425$) included 100 military officers, 95 normal fathers, 46 other normal adult males, 34 campus police applicants, 50 industrial job applicants, and 100 normal college students. The female composite sample ($n = 285$) was made up of 126 college students, 110 normal mothers, and 49 other adult normal females. The data from these composite samples should be used in converting raw scores on the cluster scales to T-scores. Tables to be used in making the T-score conversions are presented (separately for males and females) in Appendix L of this *Guide*. Whereas no profile sheets are commercially available for use with the cluster scales, they can be constructed from the data presented in Appendix L.

Reliability of the TSC Cluster Scales

Tryon (1966) presented internal consistency (α) coefficients for the seven TSC scales (see Table 7.7). An examination of the values in Table 7.7 reveals that all seven of the scales have a high degree of internal consistency.

Validity of the TSC Cluster Scales

Lorr (1968) attempted to cross-validate the TSC clusters in a shortened version of the MMPI. He selected for each cluster scale the 11 items with the highest loadings for that cluster. The responses of 774 male Veterans Administration Mental Hygiene Clinic patients to these 77 MMPI items were intercorrelated, and the resulting matrix was factor-analyzed. Seven major factors were identified, five of which were virtually identical to the TSC clusters. The clusters labeled Depression and Tension appeared as a single factor in the Lorr analysis. In addition, the Lorr analysis identified a Gastrointestinal Complaints factor that was separate from the Body Symptoms factor and was not represented in the TSC clusters.

Stein (1966) reported intercorrelations between the TSC cluster scale scores and scores from the Omnibus Personality Inventory and the Edwards Personal Preference Schedule for normal college students. The correlations were judged as providing construct validity for the cluster scales. Stein also correlated cluster scores with scores from the Strong Vocational Interest Blank for college counselees. Some reliable relationships were identified between cluster scale scores and occupational interests. For example, scores on the Introversion cluster scale were positively correlated with interest in biological sciences and engineering and negatively correlated with interest in social service, business administration, and sales activities.

Chu (reported in Stein, 1968) correlated scores on the cluster scales with scores on other MMPI scales. These intercorrelations are summarized in Table 7.9. For most of the cluster scales, high correlations were found with other MMPI scales that seem to be assessing similar characteristics. For example, the correlations between scores on the Introversion cluster and scores on scale 0 (Social Introversion) was .92; the correlation between scores on the Body Complaints cluster scale and on scale 1 (Hypochondriasis) was .97; the correlation between scores on the Depression cluster and on scale 2 (Depression) was .81; and the correlation between the Tension cluster scale and scale 7 (Psychasthenia) was .93. However, some unexpected correlations also were found. For example, the Suspicion cluster scale correlated only .16 with scale 6 (Paranoia). It appears that for some cluster scales little information is yielded that is not also available from the analysis of the standard clinical scales, but other cluster scales seem to be assessing characteristics not reflected in the standard scales.

Table 7.9. Correlations of the TSC cluster scales and 17 standard and special MMPI scales[a]

Cluster scale	MMPI scales																
	L	F	K	Hs	D	Hy	Pd	Mf	Pa	Pt	Sc	Ma	Si	Es	A	R	SD
Social Introversion	-.21	.54	-.55	.45	.71	.27	.40	.35	.42	.77	.67	-.06	.92	-.61	.76	.35	-.78
Body Complaints	-.11	.48	-.45	.97	.68	.77	.40	.14	.35	.71	.63	.14	.52	-.79	.63	.15	-.70
Suspicion and Mistrust	-.27	.38	-.73	.33	.15	-.05	.34	.04	.16	.47	.52	.53	.30	-.42	.52	-.34	-.51
Depression	-.22	.68	-.64	.57	.81	.47	.68	.43	.50	.91	.85	.20	.76	-.72	.93	.14	-.89
Resentment	-.38	.60	-.79	.52	.51	.24	.61	.31	.38	.81	.79	.39	.60	-.62	.81	-.14	-.79
Autism	-.31	.58	-.70	.57	.47	.34	.51	.31	.35	.79	.82	.41	.49	-.71	.78	-.09	-.75
Tension	-.21	.63	-.68	.73	.76	.56	.62	.32	.49	.93	.85	.25	.70	-.81	.88	.10	-.90

[a] Reproduced with permission from K. B. Stein. The outcome of a cluster analysis of the 550 MMPI items. In P. McReynolds (Ed.), Advances in psychological assessment. Vol. I. Palo Alto, Calif.: Science and Behavior Books, 1968. Copyright 1968 by Science and Behavior Books, Inc.

Data have been reported by Stein (1968) concerning the relationship between demographic variables and scores on the TSC cluster scales. In general, few significant relationships were found between scores on the cluster scales and age, education, family size, or grade-point average for normal college students. However, more intelligent persons tended to score lower than less intelligent persons on all of the cluster scales.

Stein (1968) presented data comparing several different criterion groups on the cluster scales. In one such comparison, the following groups were studied: (1) military enlisted men who were discharged for admitted homosexuality; (2) military enlisted men who were discharged for ineptness; (3) military recruits who successfully completed training; and (4) well adjusted military officers. The two groups of discharged men had higher scores than the other two groups for six of the seven cluster scales, and they had very similar patterns of scores. The well adjusted officers scored lower (near the mean) than all other groups for all seven cluster scales. Stein also reported comparisons among groups of psychiatric inpatients, psychiatric outpatients, medical patients, and normal controls. In general, the more pathological groups scored higher on the cluster scales than the less pathological groups. In addition, the groups differed in the patterns of their scores, lending additional validity support to the cluster scales.

Boerger (1975) attempted to identify empirical extra-test correlates for high and low scores on the TSC scales for a sample of hospitalized psychiatric patients. He defined high scores as those falling within the upper 25% of scores for his patient sample and low scores as those falling in the lower 25% for the patient sample. For each cluster scale, high scorers were compared with other scorers on the scale and low scorers were compared with other scorers on the scale. The groups were compared in terms of psychiatric diagnosis, reasons for hospital admission, psychiatrists' ratings of patients at admission, and nurses' ratings of patients at admission. Although Boerger was able to identify numerous extra-test correlates for high scores on some of the cluster scales, very few correlates were identified for low scores on the cluster scales. The specific results of Boerger's study are incorporated into the interpretive descriptions of the cluster scales that are presented in the next section.

Interpretation of High and Low Scores on the TSC Cluster Scales

Because limited interpretive information for the TSC scales has appeared in the literature, any descriptions given here of high or low scorers on the cluster scales should be considered to be tentative and preliminary. In addition to the data from the Boerger (1975) study described above, and the limited inferences that can be drawn from the other correlational studies reviewed in the previous section, the interpretive descriptions presented below also are based on a careful examination of the content of the items that have the highest factor loadings on each cluster scale.

As with other scales that are not frequently used in routine clinical interpretation of MMPI protocols, no strong tradition exists concerning cutoff scores to be used in considering cluster scales as high or low. The Boerger (1975) study defined high scores as those falling within the upper

25% of the scores for his patient sample and low scores as those falling in the lower 25%. Using the normative data presented by Stein (1968), most of the high cutoff scores used by Boerger were within a T-score range of 65 to 80, whereas most of his low cutoff scores were within a T-score range of 45 to 60. Although the clinician experienced in using the TSC cluster scales will come to develop his/her own cutoff scores for the settings in which he/ she uses the scales, the individual who is just beginning to use the cluster scales in MMPI interpretation will find it useful to consider T-scores greater than 70 on the cluster scales as high and T-scores less than 40 as low.

I. Social Introversion

A high score on the Social Introversion cluster scale is indicative of an individual who (is):
1. feels shy, embarassed, and bashful in social situations
2. does not mix well socially; avoids social gatherings
3. finds it difficult to talk to other people
4. self-conscious; tries to avoid being the center of attention
5. does not make friends easily
6. lacks self-confidence
7. does not express opinions and attitudes to others
8. does not stick up for his own rights
9. extremely sensitive to the reactions of others; easily hurt by criticism

A low score on the Social Introversion cluster scale is indicative of an individual who (is):
1. socially extroverted
2. enjoys social situations; is comfortable around other people
3. has no difficulty talking to other people
4. makes friends easily
5. self-confident
6. expresses his/her attitudes and opinions to others
7. sticks up for his/her own rights
8. not particularly sensitive to criticism from others
9. if a psychiatric patient, less likely than other patients to have grandiose ideas

II. Body Symptoms

A high score on the Body Symptoms cluster scale is indicative of an individual who (is):
1. preoccupied with bodily functioning
2. denies good health
3. feels weak, tired, or fatigued much of the time
4. reports a wide variety of specific somatic symptoms including:
   a. pain in head, chest, or neck
   b. heart pounding; shortness of breath
   c. dizzy spells
   d. nausea, vomiting
   e. excessive sweating

f. poor appetite

g. diarrhea

h. strange muscle or skin sensations

5. if psychiatric patient, more likely than other patients to be slow moving and sluggish

A low score on the Body Symptoms cluster scale is indicative of an individual who (is):

1. not preoccupied with bodily functioning

2. claims to be in good physical health

3. feels fresh, rested, and energetic

4. does not report the wide variety of specific somatic symptoms characteristic of high scorers on this scale

5. if a psychiatric patient, shows less anxiety, depression, and motor retardation than other patients

III. Suspicion and Mistrust

A high score on the Suspicion and Mistrust cluster scale is indicative of an individual who (is):

1. sees other people as dishonest, selfish, and demanding

2. feels misunderstood by other people

3. questions the motivation of others; is unable to trust other people

4. projects own impulses and shortcomings onto others

5. because of his/her perceptions of others, feels that his/her own aggression and hostility are justified

6. if a psychiatric patient, likely to be very disturbed and to manifest some or all of the following:

    a. paranoid suspiciousness

    b. hostility; uncooperativeness

    c. thinking disturbance; unusual thought content

    d. hallucinations

    e. delusions of persecution

    f. mannerisms or posturing

A low score on the Suspicion and Mistrust cluster scale is indicative of an individual who (is):

1. feels understood

2. sees others in naively positive terms (altruistic, honest, helpful, etc.)

3. feels that other people can be trusted

4. does not tend to stand up for his/her opinions and attitudes

5. denies hostility and aggression

IV. Depression and Apathy

A high score on the Depression and Apathy cluster scale is indicative of an individual who (is):

1. feels depressed, unhappy, sad, blue

2. may show psychomotor retardation

3. feels anxious much of the time

4. lacks energy to cope with everyday activities

5. feels that problems have piled up to the point that he/she can no longer cope with them

6. feels that everyday activities are not interesting or rewarding
7. may have given up hope of solving problems; may wish he/she were dead
8. lacks self-confidence
9. feels like a failure; guilty; useless
10. may feel that he/she is losing his/her mind but cannot tell others about this fear

A low score on the Depression and Apathy cluster scale is indicative of an individual who (is):

1. finds daily life interesting and rewarding
2. faces up to problems and difficulties
3. feels happy and comfortable most of the time
4. self-confident
5. optimistic about the future

V. Resentment and Aggression

A high score on the Resentment and Aggression cluster scale is indicative of an individual who (is):

1. irritable, cross, and grouchy much of the time
2. impatient with other people
3. resents having demands made on him/her
4. harbors intense hostility toward other people
5. fears loss of control of hostile, aggressive impulses
6. harbors grudges; seeks revenge for perceived mistreatment
7. occasionally has angry outbursts
8. feels guilt and remorse after expression of negative impulses
9. lacks self-confidence
10. indecisive

A low score on the Resentment and Aggression cluster scale is indicative of an individual who (is):

1. denies angry and aggressive feelings toward other people
2. patient, tolerant
3. feels in control of his/her impulses
4. does not feel guilt or remorse if he/she expresses negative feelings
5. self-confident, decisive

VI. Autism and Disruptive Thoughts

A high score on the Autism and Disruptive Thoughts cluster scale is indicative of an individual who (is):

1. has strange thoughts that are disturbing and frightening to him/her
2. dreams or daydreams about things (including sexual matters) that he/she is reluctant to tell other people about
3. irritable, impatient
4. indecisive
5. forgetful
6. has trouble concentrating
7. has feelings of unreality
8. if a psychiatric patient, likely to have thinking disturbance

A low score on the Autism and Disruptive Thoughts cluster scale is indicative of an individual who (is):

1. denies strange or disturbing thoughts
2. denies dreams or daydreams that are disturbing or frightening
3. does not admit to being irritable, impatient, indecisive, or forgetful
4. denies feelings of unreality or difficulty in concentrating

VII. Anxiety, Worry, Fears

A high score on the Anxiety, Worry, Fears cluster scale is indicative of an individual who (is):

1. feels anxious, tense, nervous
2. high-strung, jumpy
3. worries excessively about many things
4. has sleep disturbances
5. cries; easily upset
6. has difficulty in concentrating
7. has periods of restlessness, excitability
8. uncomfortable in unfamiliar surroundings
9. fears that he/she might be losing his/her mind
10. may express specific fears including high places, small places, disease, or natural disasters (earthquakes, etc.)

A low score on the Anxiety, Worry, Fears cluster scale is indicative of an individual who (is):

1. feels calm and comfortable most of the time
2. denies problems in sleeping or concentration
3. denies excessive worry or anxiety
4. does not express specific fears of such things as high places, small places, disease, or natural disasters (earthquakes, etc.)

CONCLUDING COMMENTS

This chapter has discussed the development and interpretation of MMPI scales derived by the logical keying and homogeneous keying approaches, as opposed to the empirical keying approach that was utilized in the development of the standard validity and clinical scales of the MMPI. Whereas interpretation of scores on these additional scales can lead to hypotheses about the examinee, there is limited *empirical* data concerning extra-test correlates of the scales. Thus, inferences based on these additional scales should be considered as tentative and should be validated against other test and clinical data. Also, the reader again is reminded that the scales discussed in this chapter should be used in conjunction with the standard validity and clinical scales and not instead of them.

8

A General Interpretive Strategy

In 1956 Paul Meehl made a strong plea for a "good cookbook" for psychological test interpretation. Meehl's proposed cookbook was to include detailed rules for categorizing test responses and was to provide empirically determined extra-test correlates for each category of test responses. The rules could be applied automatically by a nonprofessional worker (or by a computer) and the interpretive statements could be selected for a particular type of protocol from a larger library of statements. Although some efforts have been made to construct such a cookbook (e.g., Gilberstadt & Duker, 1965; Marks & Seeman, 1963; Marks et al., 1974), the current status of psychological test interpretation is far from Meehl's ideal automatic process. All tests, including the MMPI, provide opportunities for standardized observation of current behavior of examinees. On the basis of these test behaviors, inferences are made about other extra-test behaviors of the examinees. The clinician serves as an information processor and as a clinical judge in the assessment process. The major purpose of this chapter is to suggest one approach (but by no means the only one) that clinicians can utilize in translating MMPI protocols into meaningful inferences about examinees.

It should be clearly understood that the MMPI should be used to generate *hypothesis* or *inferences* about an examinee. The interpretive data presented in earlier chapters of this *Guide* will not apply completely and unfailingly to each and every person with a specified MMPI protocol. In interpreting MMPI's, one must deal in probabilities. Some particular extra-test characteristic is *more likely* than some other characteristic to hold true for a person with a particular type of MMPI protocol, but one can never be completely sure that the more likely characteristic will in fact be found for that person. The inferences generated from an individual's MMPI protocol should be validated against other test and nontest information available about him/her. The MMPI is most valuable as an assessment tool when it is used in conjunction with other psychological tests, with interview and observational data, and with appropriate background information. Although blind interpretation of MMPI's is certainly possible, and in fact is the procedure involved in computerized interpretations of the MMPI, such interpretations should be used only to generate hypotheses, inasmuch as more accurate person-specific inferences are likely to occur when the MMPI is viewed in the context of all information available for an individual. This position is consistent with research findings by investigators such as Kostlan (1954) and Sines (1959).

In general, two kinds of interpretive inferences can be made on the basis of MMPI data. First, some characteristics of an examinee with a particular kind of MMPI protocol are ones that, with better than chance probability, differentiate that examinee from other persons in a particular setting (e.g., hospital, clinic, etc.). For example, one might infer from a hospitalized patient's MMPI profile that he/she is likely to be a serious suicidal risk. Because most patients are not actually suicidal, this inference clearly differentiates this particular patient from other patients. A second kind of inference is one that involves a characteristic that is common to many individuals in a particular setting. For example, the inference that a hospitalized psychiatric patient does not know how to handle stress in an effective manner is one that probably is true for most patients in that setting. Although the differential, patient-specific inferences tend to be more useful than the more general ones, the latter are important in understanding an individual case, particularly for clinicians and others involved in the treatment process who might not have a clear understanding of what behaviors are shared by most persons in a particular setting.

Whereas Meehl envisioned the assessment process as dealing exclusively with nontest behaviors that are directly and empirically tied to specific aspects of test performance, the current status of the assessment field is such that only limited relationships of this sort have been identified. Often it is possible and/or necessary to make higher order inferences about examinees based on a conceptualization of his/her personality. For example, there currently are no hard data indicating that a particular MMMP profile is predictive of a future suicide attempt. However, if we have inferred from an individual's MMPI that he/she is extremely depressed, agitated, and emotionally uncomfortable, is impulsive, and shows poor judgment much of the time, the higher order inference that such a person has a higher risk of suicide than patients in general is a logical one. Although it is legitimate to rely on such higher order inferences in interpreting MMPI's, one should probably have greater confidence in the inferences that are less inferentially and more directly related to MMPI performance.

A GENERAL STRATEGY

In his clinical work the author utilizes an approach to MMPI interpretation which involves trying to answer the following questions about each MMPI protocol:

1. What was the test-taking attitude of the examinee, and how should this attitude be taken into account in interpreting the protocol?

2. What is the general level of adjustment of the person who produced the protocol?

3. What kinds of behaviors (symptoms, attitudes, defenses, etc.) can be inferred about or expected from the person who produced the protocol?

4. What etiology or set of psychological dynamics underlies the behaviors described above?

5. What are the most appropriate diagnostic labels for the person who produced the protocol?

6. What are the implications for the treatment of the person who produced the protocol?

Test-Taking Attitude

The ideal examinee is one who approaches the task of completing the MMPI in a serious and cooperative manner. He/she reads each MMPI item and responds to the item in an honest, direct manner. When such an ideal situation is realized, the examiner can feel confident that the test responses are a representative sample of the examinee's behavior and can proceed with the interpretation of the protocol. However, as suggested in Chapter 3, for various reasons examinees may approach the test-taking task with an attitude that deviates from the ideal situation described above. Specification of test-taking attitude for each individual examinee is important because such differential attitudes must be taken into account in generating inferences from the MMPI protocol. In addition, such attitudes may be predictive of similar approaches to other nontest aspects of the examinee's life situation.

Qualitative aspects of an examinee's test behavior often serve to augment inferences based on the more quantitative scores and indices. One such factor is the amount of time required to complete the MMPI. As stated in Chapter 2, the typical examinee takes between 1 and 1¹/₂ hr to complete the test. Excessively long testing times may be indicative of indecisiveness, psychomotor retardation, confusion, or passive resistance to the testing procedures. Extremely short times suggest that either the examinee was quite impulsive in responding to the test items or he/she did not read and consider each individual item.

Examinees occasionally become very tense, agitated, or otherwise upset in the MMPI test-taking situation. Such behavior may be predictive of similar responses in other stressful situations. Some examinees, who are obsessive in their thinking and/or indecisive, write qualifications to their true-false responses in the margins of the answer sheet. This author is even aware of one case in which the examinee attempted to eat the Box Form cards. Needless to say, such behavior has important diagnostic significance.

Although the qualitative features of test performance discussed above can offer important information about an examinee, the four validity indicators (?, L, F, K) are the primary objective sources of inferences about test-taking attitude. The Cannot Say (?) scale indicates the number of items omitted by the examinee. A large number of omitted items may indicate indecisiveness, ambivalence, or an attempt to avoid admitting negative things about oneself without deliberately lying. Examinees who answer all or most of the items are not availing themselves of this simplistic way of attempting to present a positive picture of themselves.

In judging test-taking attitude from the L scale, the examinee's educational or socioeconomic status must be taken into account (see Chapter 3). If the L scale is higher than what is expected for an individual when these factors are considered, one should consider the possibility that the examinee is using a rather naive and global denial of problems and shortcomings in an attempt to present himself/herself in a favorable light.

Scores on the F scale reflect the extent to which an examinee's responses to a finite pool of deviant items distributed throughout the MMPI compare to those of the Minnesota normal standardization groups, with a higher F scale score reflecting greater deviance. Scores that are considerably higher than average suggest that the examinee is admitting to many clearly deviant behaviors and/or attitudes. Although there are several possible reasons for such an admission (see Chapter 3), one possibility is that the examinee is emotionally disabled and is using the MMPI as a vehicle to express a cry for help. Another possibility is that he/she is functioning in a healthy range but on the basis of subjective self-appraisal is using the test-taking task as a vehicle for being extremely self-critical and self-derrogatory. F scale scores that are considerably below average indicate that the examinee is admitting fewer than an average number of deviant attitudes and behaviors. He/she may be overly defensive and trying to create an unrealistically positive picture of himself/herself. F scale scores in the average range indicate that the examinee has been neither hypercritical of himself/herself nor overly defensive and denying in responding to the test items.

The K scale can serve as another index of defensiveness, but education and socioeconomic status must be taken into account in interpreting this scale (see Chapter 3). If the score on the K scale is significantly higher than one would expect from a person of a given educational and socioeconomic background, one should suspect that the examinee has been rather defensive in describing himself. Scores lower than would be expected for a person with a given educational and socioeconomic background indicate a lack of defensiveness and a hypercritical attitude toward oneself. K scale scores in the middle range suggest that the examinee has been neither overly defensive nor overly self-critical in endorsing the MMPI items.

As discussed in Chapter 3, the profile configuration of the validity scales is important for understanding the examinee's test-taking attitudes. In general, persons who are approaching the test with the intention of presenting themselves in an overly favorable way have L and K scale scores greater than the F scale score, producing a V-shape in the validity scale portion of the profile. On the other hand, an examinee who is using the test to be overly self-critical and/or to exaggerate his/her problems produces an inverted V-shape in the validity scales (i.e., the L and K scale scores will be significantly lower than the F scale score). In interpreting the clinical scales profile, therefore, the clinician must take into account the validity scales, adjusting the meanings of the profile as he/she feels necessary.

Adjustment Level

There are two important components to psychological adjustment level. First, there is the matter of how emotionally comfortable or uncomfortable an individual is. Second, there is the matter of how well the individual carries out the responsibilities of his/her life situation irrespective of how conflicted he/she might be. For most people these two components are very much related. Persons who are psychologically comfortable tend to function well and vice versa. However, for some individuals (e.g., some neurotics), a great deal of discomfort and turmoil can be present but adequate functioning continues. For other persons (e.g., chronic schizophrenics), quite serious impairment in coping with responsibilities can be found without an accompanying emotional discomfort. Clinical experience and some research findings suggest that the MMPI potentially can permit inferences about both of these aspects of adjustment level.

The F scale seems to be the single best MMPI index of degree of psychopathology. If one rules out the possibility of deviant response sets or styles that can invalidate the protocol (e.g., the angry adolescent who decides to answer true to all of the deviant items), high F scale scores suggest intense emotional turmoil and/or serious impairment in functioning. For example, most acutely psychotic subjects tend to obtain high scores on the F scale. However, some neurotic individuals and persons undergoing severe situational stress also achieve high F scale scores. On the other hand, some clearly psychotic (or neurotic) individuals, particularly those in whom the disorder has been present for quite some time, do not achieve very high F scale scores.

A second simple but meaningful index of adjustment has to do with the overall elevation of the clinical scales. In general, as more of the clinical scales are elevated (and the greater the degree of elevation) the greater the probability that some serious psychopathology and poor levels of functioning are present. To obtain a crude, quantitative index of degree of this psychopathology, some clinicians find it useful to compute a mean T-score for eight clinical scales (excluding scales 5 and 0). Others simply count the number of clinical scales with T-scores above 70. Higher mean scores and more scores above 70 are indicative of greater psychopathology.

The *slope* of the profile also yields important inferences about adjustment level. If the clinical scales are elevated and a positive slope (left side low, right side high) is present, the likelihood of severe psychopathology, and perhaps even psychosis, should be considered. A negative slope (left side high, right side low) is more indicative of a neurotic individual or one who is internally conflicted and miserable but who still is able to function fairly well.

Scores on several of the standard clinical and special scales also can serve as indices of level of adjustment. Welsh's Anxiety (A) and Barron's Ego Strength (Es) scales are measures of general maladjustment. High scorers on A and low scorers on Es tend to be rather disturbed emotionally. The A scale seems to be more sensitive to subjective emotional turmoil than to inability to cope behaviorally. Thus some hospitalized psychotics who cannot cope at all well are free of serious emotional distress and do not achieve elevated scores on the A scale. The Es scale indicates an individual's ability to cope with stresses and problems of everyday life, with high scorers generally better able to cope than low scorers. Scale 2 (Depression) is a good indicator of a person's dissatisfaction with his/her life situation. As scores on scale 2 become higher, greater dissatisfaction is suggested. Scale 7 (Psychasthenia) is perhaps the single best measure of feelings of anxiety and agitation. High scale 7 scorers usually are overwhelmed by anxiety, tension, fear, apprehension, etc.

Goldberg (1965) derived a linear regression equation for discriminating psychotic and neurotic MMPI profiles. In addition to serving this diagnostic function, the Goldberg index also seems to be related to level of maladjustment, with higher values indicating greater maladjustment. To compute the Goldberg index, one simply inserts T-score values into the following formula: $L + Pa + Sc - Hy - Pt$. Goldberg found for his samples that a cutoff of 45 on his index provided the best discrimination between psychotic and neurotic profiles. Whereas a considerable amount of experience in applying the formula to actual cases is necessary before the values yielded by the formula take on significance concerning adjustment level, in the author's own clinical experience, higher Goldberg values suggest greater psychopathology.

Grayson (1951) suggested that it is helpful to check item responses to 38 items in the MMPI that are suggestive of special clinical difficulties. The items include a number of blatantly psychotic behaviors and attitudes as well as items dealing with sexual deviation, excessive use of alcohol, and homicidal and/or suicidal impulses. The critical items are reproduced in Appendix M of this *Guide*.

Characteristic Traits and Behaviors

At this point in the interpretive process, the clinician's goal is to describe the examinee's symptoms, traits, behaviors, attitudes, defenses, etc. in enough detail to allow an overall understanding of the kind of person that he/she is. Although not every protocol permits inferences about all of the points listed below, in general the author tries to make some statements or inferences about each of them:

1. symptoms
2. major needs (e.g., dependency, achievement, autonomy, etc.)
3. perceptions of the environment, particularly of significant other people in the examinee's life situation
4. reactions to stress (coping strategies, defenses, etc.)
5. self-concept
6. sexual identification
7. emotional control
8. interpersonal relationships
9. psychological resources

Inferences about the above features are based primarily on analysis of individual validity and clinical scales (high and low scores) and on two-point configurations of the clinical scales (see Chapters 3, 4, and 5). In addition, the special scales discussed in Chapters 6 and 7 often add important information about the examinee. One way for the beginner with the

MMPI to utilize the standard and special scales is to consider each high scale, low scale, or configuration of scales in turn, to consult the appropriate interpretive sections in earlier chapters of this *Guide,* and to write down appropriate hypotheses or inferences for each scale or configuration. Greater confidence should be placed in inferences that occur for several scales or configurations and that are consistent with other test and nontest data available for the examinee. At this point the inferences can be organized into the categories suggested above or others that suit the needs of the examiner. As mentioned earlier in this chapter, some inferences about an examinee do not result directly from scores on a scale or scales. Rather, they are higher order inferences generated from a basic understanding of the examinee. For example, there are no data indicating that scores on particular MMPI scales are predictive of success as a real estate salesperson. However, one might predict that an examinee whose MMPI scores have led to inferences of strong achievement needs, competitiveness, and ability to create a good impression would be likely to be successful in real estate sales.

Dynamics and Etiology

In most assessment situations it is desirable to go beyond a description of an individual's behavior and to make inferences about the dynamics underlying the behavior or about the etiology of a particular problem or condition. For some MMPI scales and configurations of scales, the interpretive information presented in previous chapters of this *Guide* includes some statements about these underlying factors. In addition, it is possible and/or necessary to make some higher order inferences about dynamics. For example, if one infers from an examinee's MMPI protocol that he/she is afraid of becoming emotionally involved with other people because of a fear of being hurt or exploited, one might then speculate that the person has been hurt and/or exploited in earlier emotional relationships. Or if one interprets an MMPI protocol as indicating strong resentment of authority, it is reasonable to infer than the resentment has its origins in parent-child relationships. The higher order inferences often are based on MMPI data combined with other test and nontest (interview, history, etc.) data.

Diagnostic Impressions

Although the usefulness of psychiatric diagnosis per se has been questioned by many clinicians, referral sources often request information about diagnosis. In addition, it often is necessary to assign diagnostic labels for purposes such as insurance claims, disability status, competency status, etc. Many of the interpretive sections in earlier chapters of this *Guide* present diagnostic information for the individual clinical scales and for the two-point code types. In addition, it is useful to consider the slope of the MMPI profile. A negative slope (left side high, right side low) is suggestive of a neurotic disorder, whereas a positive slope (left side low, right side high) is suggestive of a psychotic disorder. Scores on some of the supplementary MMPI scales discussed in Chapters 6 and 7 of this *Guide* also can be examined to add diagnostic information. For example, among psychiatric patients low Es scores tend to be associated with psychotic disorders and high Es scores tend to be associated with neurotic disorders. If scores on scales such as Persecutory Ideas (Pa1), Bizarre Sensory Experiences (Sc3), Psychoticism (PSY), or Autism (TSC VI) are high, the likelihood of a psychotic disorder becomes greater. As with all other aspects of MMPI interpretation, other data (history, observation, etc.) must be taken into account in arriving at a diagnostic label for an individual.

Treatment Implications

A primary goal in most assessments is to be able to make meaningful recommendations about treatment. Sometimes, when demand for treatment exceeds the resources available, the decision simply is whether or not to accept a particular person for treatment. Such a decision may involve clinical judgment about how badly the person is in need of treatment as well as about how likely he/she is to respond favorably to available treatment procedures. When differential treatment procedures are available, the assessment may be useful in deciding which procedures are likely to be most appropriate for a specific person. Even when the decision has been made before the assessment that a person will receive a particular treatment procedure, the assessment can be valuable by providing information about problem areas to be considered in treatment and by alerting the therapist (or others involved in treatment) to assets and liabilities that could facilitate or hinder progress in therapy.

The Ego Strength (Es) scale is the only scale discussed in this *Guide* that was designed specifically to predict response to psychotherapy (see Chapter 6). If one is dealing with a neurotic individual, a high Es score is likely to mean that such a person will benefit from traditional, individual psychotherapy. With other kinds of persons and/or treatment procedures the relationship between Es scores and treatment outcome is less clear, but in general higher Es scores can be interpreted as suggestive of psychological resources that can be tapped in treatment procedures.

The Control (Cn) scale (see Chapter 6) was designed to identify patients who, in spite of serious psychopathology, are able to be treated as outpatients rather than having to be hospitalized. High Cn scores indicate an ability to avoid displaying pathology to others. Whereas this ability may permit an individual to avoid hospitalization, it also can be a liability in treatment if the person chooses to keep his pathology from his/her therapist or others involved in the treatment process.

As was discussed above in relation to characteristic traits and behaviors, many of the inferences about treatment will not come directly from scores on specific MMPI scales or configurations of scales. Rather, they are higher order inferences based on other inferences that have already been made about the examinee. For example, if one has inferred from the MMPI that an examinee is in a great deal of emotional turmoil, it can now be further inferred that he/she is likely to be motivated enough to change in psychotherapy. On the other hand, if one has inferred that a person is very reluctant to accept responsibility for his/her own behavior and blames problems and shortcomings on other people, the prognosis for traditional psychotherapy is very poor. A person who is very suggestible is apt to respond more favorably to direct advice-giving than to insight-oriented therapy. A psychopathic individual (high scores on MMPI scales 4 and 9) who enters therapy rather than going to jail is likely to terminate therapy prematurely. Obviously, there are many other examples of higher order inferences related to treatment.

SOME SPECIFIC REFERRAL QUESTIONS

In addition to a rather comprehensive understanding of the examinee, an MMPI interpretation often must address itself to questions asked by the referral source (e.g., Is this patient suicidal? Is this person dangerous to others?). Whereas it is not possible to anticipate all such referral questions and to address each of them in this section, several of the more frequently asked questions are considered below.

Suicide

The clinician often is faced with the difficult problem of trying to predict suicidal behavior from the MMPI. Although some persons in psychiatric settings admit to suicidal thoughts and ideas of varying intensities, only a small proportion of these persons actually attempts suicide. Because of the obvious implications of suicidal attempts, there is a sense of urgency in trying to identify persons who are likely to make such attempts.

Suicidal ideation almost always is associated with serious depression; therefore, extreme elevations on scale 2 are almost always present in the MMPI's of persons who have suicidal ideas. Often scale 7 is the second highest scale in the profile, suggesting anxiety, agitation, and rumination or brooding. The 27/72 two-point code, then, is the most commonly found one for persons who have suicidal ideas.

Obviously, not all persons with elevations on scales 2 and 7 will attempt suicide. Persons who actually attempt suicide, as opposed to those who only think about it, tend to be rather impulsive, to prefer action to thought, and to have poor judgment. These characteristics often are reflected in elevations on scales 4, 8, and 9. Traditionally, scores on scale 9 have been thought to have especially great significance in identifying suicidal individuals. If a person is depressed and extremely uncomfortable, as suggested by elevations on scales 2 and 7, he/she may be thinking about suicide. If scale 9 is low, he/she may not have the energy to act on these ideas. However, if scale 9 also is elevated, the likelihood of the person's acting on the suicidal ideas increases. Elevations on scales 4 and 8 are suggestive of an individual who is impulsive and who shows poor judgment. When such a person also is depressed and miserable, as indicated by elevations on scales 2 and 7, the likelihood of suicide attempts increases.

There is some clinical evidence that among seriously depressed individuals suicide attempts are more likely when the depression starts to clear. If multiple administrations of the MMPI are available, significant decreases on scale 2 for persons who have been seriously depressed should alert the clinician that suicide attempts may become more likely.

In summary, elevations on scales 2 and 7 are suggestive of depression and discomfort that can give rise to suicidal *ideas*. If scales 4, 8, and 9 also are very elevated, the likelihood of suicide *attempts* increases. However, the prediction of suicide attempts from the MMPI alone is not very precise. Obviously, other data such as self-report, previous suicide attempts, familial and/or occupational crises and related situational variables, and so forth, must also be considered. However, there are some MMPI signs that can serve as valuable additional information in the attempt to make this extremely important clinical prediction. For a complete list of references relevant to predicting suicide from the MMPI the reader is referred to Chapter 1 of Volume 2 of *An MMPI Handbook* (Dahlstrom et al., 1975).

Acting Out Behavior

Another important prediction with which the clinician often is involved is that of acting out behavior. Whereas a wide array of behaviors, ranging from verbal hostility to physical assaultiveness, can be acted out, it is the physical harm to other people that is most important to predict. In talking about predicting aggressive acting out behavior from the MMPI it is important to differentiate between two different kinds of people. First, there is the person who is chronically hostile and aggressive and who gets into repeated difficulties because he acts out these impulses. Second, there is the person who usually is overcontrolled but who occasionally lashes out in dangerous and destructive ways (i.e., overcontrolled hostility). Persons in this latter category tend to be involved in harmful and destructive acts (e.g., physical assault, murder, etc.) more often than those in the former category.

The clinical scales of the MMPI can be divided into two categories: those that suggest lack of impulse control (scales 4, 6, 8, and 9) and those that suggest control and inhibition of impulses (scales 1, 2, 3, 5, 7, and 0). When the former scales are more elevated than the latter ones, one should predict problems in impulse control and chronic acting out. When the latter scales are more elevated than the former scales, one should predict adequate control of impulses.

In the MMPI literature, elevations on scale 4 and/or scale 9 have been associated with difficulties in impulse control. Such elevations are suggestive of asocial or antisocial tendencies. The 49/94 two-point code indicates impulsivity and striving for immediate gratification of needs, but it does not necessarily suggest physical harm to others. In the early MMPI literature the 48/84 two-point code type was described as suggesting senseless, vicious, poorly planned, poorly executed, and savage acting out behavior, including sexual and/or homicidal assault. More recently, evidence has emerged that indicates that the 43 code is the two-point code most associated with violent, assaultive behavior (Davis & Sines, 1971; Persons & Marks, 1971). The 43 person usually is overcontrolled, but periodic outbursts of aggressive, assaultive behavior may occur. As both scales 4 and 3 become more elevated, the likelihood of such episodes increases. In any profile configuration, the relative elevations of scales 3 and 4 are related to impulse control. As scale 4 becomes greater than scale 3, problems with impulse control are predicted, and as scale 3 becomes greater than scale 4 adequate control and inhibition are likely.

High scores on the Hy5 Harris subscale (Inhibition of Aggression) are predictive of adequate control of aggressive impulses. High scores on the Wiggins Manifest Hostility (HOS) content scale are suggestive of inadequate control and of acting out behavior. Similarly, loss of control is suggested by high scores on the Sc2C Harris subscale (Lack of Ego Mastery, Defective Inhibition).

Many additional scales have been developed from the MMPI item pool specifically to assess aggressive acting out behavior. The interested reader will find a complete list of references to studies that have involved prediction of aggressive acting out behavior from the MMPI in Chapter 3 of Volume 2 of *An MMPI Handbook* (Dahlstrom et al., 1975).

Psychosis

In many settings the identification of psychotic individuals from their MMPI protocols is an important assessment goal. Although such an emphasis on diagnosis is viewed by many clinicians as inappropriate, there are many settings in which such identification is routinely undertaken and in which important decisions about individuals (e.g., form of chemotherapy, etc.) are based on such identification.

Initially, Hathaway and McKinley hoped that accurate diagnostic classification could be accomplished by noting an examinee's highest clinical scale. Thus, if scale 8 (Schizophrenia) was highest, the examinee could be diagnosed as schizophrenic. As discussed in Chapter 1, however, this initially oversimplistic view of diagnosis from the MMPI was not realized. Examinees often have equally high scores on more than one of the clinical scales. In addition, some normal subjects achieve elevations on one or more of the clinical scales, whereas some abnormal subjects are able to achieve reasonably normal scores on the clinical scales. In spite of these problems, however, scores on scale 8 seem to be related to psychosis. If an extremely high score (T > 80) is achieved on scale 8, and if a deviant response set can be ruled out (see Chapter 3), the possibility of a psychotic disorder must be considered. Of course, other test and notest data should be examined before labeling an examinee as schizophrenic.

The relative scores on scales 7 and 8 seem to be related to psychosis. If the scale 8 T-score is greater than the scale 7 T-score, psychosis is more likely than if the reverse is true. As scale 8 becomes much higher than scale 7, the probability of psychosis is greater. At all T-score ranges, scale 8 scores greater than scale 7 scores are suggestive of some loss of control of cognitive processes.

An MMPI profile in which scales 6 and 8 are quite elevated and both are considerably higher than scale 7 (the so-called "paranoid valley") is suggestive of a psychotic disorder. Of course, one must rule out deviant response sets, in which this pattern also may occur (see Chapter 3).

Several of the additional MMPI scales that were discussed in Chapter 7 also seem to be related to psychosis. High scores on the Harris Persecutory Ideas (Pa1), Lack of Ego Mastery, Cognitive (Sc2A), and Bizarre Sensory

Experiences (Sc3) subscales may be indicative of a psychotic disorder. Likewise, psychosis is suggested by high scores on the Wiggins Psychoticism (PSY) scale and the TSC cluster VI (Autism) scale.

Many efforts have been made to develop configural rules for classifying profiles as psychotic or nonpsychotic. One of the most promising efforts is that of Goldberg (1965), which was discussed earlier in this chapter. After trying numerous different indices and sets of rules for classifying profiles as neurotic or psychotic, Goldberg concluded that a simple linear combination of T-scores on five MMPI scales yields the best discrimination of profiles. As stated above, to compute the Goldberg index, one simply inserts T-score values into the following formula: L + Pa + Sc − Hy − Pt. Goldberg found for his samples that a cutoff score of 45 on this index yielded correct placement of profiles for about 70% of his cases. Obviously, the clinician who uses this index in clinical work should determine empirically the optimal cutoff scores for each setting in which the index is used.

Other sets of rules for classifying profiles diagnostically have been developed by Henrichs (1964, 1966), Meehl and Dahlstrom (1960), Peterson (1954), and Taulbee and Sisson (1957). Because Goldberg's simple linear combination of scores seems to work as well as or better than these other more complicated and time-consuming approaches, they will not be discussed here. Dahlstrom et al. (1975) presented a detailed list of references dealing with differential diagnosis from the MMPI in Chapter 1 of Volume 2 of *An MMPI Handbook*.

Functional versus Organic Etiology

There are many somatic symptoms that can be either functional or organic in nature (e.g., paralysis, headaches, chest pain, etc.), and sometimes the clinician is called upon to assist in making the discrimination. Obviously, the MMPI should not be the only, or even the primary, diagnostic tool used in making such a determination. Whenever physical or somatic symptoms are presented by a client, appropriate medical evidence should be collected and evaluated. If no physical basis for the symptoms can be identified, one can then turn to the MMPI, social history, and other data to determine whether the person's psychological makeup is consistent with a functional etiology of the symptoms.

Scale 3 (Hysteria) of the MMPI is sensitive to tendencies to develop physical symptoms in reaction to stress (see Chapter 4). Whereas persons with bona fide physical problems obtain somewhat elevated scores on scale 3, very elevated scores (T > 70) are more likely to be suggestive of somatization reactions.

The profiles of persons reporting physical problems that are of functional origin tend to have a marked negative slope. The neurotic scales (1, 2, 3) tend to be much more elevated than the psychotic scales (8 and 9). The relative positions of scales 1, 2, and 3 have relevance to the discrimination of symptoms with functional versus organic etiology. If scales 1 and 3 are significantly higher than scale 2 (the so-called "conversion valley" pattern), particularly if all three scales are elevated in relation to the other scales in the profile, the likelihood of a conversion reaction (i.e., physical symptoms for which psychological factors are preeminent) is great. Such persons tend to report a variety of physical symptoms for which no physical basis can be identified, and they may display a classic hysterical indifference or lack of concern about their symptoms.

Hanvik (1949, 1951) developed the Lb scale (see Chapter 6) to differentiate between persons complaining of low back pain for which no physical cause can be identified (high scores) and persons with similar pain for which there is an identifiable physical basis (low scores). When the Lb scale is used along with appropriate medical evidence, it offers assistance in making the determination of functional versus organic etiology of low back pain. A detailed list of references to studies dealing with the relationship between physical problems and MMPI performance can be found in Chapter 2 of Volume 2 of *An MMPI Handbook* (Dahlstrom et al., 1975).

Alcoholism and Drug Addiction

Excessive use of alcohol as a way of reacting to stress is very common in our society, and alcoholism is found among persons of diverse personality types and with different kinds of problems. However, the literature that has dealt with the relationship between MMPI performance and excessive use of alcohol has suggested that a strong psychopathic element is present in many alcoholics. This is in agreement with data indicating that scale 4 (Psychopathic Deviate) of the MMPI often is elevated among alcoholics. In addition, several two-point codes which include scale 4 (49/94, 14/41, 24/42, 34/43, 46/64) tend to be associated with alcoholism.

Most of the studies of the MMPI performance of alcoholics have dealt with individuals who already have become alcoholics. Obviously, it would be more useful to identify such persons before they actually become alcoholics. Some data are available about the MMPI's of prealcoholics who later became alcoholics (Hoffman et al., 1974; Kammeier et al., 1973; Loper et al., 1973). MMPI's administered during college to men who later became alcoholic were compared with MMPI's of a control group of men who did not become alcoholic. The prealcoholic group had significantly higher elevations on the F scale, scale 4, and scale 9, indicating that they were more gregarious, impulsive, and less conforming than the controls even before they became alcoholics. When the college MMPI's of the alcoholics were compared with MMPI's administered later in life when they entered treatment for their alcoholism, it was found that the same basic profile configuration was present both times. However, at the latter time the elevations on scales 4 and 9 were much more extreme. It appears, then, that the MMPI's of alcoholics, both before and after they become alcoholics, are characterized by elevations on scales 4 and 9. Obviously, not all persons who have such profiles are or will become alcoholic, but the likelihood of alcoholism is greater for persons with such configurations.

The original MMPI item pool has been used to develop a number of scales for identifying alcoholics. Most of these scales effectively differentiate alcoholics from nonalcoholic controls, but they do not differentiate alcoholics from nonalcoholic psychiatric patients. However, one alcoholism scale (MacAndrew, 1965) makes this latter discrimination effectively.

MacAndrew compared item responses of 300 male alcoholics and 300 male psychiatric outpatients. He identified 51 items that differentiated these two groups (see Table 8.1). For a cross-validational sample, a raw score cutoff of 24 correctly identified 84% of the cases, with about equal numbers of false positives and false negatives among the incorrectly identified cases. There also is some evidence that the MacAndrew scale is effective in identifying prealcoholic persons who later become alcoholic (Hoffman et al., 1974).

Much less information is available in the literature concerning the MMPI performance of drug users than of alcoholics. The data that are available suggest that persons who are alcoholic and those who are addicted to drugs produce similar kinds of MMPI protocols.

There is a strong component of sociopathy in the test performance of drug addicts. They almost always have high scores on scale 4 (Psychopathic Deviate), and elevations also often are found on scales 8 and 9. The 49/94, 48/84, and 89/98 two-point code types are the most frequent ones found for drug addicts. These aspects of MMPI performance suggest that addicts tend to be impulsive, socially nonconforming, and rejecting of traditional values and restrictions. Whereas most studies have used heroin addicts as subjects, some data exist suggesting that the MMPI's of LSD users are similar to those of addicts.

Addicts also tend to score low on the Ego Strength (Es) scale, suggesting limited resources for dealing with problems and stress. They also achieve high scores on the Pd1 (Familiar Discord), Pd2 (Authority Conflict), and Pd4A (Social Isolation) subscales of Harris and on the AUT (Authority Conflict) and FAM (Family Problems) content scales (see Chapter 7). These high scores indicate that the addict has stormy family relationships, has rebelled against family authority, and feels isolated and estranged socially.

Whereas some efforts have been made to use the MMPI item pool to develop scales for identifying addicts, none has been particularly successful. There is some clinical evidence that the MacAndrew alcoholism scale, which was discussed above in relation to alcoholism, may also be sensitive to drug addiction. However, further research is needed before the MacAndrew scale can be used routinely for identifying addicts or potential addicts. Dahlstrom et al. (1975) presented a detailed list of references concerning the relationship between alcoholism and drug addiction and MMPI performance in Chapter 1 of Volume 2 of *An MMPI Handbook*.

Table 8.1.   MacAndrew's Alcoholism scale items[a]

An-swer	Item
True	6, 27, 34, 50, 56, 57, 58, 61, 81, 94, 116, 118, 127, 128, 140, 156, 186, 215, 224, 235, 243, 251, 263, 283, 309, 413, 419, 426, 445, 446, 477, 482, 483, 488, 500, 507, 529, 562
False	86, 120, 130, 149, 173, 179, 278, 294, 320, 335, 357, 378, 460

[a] From C. MacAndrew. The differentiation of male alcoholic outpatients from nonalcoholic psychiatric patients by means of the MMPI. *Quarterly Journal of Studies on Alcohol*, 1965, *26*, 238–246. Copyright 1965 by Quarterly Journal of Studies on Alcohol. Reproduced with permission.

AN ILLUSTRATIVE CASE

In order to help the reader to understand the strategy discussed above, an actual case is now considered and a step-by-step analysis of the MMPI protocol is presented.* As a practice exercise the reader can interpret the profile (Fig. 8.1) and supplementary scores (Table 8.2) and then compare his/her interpretation with the one that is presented below.

Background Information

This 27-year-old barber (J. A. K.) came to an outpatient psychological clinic complaining of depression, irritability, moodiness, lack of self-confidence, and extreme difficulty in making decisions. He dated the onset of his problems to 5 years earlier when he was discharged from military service and felt "on his own" for the first time in his life. J. A. K. was the older of two male children. He described his 25-year-old brother as being the opposite of him. Whereas J. A. K. was interested in art, literature, and other aesthetic things, his brother was interested in sports and other stereotypic masculine activities. J. A. K.'s father died about 5 years before he was seen in the clinic, and his mother had been dead for 8 years. He described his childhood as pleasant. Although his parents did not show much affection toward him, neither did they make many demands on him. After graduation from high school, J. A. K. gave in to pressure from his father that he go to college. However, he could not concentrate on his studies, and he was dismissed after 1 year. He enlisted in the Army, where he served as a clerk for 3 years. He liked military life because "everything is laid out for you." After leaving the service, he became a partner in a barber shop with a boyhood friend. At the time that he was seen in the clinic, he expressed some ambivalence about barbering, and he talked about getting a job as a photographer. J. A. K. had been married for a little over 1 year, and his wife was pregnant with their first child. He was pleased at the prospect of being a father, but he also was afraid of the increased responsibility. At the time of the MMPI administration, he was described by the examiner as cooperative and friendly, and as eager to "do well" on the test. Few overt signs of anxiety, depression, or other emotional distress were observed. He completed the MMPI in about 1½ hr.

Test-taking Attitude

J. A. K. completed the MMPI in about an average length of time, indicating that he was neither excessively indecisive nor impulsive in responding to the items. He omitted no items, suggesting that he was cooperative and did not use this rather simple way of avoiding unfavorable self-statements. His raw score of 3 on the L scale is what would be expected for someone of his educational and socioeconomic background, so we may infer that he was not blatantly defensive and denying in his approach to the test. J. A. K.'s F scale T-score of 62 suggests that he was admitting to

---

* This protocol also was submitted for scoring and interpretation to six computerized services. The interpretive sections of the six reports that were returned are presented in Chapter 9 of this *Guide*.

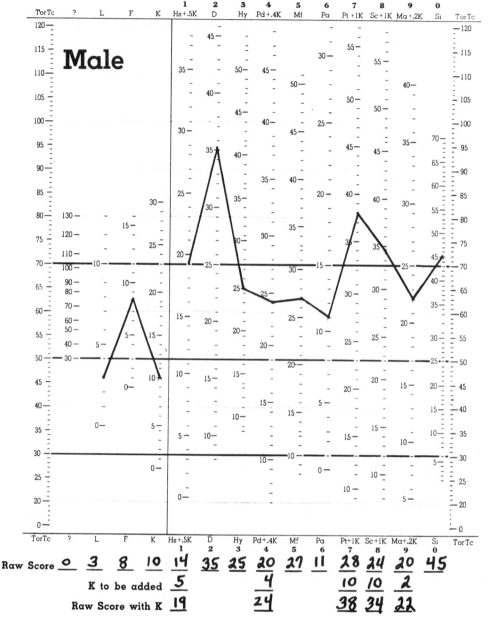

TorTc	?	L	F	K	1 Hs+.5K	2 D	3 Hy	4 Pd+.4K	5 Mf	6 Pa	7 Pt+1K	8 Sc+1K	9 Ma+.2K	0 Si

Male

Raw Score: 0 3 8 10 14 35 25 20 27 11 28 24 20 45

K to be added: 5   4   10 10 2

Raw Score with K: 19   24   38 34 22

Fig. 8.1. MMPI profile for illustrative case (J. A. K.). MMPI profile sheet copyrighted 1948 by the Psychological Corporation. Reproduced by permission granted in test catalog.

more than an average number of deviant attitudes and behaviors, but it is not high enough to indicate some invalidating response set. In all likelihood he simply was being candid in describing himself on the MMPI.

For a person of his educational and socioeconomic level, we would expect a K scale score in a range of 55 to 60. J. A. K.'s score of 45 on the K scale

Table 8.2.   Supplementary MMPI scores for illustrative case (J. A. K.)

	Scale	Raw score	T-score
A	(Anxiety)	28	70
R	(Repression)	20	59
Es	(Ego Strength)	47	54
MAS	(Manifest Anxiety)	31	97
Lb	(Low Back Pain)	13	66
Ca	(Caudality)	21	71
Dy	(Dependency)	34	66
Do	(Dominance)	13	45
Re	(Responsibility)	20	50
Pr	(Prejudice)	13	52
St	(Social Status)	21	58
Cn	(Control)	29	61
D1	(Subjective Depression)	22	93
D2	(Psychomotor Retardation)	10	76
D3	(Physical Malfunctioning)	4	56
D4	(Mental Dullness)	8	80
D5	(Brooding)	6	71
Hy1	(Denial of Social Anxiety)	1	36
Hy2	(Need for Affection)	3	42
Hy3	(Lassitude-Malaise)	10	83
Hy4	(Somatic Complaints)	7	67
Hy5	(Inhibition of Aggression)	3	53
Pd1	(Familial Discord)	2	51
Pd2	(Authority Problems)	5	55
Pd3	(Social Imperturbability)	4	35
Pd4A	(Social Alienation)	6	52
Pd4B	(Self-alienation)	10	74
Pa1	(Persecutory Ideas)	1	46
Pa2	(Poignancy)	5	68
Pa3	(Naivete)	2	41
Sc1A	(Social Alienation)	5	56
Sc1B	(Emotional Alienation)	4	66
Sc2A	(Lack of Ego Mastery, Cognitive)	4	66
Sc2B	(Lack of Ego Mastery, Conative)	10	94
Sc2C	(Lack of Ego Mastery, Defective Inhibition)	3	60
Sc3	(Bizarre Sensory Experiences)	7	69
Ma1	(Amorality)	4	67
Ma2	(Psychomotor Acceleration)	6	66
Ma3	(Imperturbability)	3	47
Ma4	(Ego Inflation)	2	46
Mf1	(Narcissism-Hypersensitivity)	9	95
Mf2	(Stereotypic Feminine Interests)	5	61
Mf3	(Denial of Stereotypic Masculine Interests)	7	81
Mf4	(Heterosexual Discomfort-Passivity)	1	33
Mf5	(Introspective-Critical)	3	46
Mf6	(Socially Retiring)	3	42
Si1	(Inferiority-Personal Discomfort)	19	96
Si2	(Discomfort with Others)	5	55
Si3	(Staid-Personal Rigidity)	9	50
Si4	(Hypersensitivity)	5	65
Si5	(Distrust)	8	71
Si6	(Physical-Somatic Concerns)	2	53

Table 8.2—Continued

Scale		Raw score	T-score
SOC	(Social Maladjustment)	17	67
DEP	(Depression)	20	75
FEM	(Feminine Interests)	14	66
MOR	(Poor Morale)	15	64
REL	(Religious Fundamentalism)	6	49
AUT	(Authority Conflict)	12	56
PSY	(Psychoticism)	7	48
ORG	(Organic Symptoms)	11	63
FAM	(Family Problems)	3	47
HOS	(Manifest Hostility)	16	63
PHO	(Phobias)	11	64
HYP	(Hypomania)	11	48
HEA	(Poor Health)	7	55
TSC I	(Social Introversion)	22	83
TSC II	(Body Complaints)	16	93
TSC III	(Suspicion and Mistrust)	10	54
TSC IV	(Depression)	20	94
TSC V	(Resentment)	12	70
TSC VI	(Autism)	9	63
TSC VII	(Tension)	19	77

indicates that he was somewhat self-critical in responding to the items. J. A. K.'s configuration on the validity scales resembles the inverted V-shape discussed above. Whereas it is possible that he was exaggerating his problems as a cry for help, the moderate level of the F scale and the position of the L and K scales near the mean indicate that more likely he was honestly describing a moderate discomfort and psychopathology. In summary, J. A. K seems to have approached the MMPI in an honest and open manner, and although he was moderately self-critical in responding to the test items, there is no reason to believe that the test behavior is not a representative sample of his behavior.

Adjustment Level

J. A. K.'s F scale T-score of 62 indicates a moderate degree of emotional discomfort; it is at a level that indicates that he is able to cope with many aspects of his life situation, but at some great psychological cost to him. In general, his scores on the clinical scales are quite elevated. The mean T-score on the clinical scales (excluding scales 5 and 0) is about 70. Such a mean score indicates moderate to severe psychopathology and somewhat serious problems in functioning in everyday activities. He has four clinical scales equal to or greater than a T-score of 70, further supporting the inference of moderate to severe disturbance. Although the slope of his profile is not dramatic, it tends to be somewhat negative, suggesting internal conflict and discomfort but not severe impairment in functioning. His T-score of 67 on the Anxiety scale indicates that he is in a good deal of emotional turmoil. The rather extreme elevations on scales 2 and 7 further suggest turmoil, including anxiety, depression, and feeling overwhelmed and unable to cope. His Es scale score is about at the mean, further suggesting moderate maladjustment. J. A. K. endorsed only 6 of the 38 critical items (see Appendix M of this *Guide*), and none of them was a blatantly psychotic item. The critical items that he endorsed in the pathological direction deal with head discomfort, impulses to hurt himself or someone else, periods of activity that he later could not remember, peculiar odors, feelings of unreality, and wishing that he were dead. In summary, it appears that J. A. K. is in a great deal of personal discomfort. However, his discomfort level is somewhat greater than his actual inability to function in everday activities. He is likely to feel terrible much of the time, but he continues to function in spite of how he feels.

Characteristic Traits and Behaviors

A first step in trying to generate inferences in this area is to examine each of J. A. K.'s validity scale scores and to consult Chapter 3 for appropriate hypotheses or inferences.

L (T = 46)

This score is about what is expected for someone of his educational and socioeconomic background; not particularly defensive or denying.

F (T = 62)

This score is somewhat higher than in most persons with his background; he admitted to some but not very many deviant behaviors and/or ideas; he endorsed items dealing with passivity, tendency to withdraw from problems, difficulties in sleeping, impulses to injure himself or other people, and periods of activity during which he was not aware of what he was doing; he functions adequately in many aspects of his life situation even though he is very unhappy and uncomfortable.

K (T = 46)

This score is somewhat lower than expected for someone who completed 1 year of college; he is self-critical, self-dissatisfied; he may be exaggerating his problems somewhat as a cry for help; he is somewhat ineffective in dealing with problems of everyday life; he has little insight into his own motives and behaviors; socially awkward; he is socially conforming and overly compliant with authority; he is inhibited, retiring, shallow, has slow personal tempo, is critical of other people, is suspicious of motivations of others, is cynical, skeptical, caustic, and has a disbelieving outlook.

Next, clinical scales on which J. A. K. achieved T-scores equal to or greater than 70 are identified, and appropriate sections of Chapter 4 are consulted for hypotheses.

Scale 2 (T = 94)

This is a very high score, suggestive of serious depression; he feels blue, depressed, unhappy, dysphoric; he is pessimistic about future, self-depreciatory; he harbors guilt feelings. Depressive diagnosis is likely; he has somatic complaints, weakness, fatigue, loss of energy; he is agitated, tense, irritable, high-strung, prone to worry; he lacks self-confidence, feels useless and unable to function; feels like a failure on job; is introverted, shy, retiring, timid, seclusive, secretive, aloof; maintains psychological distance; avoids interpersonal involvement. He is cautious and conventional in approach to problems; has difficulty in making decisions; is nonaggressive and overcontrolled; denies impulses, avoids unpleasantness, makes concessions to avoid confrontations and is motivated for therapy because of intense discomfort.

Scale 7 (T = 81)

This score suggests a great deal of discomfort and turmoil. He is anxious, tense, agitated, worried, apprehensive, high-strung, jumpy; he has difficulties concentrating; is introspective, ruminative, obsessive, compulsive. He feels insecure and inferior; lacks self-confidence; has self-doubts; is self-critical, self-conscious, self-derogatory; is rigid, moralistic; sets high standards for self and others; is perfectionistic, conscientious, guilty, depressed, neat, orderly, organized, meticulous, persistent, reliable. He lacks ingenuity in approach to problems, is dull, formal; he vacillates, is indecisive; distorts importance of problems, overreacts; does not interact socially; is hard to get to know; worries about popularity and acceptance; is sentimental, peaceable, soft hearted, trustful, sensitive, kind, dependent, individualistic, unemotional, and immature. He has physical complaints (heart, gastrointestinal, genitourinary, fatigue, exhaustion, sleep disturbance); he is not responsive to brief psychotherapy; he has some insight into problems but intellectualizes and rationalizes; he is resistant to interpretations in therapy; he will develop excessive hostility toward therapist; he will remain in therapy longer than many patients, and make slow but steady progress; in therapy he will discuss difficulties with authority figures, poor work or study habits, and fear of homosexual impulses.

Scale 8 (T = 73)

At this level many of the blatantly psychotic items are not endorsed. He has a schizoid life style; feels as if he is not part of social environment; feels isolated, alienated, misunderstood, unaccepted; is withdrawn, seclusive, secretive, inaccessible; avoids dealing with people and with new situations; is described by others as shy, aloof, uninvolved; has generalized anxiety; is resentful, hostile, aggressive, but unable to express such feelings; responds to stress by withdrawal into daydreams and fantasies; has self-doubts; feels inferior, incompetent, dissatisfied; has sexual preoccupation and sex role confusion. Others see him as nonconforming, unusual, unconventional, eccentric; his physical complaints are vague and long-standing; he is stubborn, moody, opinionated, generous, peaceable, sentimental, immature, impulsive, adventurous, sharp witted, conscientious, high-strung. He has a wide range of interests, is creative and imaginative; his goals are abstract and vague; he lacks basic information that is required for problem solving; his prognosis for therapy is poor because of long-standing problems and reluctance to relate in a meaningful way; he stays in therapy longer than most patients, and eventually may come to trust the therapist.

Scale 0 (T = 72)

He is socially introverted; insecure and uncomfortable in social situations; shy, reserved, timid, retiring; feels more comfortable alone or with a few close friends; does not participate in many social activities; is especially uncomfortable around members of opposite sex; lacks self-confidence; is self-effacing; is hard to get to know; is seen by others as cold and distant; is sensitive to what others think of him; is troubled by lack of involvement with other poeple; is overcontrolled; does not display feelings openly; is submissive, compliant, overly accepting of authority; has a slow personal tempo; is reliable, dependable; is cautious, conventional and unoriginal in approach to problems; is rigid and inflexible in attitudes and opinions; has difficulty in decision-making; enjoys work; gets pleasure from personal achievement; worries; is irritable; anxious, moody; has guilt, depression.

Scale 1 (T = 70)

This score is indicative of bodily concern. He has vague, nonspecific physical complaints, epigastric complaints, chronic fatigue, pain, weakness. He is given a neurotic diagnosis; acting out is unlikely; he is selfish, self-centered, narcissistic, pessimistic, defeatist, cynical, dissatisfied, unhappy; he makes others miserable, and complains in a whiny manner; he is critical and demanding; expresses hostility indirectly; is dull, unenthusiastic, unambitious; lacks ease of oral expression; does not manifest much anxiety; shows no signs of major incapacity; is functioning at reduced level of efficiency; has long-standing problems; is cynical; lacks insight; is not very responsive to traditional therapy; is critical of therapist.

Next, J. A. K.'s two-point code is identified. Chapter 5 is consulted and hypotheses appropriate for the 27/72 code are generated: anxious, nervous, tense, high-strung, jumpy; worries excessively; vulnerable to real or imagined threat; anticipates problems before they occur; overreacts under stress; has somatic symptoms; has chronic fatigue, tiredness, exhaustion; depressed, but may not feel especially sad; shows clinical signs of depression (slowed speech, weight loss, slow personal tempo, etc.); pessimistic about world in general and more specifically about the likelihood of overcoming his problems; broods, ruminates about his problems; has strong need for achievement and for recognition for accomplishments; has high expectancies for self; feels guilty because he has fallen short of his goals; indecisive; feels inadequate, insecure, inferior; intropunitive, blames self for problems; rigid in thinking and problem solving; meticulous, perfectionistic in daily activities; excessively religious and moralistic; docile and passive-dependent in relationships; has capacity for deep emotional ties; becomes clinging and dependent in times of stress; not aggressive or belligerent; elicits nurturance and helping behavior in others; motivated for therapy because of intense discomfort; remains in therapy and considerable improvement likely; receives neurotic diagnosis.

An examination of J. A. K.'s high and low scores on the supplementary scales discussed in Chapters 6 and 7 of this *Guide* leads to still more hypotheses about J. A. K.

A — Anxiety (T = 70)

He is anxious, uncomfortable; has slow personal tempo; is pessimistic, apathetic, unemotional, unexcitable, shy, retiring, lacks confidence in own abilities; hesitates, vacillates, is inhibited, overcontrolled; is influenced by diffuse personal feelings; is defensive; rationalizes, blames others for difficulties; lacks poise in social situations; is accepting of authority, conforming, submissive, compliant, suggestible, cautious, fussy, effeminate, cool, distant, uninvolved; he becomes confused, disorganized, maladaptive under stress, and is uncomfortable enough to change in therapy.

MAS — Manifest Anxiety (T = 97)

He is predisposed to experience great emotional discomfort in stressful situations; feels anxious, tense, jumpy; experiences physiological changes under stress (e.g., excessive perspiration, increased pulse rate, etc.); perceives his environment as threatening; feels at mercy of forces beyond his control; emphasizes present more than the future; bases expectations on immediate past experiences; has somatic complaints; feels excited, restless some of the time; has difficulties in concentrating; lacks self-confidence; is overly sensitive to reactions of others; feels unhappy, useless.

Do — Dominance (T = 45)

He is submissive, unassertive, unable to stand up for his own rights and opinions, easily influenced by others; he lacks self-confidence; is pessimistic, inefficient and stereotyped in approach to problems; gives up easily; does not feel sense of duty to others; does not face up to realities of his life situation.

D1 — Subjective Depression (T = 93)

He is unhappy, blue, depressed; lacks energy for coping with problems in his life situation; is not interested in what goes on around him; feels nervous, tense; has problems in concentrating and attending, poor appetite, sleep disturbance; broods, cries; lacks self-confidence; feels inferior, useless; is easily hurt by criticism, uneasy, shy, embarassed in social situations; tends to avoid social interactions. Depressive neurosis is the most likely diagnosis.

D4 — Mental Dullness (T = 80)

He lacks energy to cope with problems of everyday life; is tense; has difficulty in concentrating, poor memory and judgment; lacks self-confidence; feels inferior to others; gets little enjoyment out of life; feels life is no longer worth living.

D5 — Brooding (T = 71)

He broods, ruminates, cries; lacks energy to cope with problems; feels that life is no longer worthwhile; feels inferior; is unhappy, easily hurt by criticism; feels he is losing control of his thought processes.

Hy1 — Denial of Social Anxiety (T = 36)

He is socially introverted, shy and bashful in social situations; finds it difficult to talk to people; is greatly influenced by social standards and customs.

Hy3 — Lassitude-Malaise (T = 83)

He feels uncomfortable; says he is not in good health; is weak, tired, fatigued but may not report specific somatic symptoms; has difficulty concentrating, poor appetite, sleep disturbance; is unhappy, blue, sees home environment as unpleasant and uninteresting.

Pd3 — Social Imperturbability (T = 35)

He feels uncomfortable in social situations; does not like to interact with other people; finds it difficult to talk with others; avoids being center of attention; does not express his opinions or defend them.

Pd4B — Self-Alienation (T = 74)

He is uncomfortable, unhappy; has problems in concentrating; finds daily life uninteresting; verbalizes regret, guilt, remorse for past misdeeds but is vague about nature of these misdeeds; finds it hard to settle down; may use alcohol excessively.

Sc2B — Lack of Ego Mastery, Conative (T = 94)

He feels that life is a strain; has depression, despair, difficulty in coping; worries excessively; withdraws into fantasy and daydreaming; finds daily life uninteresting; has given up hoping that things will get better; may wish that he were dead.

Mf1 — Narcissism-Hypersensitivity (T = 95)

He is self-centered, narcissistic; concerned about his physical appearance; extremely sensitive and easily hurt; lacks self-confidence. He is also preoccupied with sexual matters; expresses resentment and hostility toward family members; sees others as insensitive, unreasonable, dishonest; worries excessively.

Mf3 — Denial of Stereotypic Masculine Interests (T = 81)

He is not interested in culturally masculine occupations, does not enjoy culturally masculine activities and interests.

Mf4 — Heterosexual Discomfort-Passivity (T = 33)

He denies being attracted to members of his own sex; he is comfortable talking about sex, is assertive and aspiring.

Si5 — Distrust (T = 75)

He has a negative perception of others; sees others as selfish, dishonest, insensitive, untrustworthy; feels overwhelmed by problems and responsibilities; is indecisive and obsessive; lacks self-confidence.

DEP — Depression (T = 75)

He feels depressed, experiences guilt, regret, worry, unhappiness. Life has lost its zest for him; he has little motivation to pursue things, difficulties in concentration. He is anxious, apprehensive about the future; feels misunderstood; is convinced of his unworthiness; believes he deserves to be punished.

TSC I — Social Introversion (T = 83)

He is shy, embarassed, bashful in social situations; does not mix well socially; avoids social gatherings; has difficulty in talking to people in social situations; is self-conscious, tries to avoid being the center of attention; does not make friends easily; lacks self-confidence; does not express opinions to others; does not stick up for his own rights; is sensitive to reactions of others and easily hurt by criticism.

TSC II — Body Symptoms (T = 93)

He is preoccupied with bodily functions; denies good health; feels weak, tired, fatigued; has a wide variety of somatic symptoms.

TSC IV — Depression and Apathy (T = 94)

He is depressed, unhappy, sad, blue; demonstrates psychomotor retardation; is anxious; lacks energy to cope with everyday activities; feels that problems have piled up so high that he can no longer cope with them; finds everyday activities uninteresting; has given up hope of solving his problems; feels like a failure, guilty, useless; feels that he may be losing his mind, but he can't tell others about it.

TSC VII — Tension, Worry, Fears (T = 77)

He feels anxious, tense, nervous, high-strung, jumpy; worries excessively; has sleep disturbances; cries, is easily upset; has difficulties in concentrating, periods of restlessness, excitability; is uncomfortable in unfamilar surroundings; fears that he may be losing his mind; may report some phobias.

A careful examination of the numerous hypotheses generated about J. A. K. from his scores on the various scales reveals that there is remarkable overlap and agreement among the hypotheses generated from different scales. Only a few of the hypotheses are generated from a single scale. The reader will note a few inconsistencies among the hypotheses. Obviously, the greatest emphasis should be placed on those hypotheses that result from several or more scales. Hypotheses resulting from a single scale should be discarded or treated as very tentative. In dealing with the inconsistent hypotheses, several factors should be considered. If inconsistent hypotheses result from two scales and one of the scales has a more extreme score (higher or lower) than the other, greater emphasis should be placed on the hypotheses associated with the scale with the more extreme score. Also, one should consider whether the hypotheses resulted from empirical data or whether they were more subjectively generated (e.g., from item content). Greater weight should be given to those hypotheses that are of empirical origin.

After considering these matters, the next step in the interpretive process is to group the hypotheses into some meaningful categories (either those suggested earlier in this chapter or others that have meaning for the MMPI user).

Symptoms

There is rather clear agreement from various aspects of the MMPI protocol that J. A. K. is likely to be very depressed. He feels blue, unhappy, and dysphoric much of the time. Most of the time he is likely to be rather unemotional and unexcitable and to have a slow personal tempo, but he may also experience episodes of unexplainable excitement and restlessness. He tends to be very moody, and he may brood and ruminate over his problems. He is very pessimistic about the possibility that things will get better, and he may have concluded that life is no longer worthwhile. Although frequent suicidal thoughts are likely, he does not seem to be more likely to attempt suicide than other very depressed patients. He lacks energy to cope with everyday problems, and he is not very interested in or stimulated by his daily life. He may express guilt, remorse, or regret for past misdeeds, but he is vague about the nature of these misdeeds.

J. A. K. clearly also is experiencing a great deal of turmoil and discomfort. He is likely to feel tense, agitated, and anxious. He has a strong tendency to experience great emotional discomfort under stress, and at these times he may manifest physiological signs of anxiety (e.g., excessive perspiration, increased pulse rate, etc.). He tends to be very irritable, highstrung, jumpy, and apprehensive, and he is extremely vulnerable to real or imagined threat.

J. A. K. is likely to be quite concerned about bodily functioning, and may feel that he is in poor physical health. He may report a large number of very specific somatic symptoms, or his complaints may be very vague and nonspecific in nature. Chronic weakness, tiredness, fatigue, or exhaustion are probable. Sleep disturbances and poor appetite also may occur.

Difficulties with concentration and attention may also be reported by J. A. K. He is likely to complain of poor memory and judgment. Ruminative and obsessive thoughts and compulsive behaviors may be present. Decisions are especially difficult for him, and he appears to others to be indecisive much of the time. He may admit to having had periods during which he was unaware of what he was doing. These episodes, coupled with obsessive and intruding thoughts, may lead him to fear that he is losing his mind, but he is afraid to tell other people of this fear.

Major needs

J. A. K. has very strong and unfulfilled dependency needs. He feels very inadequately prepared to handle problems and stresses on his own, and he is likely to turn to others for support and guidance. During periods of extreme stress he may display a rather infantile clinging behavior. He also has very strong needs for achievement and for recognition for his accomplishments. He sets high standards for himself, and he feels guilty when he fails to attain his goals, but his strong fear of failing keeps him from placing himself in directly competitive situations, and his goals are likely to be vague and poorly defined. Although he harbors strong hostile and aggressive impulses toward other people, particularly those who are perceived as not meeting his dependency needs, he is uncomfortable with these negative feelings and is not likely to express them directly. Rather, they are likely to gain expression in indirect passive-aggressive behaviors such as uncooperativeness, stubbornness, and hypercriticality of the behavior of others.

Perceptions of the environment

J. A. K. views the world as a rather threatening and nonsupportive place. He feels that he is at the mercy of forces over which he has no control. His general outlook can be characterized as pessimistic, cynical, skeptical, caustic, and disbelieving. He tends to see other people as selfish, insensitive, unreasonable, and dishonest. He feels that he has been mistreated and misunderstood and that his needs have not been adequately met.

Reactions to stress

J. A. K. feels inadequate and incompetent to cope with problems and stresses in his life situation. He feels that problems have been piling up so long that he no longer can cope with them. Although he may be able to cope with many aspects of his life situation, he does so at reduced efficiency and at great psychological cost to himself. His preferred reaction to problems is to deny their existence and to withdraw into fantasy and daydreaming. When these mechanisms fail, he may feel overwhelmed and his behavior may appear to be disorganized and maladaptive. He has a tendency to anticipate problems before they occur and to overreact to stress. He may develop somatic symptoms in reaction to stress. His approach to problem solving tends to be cautious, conventional, and unoriginal, and his thinking may be rigid and inflexible.

Self-concept

J. A. K.'s self-concept is extremely unfavorable. He sees himself as inferior to other people, and he feels inadequate to handle his own problems. He has set unrealistically high standards for himself, and he feels worthless and useless when he fails to live up to his goals. He is self-critical and self-depreciatory, and he feels unworthy and deserving of punishment. At times he is likely to harbor self-destructive impulses, but he does not appear to be more likely than other depressed patients to attempt suicide. His negative self-image is well integrated into his life style and is likely to be very resistant to change. He may selectively attend to failures and shortcomings and ignore his past accomplishments.

Sexual identification

J. A. K. harbors serious concerns about his sexual adequacy and may engage in rich sexual fantasies. Mature heterosexual relationships are difficult for him, and he probably feels quite uncomfortable around members of the opposite sex. Women are seen as sources of gratification for his intense dependency needs, and he may tend to cast them into the role of mother figures. Although he is likely to deny being attracted to members of his own sex, he may at times become extremely anxious because of transitory homosexual impulses. However, overt homosexual behavior is quite unlikely.

Emotional control

J. A. K. is very much constricted and overcontrolled most of the time. He is uncomfortable with his own feelings, both positive and negative ones, and he is not likely to express them directly. In fact, much of the time he may not even be aware of his own feelings. He harbors rather strong hostile and aggressive feelings, particularly toward parents and other authority figures, and these negative feelings find expression in rather indirect, passive-aggressive behaviors.

Interpersonal relationships

Whereas J. A. K.'s strong needs for attention and recognition may drive him into some interpersonal relationships, they are likely to be shallow and superficial. He has the capacity for developing deep emotional ties, but he prevents people from getting too close to him because of fear of rejection and/or exploitation. He is uncomfortable around people unless he knows them very well, and he does not get involved in many social activities. He is timid, shy, and retiring around other people, and he tries to avoid being the center of attention. He finds it difficult to talk to others except for a few close relatives and friends. He does not make friends easily, and he is seen by other people as secretive, aloof, cool, distant, inaccessible, and hard to get to know. He worries a great deal about being accepted by peers, and he is bothered by his lack of meaningful involvement with other people. With the few people with whom he may be involved, he tends to be very passive, submissive, and compliant. He is easily influenced by the values and standards of others, and he is overly accepting of authority. He does not express or defend his opinions and values to other people. He is very sensitive to the reactions of others and is easily hurt by even minor criticism. He is intent on avoiding unpleasantness and makes many concessions in order to avoid confrontations.

Psychological resources

J. A. K. is likely to have more resources and assets than his self-description suggests. In spite of his extreme discomfort, he is better able to cope with everyday problems than is thinks he is. Although he may not be closely involved with other people, he has the capacity for forming deep emotional ties. He has high standards for his own behavior. He tends to be neat, clean, and orderly, and he is reliable and conscientious. He is seen by others as sensitive, kind, peace-loving, and generous. He enjoys work and gets pleasure from personal achievement.

Dynamics and Etiology

Many of J. A. K.'s symptoms and problems are likely to be associated with his unrealistically high standards and goals for himself and his perceived failure to achieve them. The clinician should explore his family constellation to try to identify the sources of these unrealistic self-expectations. Often such attitudes are produced by demanding and perfectionistic parents who are almost impossible to please. As J. A. K. was the older of two male children, his parents may have had unrealistic expectations of him.

His feelings of inadequacy, dependency, and inability to cope could be related to overprotection and dominance on the part of his parents, particularly his mother. However, such insecurities also can result when an individual is not required, or at least encouraged, to accept increasing responsibilities as he is growing up. This latter inference is in keeping with J. A. K.'s report of his childhood.

One suspects that J. A. K.'s dependent, submissive style is directed at getting sympathy and support from other people. His attitudes and behaviors make it extremely difficult for people to react to him in negative or hostile ways. His avoidance of deep emotional involvement with other people ensures that he cannot be hurt seriously by them.

J. A. K.'s feeling of masculine inadequacy might be related to a faulty identification with his father. Although little is known about the father, except that he died when J. A. K. was 22, one might speculate that he might have been absent from the home a great deal, cool and aloof, very critical and demanding, or otherwise inaccessible as an acceptable male model for his son.

It is possible that J. A. K.'s anger and hostility stem from perceived failures on the part of other people to fulfill his strong dependency needs. Also, they might be related to demands placed on J. A. K. that he feels inadequately prepared to meet.

Diagnostic Impression

Persons with MMPI protocols similar to that of J. A. K. usually receive a neurotic diagnosis, with depressive neurosis and anxiety neurosis being the most common. The level of his F scale score, the rather extreme elevations on scales 2 and 7, and the 27 two-point code all are consistent with such diagnoses. Occasionally, persons with this kind of protocol receive a diagnosis of schizoid personality or schizophrenic reaction, but based on the total data available about J. A. K., these latter diagnoses do not seem to fit in this case.

Implications for Treatment

Because of his intense turmoil and discomfort, J. A. K. is likely to be receptive to counseling or psychotherapy and highly motivated to change. His Es scale T-score is 54, suggesting only moderate resources that can be tapped in treatment. His T-score of 61 on the Control scale indicates that he is able selectively to avoid displaying his psychopathology and that he probably can be treated effectively as an outpatient. This same ability, however, may lead him to keep problems from his therapist.

From his scores on the clinical scales, we can infer that J. A. K. has some characteristics that could be obstacles to successful therapy. Although he seems to have some insight into his problems, he is likely to intellectualize and to rationalize excessively. He can be expected to be resistant to interpretations in therapy. Initially, he may have difficulty in relating to the therapist in a meaningful way. Later in therapy he may develop excessive anger and hostility toward the therapist. However, he is likely to remain in therapy longer than many patients, and eventually he may come to trust the therapist. Slow but steady changes in therapy can be expected.

An initial goal in therapy would be an examination and reevaluation of his self-expectations and development of more realistic standards and goals for himself. Recognition of his negative feelings, followed by development of more effective ways of expressing them, might also be accomplished in therapy. Through the development of a meaningful relationship with his therapist, J. A. K. can come to reassess his fear of becoming emotionally involved with other people.

Specific Referral Questions

Although it is unlikely that all of the referral questions considered earlier in this chapter would be asked for a single case, they all will be considered for J. A. K. for illustrative purposes.

Suicide

J. A. K.'s rather extreme elevations on scales 2 and 7 indicate that he is likely to feel that life is no longer worthwhile and may wish that he were dead. Whereas such suicidal ideas at times may be very intense, there is no indication from the MMPI that J. A. K. is more likely than other depressed patients to attempt suicide. Although scale 8 is moderately elevated, scales 4 and 9 are not very high. Obviously, other factors such as past history of suicide attempts or situational stresses, e.g., death of a family member, job loss, divorce, etc., could make the likelihood of suicide attempts greater.

Acting out behavior

Whereas there is some evidence that J. A. K. harbors some intense hostile and aggressive impulses, there is little reason to expect that he will act out these impulses. Quite to the contrary, he tends to be much too inhibited and overcontrolled. His mean T-score for the control scales (1, 2, 3, 5, 7) is about 75, whereas the mean T-score for the acting out scales (4, 8, 9) is about 62. Scales 4 and 9, which are indicative of acting out behavior, are among the lowest clinical scales in the profile. The 43 two-point code, which may suggest overcontrolled hostility and episodes of aggressive behavior, is not present. His score on the Hy5 subscale (Inhibition of Aggression) is somewhat above average. His score on the Wiggins Manifest Hostility (HOS) scale is not high enough to suggest problems with control. Finally, his score on the Sc2C subscale (Lack of Ego Mastery, Defective Inhibition) is not suggestive of acting out problems.

Psychosis

J. A. K.'s profile is not suggestive of psychosis. Although his scale 8 score is 75, it is not high enough to warrant a diagnosis of psychosis. Scale 7 is higher than scale 8, suggesting control of cognitive processes. The Persecutory Ideas subscale (Pa1), the Lack of Ego Mastery, Cognitive, subscale (Sc2A), and the Bizarre Sensory Experiences subscale (Sc3) all are below 70, supporting the hypothesis that J. A. K. is not psychotic. When his T-scores are entered into Goldberg's index, a value of 22 is obtained. This value is considerably lower than the cutoff score of 45 that Goldberg found most effective in differentiating neurotic and psychotic profiles.

Functional versus organic etiology

Whereas persons with profiles similar to that of J. A. K. tend to present somatic complaints, it is unlikely that he would have some specific conversion symptom (e.g., paralysis, blindness, etc.). The fact that scale 2 is much higher than scale 1 contraindicates a conversion reaction. If J. A. K. were complaining of low back pain, his score on the Lb scale would be considered borderline and not particularly helpful in determining whether the pain were functional or organic in nature.

Alcoholism and addiction

Although persons with this kind of protocol may at times drink excessively, the MMPI protocol is not indicative of alcoholism or addiction. Scale 4, which is often elevated among persons with these problems, is relatively low in the profile. Also, the 27 two-point code is not one often found among alcoholics or addicts. J. A. K.'s raw score on the MacAndrew alcoholism scale is 15, which is far below the cutoff score of 24 found by MacAndrew to be most effective in identifying alcoholics.

Summary

The above analysis of this single case is extremely lengthy in its presentation because it is meant as a teaching-learning tool for the beginning MMPI clinician. The experienced MMPI clinician would write a much briefer interpretation of the protocol. Specifically, the following is what the author would write about J. A. K. in a clinic chart, or to the referring source, or for his own psychotherapy notes, from the same MMPI protocol:

There is no indication that the protocol produced by J. A. K. is not valid. He was not overly defensive in answering the MMPI items, and, in fact, he tended to be somewhat self-critical.

J. A. K. appears to be in a great deal of psychological discomfort. He feels anxious, depressed, and overwhelmed by his problems. Although he continues to function adequately in most aspects of his life situation, he does so at great psychological cost to himself. Most of the time he is likely to be rather unemotional and unexcitable and to have a slow personal tempo, but he may also experience episodes of unexplainable excitement and restlessness. He ruminates over his problems; he is very pessimistic about the possibility that things might get better; and he may have concluded that life is no longer worthwhile. He feels very guilty about perceived misdeeds, and he may harbor suicidal ideas, but he does not seem to be more likely than other depressed patients to attempt suicide. He is likely to report somatic concerns, and they may be general and vague or very specific in nature. J. A. K. is likely to have problems with concentration, attention, memory, and judgment. Decisions are especially difficult for him. He may have experienced periods during which he was unaware of what he was doing, and these episodes, coupled with obsessive and intruding thoughts, may lead him to fear that he is losing his mind.

J. A. K. has very strong unfulfilled dependency needs. He feels very inadequately prepared to handle problems and stresses on his own, and he is likely to turn to others for support and guidance. He has very strong needs for achievement, and he feels guilty when he falls short of his goals. Although he harbors strong hostile and aggressive impulses toward other people, particularly those who are perceived as not meeting his dependency needs, he is uncomfortable with these negative feelings and is not likely to express them directly.

J. A. K. views the world as a rather threatening and nonsupportive place, and he feels that he is at the mercy of forces which are beyond his control. He has a very cynical, skeptical, and disbelieving attitude, and he feels mistreated and misunderstood by other people. His preferred reaction to problems is to deny their existence and to withdraw into fantasy and daydreaming. When these mechanisms fail, he may feel overwhelmed and his behavior may appear to be disorganized and maladaptive. He anticipates problems before they occur, and he overreacts to stress.

J. A. K. has an extremely unfavorable self-concept. It is well integrated into his life style and is likely to be very resistant to change. J. A. K. is likely to have difficulty in establishing mature heterosexual relationships. He harbors doubts about his own masculinity and views women primarily as sources of gratification for his strong dependency needs. J. A. K. is very much constricted and overcontrolled most of the time, and he inhibits direct expression of negative feelings, but passive-aggressive behaviors may be expected. J. A. K.'s relationships with others tend to be very superficial and unrewarding. He needs other people and he has the capacity for developing deep emotional ties, but he is afraid of getting too involved with others because of fear of rejection and/or exploitation. He does not make friends easily, and other people see him as distant, aloof, and hard to get to know. He is very passive in interpersonal relationships, and he rarely expresses his true feelings. He is very sensitive to the reactions of others, and he is easily hurt by criticism. He makes many concessions to avoid confrontations. In spite of his extreme discomfort, he is better able to cope with everyday problems than he thinks he is. He tends to have high standards and is reliable and conscientious. He enjoys work and gets pleasure from personal achievement.

Many of J. A. K.'s problems stem from his unrealistically high standards and goals for himself and his perceived failure to achieve them. Such

itudes often are produced by demanding and perfectionistic parents who
e almost impossible to please. J. A. K.'s dependent, submissive style is
rected at getting sympathy and support from other people. His attitudes
nd behaviors make it very difficult for other people to react to him in
negative or hostile ways. His avoidance of deep emotional ties ensures that
he will not be seriously hurt by other people. One suspects that his feelings
of masculine inadequacy stem from a faulty identification with his father.
His anger probably comes from perceived failures on the part of other
people to fulfill is strong dependency needs and from their placing of
demands on him that he feels he cannot meet.

The most appropriate diagnostic label for J. A. K. is either depressive
neurosis or anxiety neurosis. Because of his intense discomfort, he is likely
to be receptive to counseling or psychotherapy. Initially, he might rationalize and intellectualize excessively and avoid relating to the therapist in a
meaningful way. However, he is likely to remain in therapy, and slow but
steady progress can be expected. An initial goal in therapy would be an
examination and reevaluation of his self-expectations and development of
more realistic goals for himself. Through the development of a meaningful
relationship with the therapist, he can come to admit his fears and conflicts and acquire more effective ways of coping with them.

ADDITIONAL PRACTICE PROFILES

Brief interpretations of two additional MMPI profiles will now be presented. As a learning exercise, the reader can write his own interpretation
of each profile and then compare his/her interpretations with the ones
presented below.

Figure 8.2 presents the MMPI profile of a 41-year-old male (D. A. V.)
who was a patient in a psychiatric hospital when he completed the test. He
was married, had completed 11 years of formal education, and was working
as a truck driver at the time of his hospitalization.

D. A. V. was very frank and candid, and perhaps even self-critical, in his
approach to the test, and he admitted to a large number of clearly deviant
behaviors. He is likely to be quite disturbed emotionally. Although he does
not experience disabling anxiety or depression, he does have problems in
attending and concentrating, and he may admit to deficits in memory. He
is likely to manifest signs of thinking disturbance. He may appear to be
confused, disoriented, and disorganized. His thinking may be fragmented,
autistic, and circumstantial, and bizarre thoughts and ideas are likely. A
clearly paranoid orientation, including suspiciousness, hallucinations, delusions of persecution and/or grandeur, and feelings of unreality, may be
present. Long-standing, vague somatic complaints also may be reported.

D. A. V. views the world as a very threatening and unsupportive place,
and he feels quite unable to respond to the demands of his daily life. He
feels very insecure and inferior, and he is guilty about his perceived
failures in life. He reacts to stress by withdrawing into daydreaming and
fantasy, and he may have difficulty in differentiating fantasy from reality.

D. A. V. has a rather cynical, pessimistic, and disbelieving attitude
toward life. He is angry and resentful because of perceived mistreatment

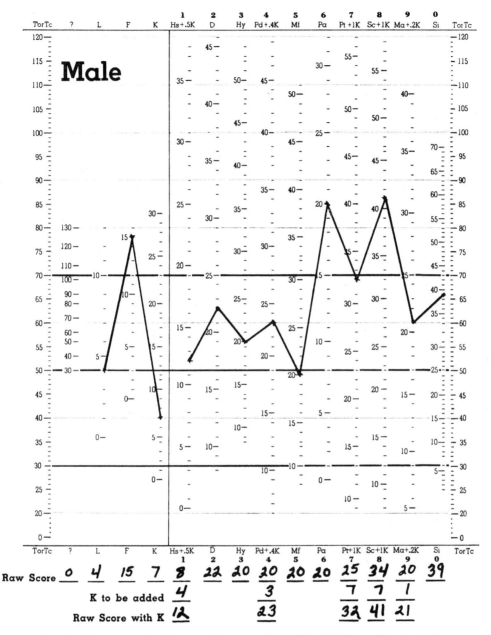

Fig. 8.2. MMPI profile for practice case (D. A. V.). MMPI profile sheet copyrighted 1948 by the Psychological Corporation. Reproduced by permission granted in test catalog.

by others, but he is unable to express these negative feelings in modulated, adaptive ways. He is not emotionally involved with other people. He is distrustful and suspicious of their motives, and he keeps them at a psychological distance. Other people perceive him as cold, aloof, and hard to get to know. Whereas D. A. V. may have many interests, his goals are vague and abstract, and his achievement level is likely to be mediocre at best. He may be preoccupied with abstract and theoretical matters to the exclusion of specific, concrete aspects of his life situation.

The most appropriate diagnosis for D. A. V. is schizophrenia, paranoid type. He appears to have little insight into his problems and behaviors, and he is reluctant to accept responsibility for his difficulties. He blames others for his failures and shortcomings. Although his reluctance to relate to the therapist in a meaningful way would be a definite liability in psychotherapy, he probably would remain in therapy and eventually could come to trust the therapist. Antipsychotic medication may be useful in alleviating overt symptomatology.

Figure 8.3 presents the MMPI profile of M. A. R., a 28-year-old housewife with a high school education. She was given the MMPI while an outpatient at a community mental health center. It appears that M. A. R. was rather honest and straightforward in her approach to the MMPI. She was neither overly defensive nor excessively self-critical in her responses. The deviant behaviors to which she admitted are likely to be concentrated in some particular problem area (e.g., sexual concerns, marital difficulties, etc.). Although she may feel bored, restless, and dissatisfied with her life situation, she probably is free of disabling anxiety and depression, and she is unlikely to manifest frankly psychotic behaviors. She is likely to deny serious emotional problems, and she may structure difficulties in terms of marital incompatability.

M. A. R. is a very immature, narcissistic, and self-indulgent person who demands sympathy and attention from other people. However, she becomes very resentful when even mild demands are made on her. She appears to be overly identified with the stereotypic female role, and she is passive, dependent, and yielding in her relationships with men. At the same time, however, she is likely to be uncomfortable with this more traditional role, and she probably harbors strong desires to be more assertive. Her feminine identification may be quite weak, and she may resort to sexual promiscuity to try to demonstrate her feminine adequacy.

Although she is likely to be rather gregarious and outgoing and to make good first impressions, she really does not relate very well to other people, particularly males, and she is rather uncomfortable in social situations. She is guarded and suspicious about the motives of other people, and she avoids deep emotional ties. She is interested in others primarily because of what they can do for her. M. A. R. tends to be rather impulsive, and she acts without considering the consequences of her actions. She has a low tolerance for frustration, and she is impatient and irritable when things do not suit her. Periodic outbursts of anger and hostility can be expected.

The prognosis for traditional psychotherapy is poor. She does not admit to serious emotional problems, and therefore she is not likely to be receptive to treatment. She may agree to treatment if she is in trouble (e.g., legal difficulty, marital problems, etc.), but she is likely to terminate treatment prematurely when the situational stresses subside. She tends to intellecutalize and to rationalize a great deal, and she blames others, particularly parents, for her problems. If situational stresses are prolonged, she may become motivated to try to change in therapy.

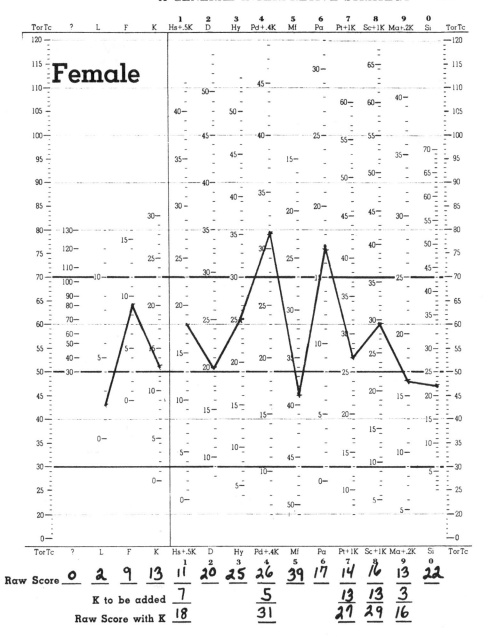

Fig. 8.3. MMPI profile for practice case (M. A. R.). MMPI profile sheet copyrighted 1948 by the Psychological Corporation. Reproduced by permission granted in test catalog.

To provide the novice MMPI user with additional opportunities to practice interpretation of MMPI profiles, six additional profiles are presented in Appendix O. Each of these protocols has been published previously. The reader may wish to interpret each profile and then go to the original source indicated for each profile and compare his/her interpretation with other information presented for each case.

A FINAL COMMENT

The purpose of this chapter has been to present one strategy for organizing inferences from MMPI data into a meaningful understanding of a specific case. Although it is recognized that many MMPI users will find other strategies more to their liking, the person who is just starting to use the MMPI in clinical work may find the strategy suggested here to be helpful until he/she has gained enough experience and skill to develop a strategy of his/her own.

9

Computerized Interpretation
Services

In an era of almost unbelievable advances in computer technology, it is not surprising that computerized interpretation of the MMPI has grown in popularity. The scoring of MMPI protocols, the classification of profiles into categories, assuming that their validity can be demonstrated, and the assignment of interpretive statements to the categories are tasks for which the computer is much better equipped than the human clinician.

A major advantage of the computerized interpretation is the speed with which the appropriate operations are performed. Whereas a clinician might have to spend over an hour in scoring a protocol, determining the appropriate interpretive statements for the resulting profile, and preparing the report, these same operations can be performed by the computer in a matter of seconds. When one considers the shortage of professional mental health manpower, this efficiency is very appealing. The computer also performs its operations in a very reliable manner. Once appropriate input is provided for the computer, virtually no variation in procedures occurs. Finally, the storage capacity of the computer far exceeds that of the human clinician. A virtually infinite number of bits of information can be stored by the computer and called upon as needed for profile interpretation. By contrast, the clinician typically has at his disposal only several bits of well learned information about the meaning of a particular type of protocol, and he must turn to various codebooks and interpretive guides for additional information.

The typical computerized interpretation process involves the following steps:

1. Rules for scoring and classifying protocols are fed into the computer. These rules may be very simple ones, dealing with various levels of scores on a single scale at a time, or they may involve complex configural analyses.

2. Interpretive statements for the various categories of protocols that can result from the classification rules also are fed into the computer.

Examples of the form of such interpretive statements can be found in earlier chapters of this *Guide*. Whereas these statements may be based on empirical research data, usually they represent the clinical judgment of MMPI experts concerning how a particular kind of protocol should be interpreted.

3. The completed answer sheet of an examinee is fed into the computer, usually by optical scanning equipment. The protocol is scored, and the appropriate classification rules are applied in order to determine the categories for the profile. The computer then searches its memory for interpretive statements appropriate for the categories and prints out a report.

If one thinks about these steps carefully, it becomes obvious that the most important part of the process centers around the interpretive statements that are available for various categories. Obviously, the final interpretive report can only be as good and as valid as the statements that are stored in the memory of the computer. Because most computerized interpretation systems base these statements on the clinical judgment of clinicians who are skilled and knowledgeable in MMPI interpretation, the services provide to their users the best clinical interpretation currently available.

Unfortunately, computers are not easily understood by most people, and there is a tendency to attribute scientific authenticity to any output coming from these formidable machines. Unless great caution is taken by the novice MMPI user to combat against it, greater validity than is warranted is likely to be attributed to computerized interpretations. Another potential difficulty with the computerized interpretations is that they tend to "fix" interpretations which in reality may not have been adequately validated. Once an interpretive statement is programmed into the system, it is likely that it will remain there even if further validational data are not reported or if such data do not support the statement's validity.

Perhaps the greatest danger of computerized interpretations is that they have come to be viewed by many persons as a substitute for a skilled clinician rather than as a valuable tool to be used by an experienced clinician. As was pointed out in Chapter 1 of this *Guide*, a skilled and experienced clinician is necessary to give meaning to test data for the individual client or subject. Most clinicians use the MMPI protocol as only one piece of information about an examinee. The inferences based on the protocol are validated against other test data, history, and observation in arriving at a meaningful formulation of the case. When the computerized interpretation of the MMPI is used instead of this more complete clinical analysis, the resulting formulation is at best incomplete and at worst inaccurate and potentially harmful to the examinee. Because some of the computerized interpretation services are used by individuals who are not psychologically sophisticated, the above concerns seem to be justified.

In spite of the potential dangers of the computerized interpretation services, if utilized as *part* of the clinical assessment process, they can be extremely helpful. They can free the individual clinician from the drudgery of scoring and classifying protocols and from the time-consuming process of determining appropriate interpretive statements for the protocols. In the past decade, many computerized interpretation services have been developed. In this chapter, six of the most widely used services are discussed. It is hoped that the information provided here will allow the clinician to make an informed choice if he decides to use such a service and will allow users of the various services to better understand and benefit from the services. Previous reviews of computerized interpretation services by Dahlstrom et al. (1972), Eichman (1972 abcde), and Kleinmuntz (1972) should also be of interest to the reader.

THE PSYCHOLOGICAL CORPORATION MMPI REPORTING SERVICE

Address

National Computer Systems
4401 West 76th Street
Minneapolis, Minnesota   55435

User Qualifications

This service is available to persons who are qualified to purchase the MMPI test materials. The MMPI is designated as a "Level C" test by the American Psychological Association and as such its use is restricted to members of APA and others who individually have demonstrated to the test publisher (The Psychological Corporation) that they have appropriate training and experience.

General Description

This service utilizes a program developed at the Mayo Clinic by Pearson, Swenson, and Rome to provide a psychiatric screening evaluation for the medical services. Although it is perhaps the least sophisticated of the current services, it has the distinction of being the pioneering effort. The report provided by the service is brief and descriptive in nature, concentrating on symptomatology and general emotional status. Although it has utility for its intended purpose, i.e., general psychiatric screening, the clinician who expects more than screening information from the MMPI will be dissatisfied with the service. A major advantage of the service is that the interpretation of individual protocols is very conservative, a very desirable feature considering the kinds of persons who are likely to use the service.

Materials

Answer sheets and test booklets to be used for the service are available from the Psychological Corporation. Either the group (booklet) form or the Form R test booklets can be used. National Computer Systems (NCS) answer sheets appropriate for the booklet selected must be used.

Turn around Time

Reports are mailed within 1 business day after answer sheets are received in Minneapolis.

The Report

This service offers users two different kinds of output, scoring of the MMPI answer sheet alone or scoring plus an interpretive section. The scoring includes raw scores, K-corrected raw scores, T-scores without the K correction, and K-corrected T-scores for the standard 4 validity and 10 clinical scales. The K-corrected T-scores are plotted on a specially designed profile form. The clinician must connect the data points to complete the profile. In addition, raw scores and T-scores are provided for the following scales, most of which were described in Chapter 6 of this *Guide*:

Anxiety (A)
Repression (R)
Ego Strength (Es)
Low Back Pain (Lb)
Caudality (Ca)
Dependency (Dy)
Dominance (Do)
Social Responsibility (Re)
Prejudice (Pr)
Social Status (St)
Control (Cn)
Tired Housewife (Th); females only
Worried Breadwinner (Wb); males only

Each of these scales is described briefly in *A User's Guide to the Mayo Clinic Automated MMPI Program* (Pearson & Swenson, 1967), which is available from the Psychological Corporation. The original answer sheet is returned with the report.

The interpretive section of the report is brief (less than one page) and consists of phrases rather than polished narrative. The population of possible statements programmed into the computer is 75, and from 6 to 15 statements are printed for any particular protocol. The statements are primarily descriptive and symptomatic, and no statements concerning diagnosis, dynamics, or treatment implications are included. The decision rules and interpretive statements have been published (Pearson & Swenson, 1967). The interpretation is based primarily on single scale analyses (See Chapter 4 of this *Guide*). Each validity and clinical scale is divided into five levels, and appropriate interpretive statements are assigned to each level. In addition, several configural analyses, including up to three scales plus age of examinee, are included.

ROCHE MMPI COMPUTERIZED INTERPRETATION SERVICE

Address

Roche Psychiatric Service Institute
Box 170
Nutley, New Jersey   07101

User Qualifications

This service is available to clinical psychologists and psychiatrists for use in clinical practice and research.

General Description

This service uses programs developed by Raymond D. Fowler, Jr., PhD. The narrative portion of the report is about one or two pages long, and its format is similar to that of a more traditional assessment report. The interpretive statements used in the report go beyond a descriptive level and deal with dynamics and implications for treatment. Most of the interpretive statements appear to be generated from configural aspects of the standard validity and clinical scales (e.g., high scores, low scores, two-point codes, etc.). Fowler (1969) reported that in writing the program for generating descriptive statements, such factors as sex, age, and marital status were taken into account. In addition to the full interpretive report, Roche offers an abbreviated report which involves scoring of the MMPI protocol only and omits the interpretive sections.

Materials

The Roche service requires that special test booklets and answer sheets developed by the service be used. These materials, along with appropriate instructions for administering the MMPI and using the report, are made available in a user's kit. The booklet is similar in format to the standard MMPI Form R booklet, but the items are in completely different order in the Roche than in the Form R booklet. The answer sheet is one that can be processed by optical scanning equipment. The entire 566-item MMPI must be administered.

Turn around Time

Complete reports are sent by return mail within 24 hr after the answer sheets are received in New Jersey.

The Report

After some basic identifying and demographic information (Roche identifying case number, age, sex, date), the first page or two of the report includes the narrative portion. This section includes statements about the validity of the protocol, diagnosis, symptoms, dynamics, and attitudes toward and prognosis for treatment. The descriptive statements appear to be based on two-point codes and on single scales that are elevated. In addition to the standard validity and clinical scales, three additional scales (Anxiety, Ego Strength, and Prejudice) are used in generating descriptive statements. In general, the interpretations tend to be conservative, and pathological terms, such as "psychosis," are not used. The narrative section of the report ends with the following caution:

> Note: Although not a substitute for the clinician's professional judgment and skill, the MMPI can be a useful adjunct in the evaluation and management of emotional disorders. The report is for professional use only and should not be shown or released to the patient.

The next several pages of the report list critical items that were answered in the deviant direction by the examinee. The items are grouped into problem areas (e.g., suspicion and ideas of reference, health and bodily concerns, sexual concerns and problems, etc.). The user is cautioned not to overinterpret specific responses and to explore these problem areas in subsequent interviews.

The next section of the report presents brief descriptions of the examinee based on Wiggins' content scales (see Chapter 7 of this *Guide*). A T-score and an indication of the degree to which the statements apply to the examinee (high, moderate, average, low) also are included for each content scale.

The next page of the report presents raw scores and T-scores for the 4 standard validity and 10 stranded clinical scales. The scores are plotted on a computer-generated profile form, but the user must connect the plotted scores to construct the profile.

On the final page of the report, the raw scores and T-scores for the standard validity and clinical scales are repeated. In addition, raw scores and T-scores are reported for the following scales:

Ego Strength (Es)
Maladjustment (Mt)
Anxiety (A)
Repression (R)
Low Back Pain (Lb)
Caudality (Ca)
Dependency (Dy)
Dominance (Do)
Responsibility (Re)
Prejudice (Pr)
Social Status (St)
Control (Cn)
Manifest Anxiety (At)
Social Desirability (SO-R)

Descriptions of these scales and other information necessary to utilize the service are included in a kit of materials provided to users. This last page of the report also includes a Welsh code for the profile and a raw score on MacAndrew's Alcoholism scale, along with a statement of similarity between the examinee and patients who abuse drugs and alcohol. Finally, a matrix of the examinee's answers to all MMPI items is presented. The service retains the original answer sheet.

CALDWELL REPORT

Address

Clinical Psychological Services, Inc.
3122 Santa Monica Boulevard
Santa Monica, California   90404

User Qualifications

This service is available to psychologists, psychiatrists, and other professional level mental health workers.

General Description

The Caldwell Report utilizes programs developed by Alex B. Caldwell,

PhD. It is the most polished of the computer services. The format is similar to that of an individualized assessment report. The report goes beyond simple symptom and behavioral description and includes inferences about dynamics, etiology, and treatment implications. Although the specific decision rules have not been published, it appears that the descriptive statements are based on analysis of individual validity, clinical, and special scales and on two- and three-point configurations of the clinical scales.

Materials

Any MMPI answer sheet can be processed. Although the service recommends that all 566 items should be administered, abbreviated forms that cover the first 399 items of Form R or the first 366 items plus the remaining K scale and scale 0 items of the booklet form can be processed.

Turn around Time

Reports are sent by return mail within 24 to 48 hr after answer sheets are received in California. Remote terminals can be arranged for high volume users. When a terminal is used, scores are sent almost immediately via teletype; the diagnostic section of the report is sent the next morning via teletype; and the entire report is mailed within 24 hr.

The Report

After the presentation of some basic identifying and demographic data (date, name, age, sex, education, marital status, referral source, date tested, and test administered – MMPI), the first two or three pages of the Caldwell report consist of the narrative portion of the report. The four sections included in the narrative portion are: (1) Test-taking Attitudes; (2) Symptoms and Personality Characteristics; (3) Diagnostic Impression; and (4) Treatment Considerations.

The next page of the report lists MMPI critical items, and the items answered in the pathological direction are circled. The critical items are arranged according to their content into problem areas (e.g., distress and depression, sexual difficulties, family discord, etc.).

The final page of the report is a standard group form profile sheet. Raw scores and T-scores are presented for 3 of the 4 standard validity and 10 clinical scales. A K-corrected profile is drawn from these scores, and the profile is coded according to the Welsh system. Raw scores and T-scores also are reported for the following additional scales:

Ego Strength (Es)
Familial Discord (Pd1)
Authority Problems (Pd2)
Persecutory Ideas (Pa1)
Poignancy (Pa2)
Naivete (Pa3)
Amorality (Ma1)
Psychomotor Acceleration (Ma2)
Imperturbability (Ma3)

Ego Inflation (Ma4)

Low Back Pain (LBP)

Finally, raw scores are presented for the Overcontrolled Hostility (OH) scale and for MacAndrew's Alcoholism (ALC) scale. Brief descriptions of these additional scales are presented in materials provided to users. The original answer sheet is returned with the report.

BEHAVIORDYNE PSYCHODIAGNOSTIC LABORATORY SERVICE

Address

Post Office Box 3689

Stanford, California   94305

User Qualifications

There are 19 different types of reports available. The highest level reports are available only to licensed psychologists and physicians, but other reports are available for use by counselors, social workers, personnel directors, probation officers, vocational counselors, pastoral counselors, etc. There also is a report that can be given to the examinee to read.

General Description

This service utilzies programs developed by Joseph Finney, PhD, and his colleagues at the University of Kentucky. Either the MMPI or the California Psychological Inventory can be used as a data source for the service. The service differs from the others discussed in this chapter in several other important ways. First, the interpretive statements are not based primarily on the standard MMPI validity and clinical scales. Instead, scores on eight factor scales developed by Finney (1961) and on a large number of additional special scales provide the basis for most interpretive statements. Second, Finney collected his own norm sample (approximately 2,000 normal men and women). In addition to the reporting of traditional T-scores based on the Minnesota norms for the standard validity and clinical scales, normalized T-scores based on the new sample are reported. Scores that have been corrected to reduce the effects of anxiety, social desirability, and rare responses are reported for the standard validity and clinical scales and for a large number of additional scales. Third, 19 different levels of reports are available depending on the qualifications of the recipient. Although the reports offered by the service include very complete and potentially useful information and the innovations introduced by the service may represent psychometric improvements over traditional MMPI usage, the clinician who is accustomed to traditional MMPI interpretation may find the reports unfamiliar and somewhat confusing.

Materials

Standard group form booklets are utilized, but special answer sheets available from the service must be used.

Turn around Time

Reports are mailed within 24 hr after answer sheets are received in

California. Special on-line computer arrangements can be made for high volume users.

The Report

As stated above, 19 different levels of reports are available. Because all 19 reports cannot be discussed here, only the detailed clinical report that is available to licensed psychologists and physicians is considered. Readers who are interested in other reports should contact the service for details and sample reports.

The first page of the report includes some basic identifyng data (age, sex, report level, date, identification numbers) and a caution that no decision should be made from the report alone, but only from consideration of case history and all of the available evidence. The next page includes a computer-generated profile form on which are plotted 2 sets of scores for 3 of the 4 standard validity and 9 of the 10 standard clinical scales (scale 0 is not included). One set of scores is in the form of T-scores based on the original Minnesota norms. The other set of scores is in the form of normalized T-scores based on Finney's sample of normal men and women and corrected to reduce the effects of social desirability, anxiety, and rare answers. For the sample case presented later in this chapter, the profile resulting from the special normalized T-scores is similar in shape to the traditional profile, but all of the clinical scales are lower than for the traditional profile.

The narrative portion of the report begins on the third page, and for the sample case discussed later in this chapter it is seven pages long. This section is rather polished in form and includes the following parts: (1) Validity and Response Attitude (including listing of critical items endorsed in the deviant direction); (2) Evidence for Psychosis or Mental Illness; (3) Basic Trust, Confidence, and Self-esteem; (4) Dependency Problems; (5) Demandingness or Oral Aggression; (6) Masochistic Dependency and Bitterness; (7) Hostility and Coping; (8) Response to Authorities; (9) Compulsive Character Features; (10) Hysterical Personality Features; (11) Identification, Ideals, and Responsibilities; (12) World of Work; (13) Diagnostic Impression (several offered in order of probability of application to the examinee); (14) Potential for Psychotherapy; and (15) Summary.

The next page reports traditional T-scores for the standard 4 validity and 10 clinical scales. The results of nine tests for psychosis (Meehl-Dahlstrom rules, Goldberg index, etc.) are given, and they are rationally combined to yield a summary score that ranges from 0 to 18 (0 to 6 = clearly normal; 7 to 9 = indeterminate; 10 to 18 = psychotic). Rankings of eight clinical scales (excluding scales 5 and 0) using four different corrected normalized T-scores are reported, and the two-point code type for each of the four different scores is identified. A count of the mismarked or omitted items is presented on this page. The last data presented on this page are addiction band and alcoholism band numbers. Scores for each band can range from 1 to 5, depending on how closely the examinee resembles people having strongly addictive or alcoholic personalities, and scores of 4 and 5 are considered high.

The next five pages of the report include research data. One of these pages contains scores for 12 special factor scales, calculation of values for the Meehl-Dahlstrom and Taulbee and Sisson rules for classifying profiles, and 28 other indices and proportions (e.g., neurotic index, counseling prediction score, job success code, etc.). The other four pages of research data are scores for 166 different scales. For each scale a raw score and four T-scores corrected for anxiety, social desirability, and rare responses are reported. Descriptions of the indices and proportions and references for the research scales are included in a user's kit that is available from the service. The final page of the report is a print-out of responses to all 566 items of the MMPI (original answer sheet is retained by the service).

INSTITUTE OF CLINICAL ANALYSIS MMPI-ICA REPORT

Address

1000 East Broadway
Glendale, California   91205

User Qualifications

This service is available to psychologists, psychiatrists, and physicians.

General Description

The report provided by this service seems to be directed at physicians and others who use the MMPI as a screening instrument. Emphasis is placed on the likelihood and level of emotional disturbance, which are assessed by special indices developed by the service. Although no explanation of the nature of these indices is presented in the report, they are discussed briefly in descriptive materials provided to users of the service. Some descriptive statements about personality traits, symptoms, and coping strategies are included in the report, and they seem to be based on analysis of single clinical scales and two-point codes. A review of symptoms is presented in the form of a listing of critical items endorsed in the deviant direction and descriptive phrases which apparently are based on endorsements of single items and clusters of items. The service appears to provide a screening-level analysis of the MMPI that should be useful to persons unsophisticated in MMPI interpretation, but the report is likely to be disappointing to users who expect more information to be extracted from the MMPI protocol.

Materials

The standard booklet form of the MMPI is used. A special optical scan answer sheet must be obtained from the service.

Turn around Time

Reports are mailed within 2 days after answer sheets are received in California.

The Report

After some basic identifying data (identification numbers, testing date, processing date, age, and sex), the first page of the report includes two indices of disturbance. The Multiphasic Index (MI) score is reported (range 65 to 150), and a severity label (e.g., moderate, marked, etc.) is indicated. Probability of significant disturbance is indicated as a percentage value.* These two indices are discussed in materials provided by the service, but no precise details about their calculations are given. A short narrative interpretation of the MI score also is given. The first page of the report also includes a brief summary of the examinee's level of disturbance, diagnostic impressions, coping ability, and recommendation concerning psychiatric evaluation. The final section of the first page describes the examinee's test-taking attitude.

The second page of the report includes the following brief narrative sections: (1) Personality Description; (2) Suggestions to Improve Coping; (3) Special Coping Problems; (4) Positive Traits; and (5) Diagnostic Impression. The remainder of page 2 and all of page 3 are devoted to a review of symptoms (e.g., anxiety, phobias and obsessions, unusual thoughts and experiences, etc.). For each symptom category, critical items endorsed in the deviant direction are printed and brief descriptive phrases, which apparently are based on endorsements of single items and clusters of items, are presented.

The next two pages of the report present raw scores and T-scores for about 100 scales and indices. These scales and indices are grouped into content categories (e.g., validity, anxiety, authority conflict, general defenses, etc.). Included in this section are scores on the Harris subscales and the Wiggins content scales. Some, but not all, of these indices are described in materials provided by the service.

The last page of the report is a special computer generated profile form on which are plotted T-scores for the standard 4 validity and 10 clinical scales. Raw scores, raw scores with the K-correction, and T-scores for the standard 4 validity and 10 clinical scales are printed at the bottom of the profile form. It should be noted that the answer sheet is retained by the service, and the examinee's responses to individual items are not reported.

VETERANS ADMINISTRATION MMPI RESEARCH LABORATORY

Address

Veterans Administration Hospital
Minneapolis, Minnesota   55417

User Qualifications

This service is available only to professional staff of Veterans Administration facilities.

General Description

This service uses programs and data compiled by the Veterans Adminsitration MMPI Research Laboratory under the direction of Harold Gilber-

---

* It should be noted that for the sample case submitted to this service no percentage value was reported.

stadt, PhD. The rules for classifying protocols and the descriptive statements associated with the rules have been published in detail in the *Comprehensive MMPI Codebook for Males* (Gilberstadt, 1970). Interpretation is based on the standard validity and clinical scales, singly and in configuration, and on special scales developed by Gilberstadt to assess profile types described in an earlier codebook (Gilberstadt & Duker, 1965). The narrative section of the report is brief (less than one page) and primarily descriptive in nature.

Materials

Standard Form R booklets and answer sheets are used. Arrangements for remote terminals can be made.

Turn around Time

Reports typically are mailed within 1 or 2 days after the answer sheets are received in Minneapolis.

The Report

The first page of the report is a computer-generated profile form on which are plotted K-corrected T-scores for 3 of the 4 standard validity and the 10 standard clinical scales. Raw scores, raw scores with the K-correction, and T-scores (K-corrected when appropriate) also are reported for these scales.

The narrative section of the report is found on the second page. A profile code based on the T-scores and a code based on Gilberstadt's special P scales appear at the top of the page. The first paragraph of the narrative section includes a statement of test-taking attitude based on scores on the L, F, and K scales and a description of current state based on an analysis of scales 2, 4, 7, and 9 singly and in configuration. The second paragraph consists of single scale and two-scale interpretations of the clinical scales. Statements in this paragraph deal with symptoms, personality traits, coping strategies, etc. Paragraph 3 presents a summary of trait and diagnostic possibilites based on configural interpretations of the clinical scales and on Wiggins' content scales. The fourth paragraph presents a summary description of the examinee based on scores on Gilberstadt's special P scales. When the profile fits one of the 19 code types defined by Gilberstadt and Duker (1965), the appropriate interpretive material from their codebook is printed as a fifth paragraph.

The third page of the report presents raw scores and T-scores for the standard validity and clinical scales, Wiggins content scales, and 29 additional special scales. Scores also are presented for Gilberstadt's codebook scales and for six special indices. All of the special scales and indices are listed and referenced in the *Comprehensive MMPI Code Book for Males* (Gilberstadt, 1970). The Grayson critical items endorsed in the deviant direction also are printed on this page.

The fourth page of the report is a print-out of individual responses to all 566 items. The last page of the report is a brief rating form to assess the accuracy of the report. The user is encouraged to complete the rating form and return it to the MMPI Research Laboratory.

SAMPLE CASE

The answer sheet for the illustrative case discussed in Chapter 8 of this *Guide* was sent to the six services discussed above. The narrative portions of the reports that were returned are presented below.

Psychological Corporation MMPI Reporting Service

Consider psychiatric evaluation.

Somewhat tense and restless.

May have poor self-concept. Probably would like to discuss emotional problems.

Severely depressed, worrying, indecisive, and pessimistic.

Rigid and meticulous, worrisome and apprehensive, dissatisfied with social relationships. Probably very religious and moralistic.

Probably somewhat eccentric, seclusive, and withdrawn. Many internal conflicts.

Probably retiring and shy in social situations.

Slightly more than average number of physical complaints. Some concern about bodily functions and physical health.

Inclines toward esthetic interests.

Independent or mildly nonconformist.

Sensitive. Alive to opinions of others.

Roche MMPI Computerized Interpretation Service

The response of this patient to the test indicates that he understood the items and that he correctly followed the instructions. However, it appears that he is somewhat self-critical. He may be somewhat more likely than the average person to admit to symptoms and psychological problems even when they are minimal. This suggests that he may be willing to accept professional assistance.

This patient shows a personality pattern which occurs frequently among persons who seek psychiatric treatment. Feelings of inadequacy, sexual conflict and rigidity are accompanied by a loss of efficiency, initiative, and self-confidence. Insomnia is likely to occur along with chronic anxiety, fatigue, and tension. He may have suicidal thoughts. Patients with this pattern are likely to be diagnosed as depressives or anxiety reactions. The basic characteristics are resistant to change and will tend to remain stable with time. Among medical patients with this pattern, a large number are seriously depressed, and others show some depression, along with fatigue and exhaustion. There are few spontaneous recoveries, although the intensity of the symptoms may be cyclic.

There are unusual qualities in this patient's thinking which may represent an original or eccentric orientation or perhaps some schizoid tendencies. Further information is required to make this determination.

He is concerned, to an unusual degree, with bodily functions and health. He may overreact to illness, and complain unreasonably about relatively minor ailments. Medical patients with this characteristic tend to be frustrating to their physicians because they complain of pains and disorders that are vague, difficult to identify, and may have no organic basis.

sometimes attempts to control its expression, but he is not greatly disturbed by the discomfort of others, even when he is its cause.

8. Family Problems (FAM) average T = 47
9. Hypomania (HYP) average T = 48
10. Social Maladjustment (SOC) high T = 70

He expresses feelings of social isolation and shyness. He is reticent and self-conscious, especially in groups, and he avoids parties and other situations which would require him to meet new people. He finds it particularly difficult to talk, even in fairly familiar situations, and he avoids expressing his opinions or letting people know very much about him.

Caldwell Report

Test-taking attitude

He was straightforward in answering the MMPI without being unduly defensive or self-critical. The profile appears valid.

Symptoms and personality characteristics

The profile indicates a moderate to severe disturbance. Tensions, worrying, self-doubts, and mutiple fears and anxieties appear to seriously interfere with his life. In a few related cases such symptoms as a blunting of affect, concreteness of thinking, morbid ruminations, or transitory ideas of reference suggested schizoid trends and the possibility of psychotic depressive or latent schizophrenic elements in the patient's makeup despite preserved reality testing and the absence of a loosening of associations. Difficulties in concentrating, obsessive ruminations, phobias, and feelings of despondency and guilt are suggested. Suicidal preoccupations are especially common with this pattern. Indecisiveness and a pervasive loss of interest would relate to the depth of his ambivalences. Shy, introverted, and withdrawing, he appears quite uncomfortable socially, keeping others at a distance and fearing close involvement.

The physical worries and complaints that he reported on the test suggest a variety of somatic symptoms lacking a sufficient organic basis. Pains in the "pit of the stomach" and related gastrointestinal distress, headaches, heart symptoms, constipation, and symptoms related to chronic physical tension would be typical, as would be undue concern about physical health and overreactions to minor physical dysfunctions. Muscle twitching, tremors, numbness, and peculiar "neurologic-like" symptoms are also common with his makeup. His overall balance of masculine and feminine interests tends mildly toward verbal or esthetic interests rather than mechanical and outdoor activities.

Typical family backgrounds involved rejection by one or sometimes both parents. Sometimes this was indirect, as by the illness or death of one parent and the resulting burdens on the other parent. Personal peculiarities often had provoked negative reactions from family members, including unfavorable comparisons to "superior" siblings or others in the family along with an excessive amount of teasing by siblings. Their interpersonal ineptness and difficulties in giving love resulted in repeated frustrations of their wishes for emotional closeness. They often studied and cultivated interests in obscure intellectual subjects such as religions and philosophies of life, typically ruminating about these with oddly personalized interpretations.

Diagnostic impression

The most typical diagnosis with this profile is of a chronic "endogenous" depression. Some patients with this pattern were seen as schizoid and a few as chronic undifferentiated schizophrenic reactions.

Treatment considerations

The profile suggests a moderate to severe suicide risk. If a significant suicidal risk was confirmed in the interview, then it could be crucial to arrange continuing human contact. This should include his knowing whom to contact and someone, family or professional, who will maintain contact with him. The treatment of similar patients has often included combinations of tranquilizers and antidepressants. These patients had only brief and limited responses to shock therapy, and the transient post-shock lifting of the depression was often followed by a flooding of intense anxieties, fears, and ruminations.

Slowness to relate and immature emotional distortions are likely handicaps in psychotherapy. He is apt to have a resistively negative self-image despite steady if not positive past accomplishments. These critical self-judgments are apt to be unrealistic but sufficiently integrated into the patient's identity so that they are slow to change. Some patients with this pattern were able to develop intellectual insights at great length, with few apparent resulting changes in their behavior.

The profile predicts a gradual response to psychotherapy—especially if his depression is not of recent onset—but most similar patients have eventually made positive responses to treatment. One study reported relatively favorable responses by patients to support from older, kindly, understanding, well adjusted, and motherly female therapists. Difficulties brought on by his rigid internal standards and ideals are apt to be a major focus in treatment. Chronic difficulties in expressing anger and particularly his guilt over anger toward family members are apt to require an extended working through. Dissatisfaction with work achievement is a likely focus, especially if it involves the frustration or the possible giving up of his life ambitions. Overreactions to any physical, intellectual, and other handicaps are also likely points of focus in therapy. In some cases increasing self-assertiveness and integrated expressions of anger were seen as particularly meaningful signs of improvement.

Thank you for this referral.

Behaviordyne Psychodiagnostic Laboratory Service

Validity and response attitude

He chooses his answers so as to give an unfavorable or sick picture of himself. It may be that he wants us to know that he needs help. He tends to mark as false the neutral-sounding items that are frank in expressing feelings. He admits being somewhat disorganized and worried, and having some urges to misbehave. He admits faults willingly. He describes himself as an unreactive, unenthusiastic person, one who firmly avoids commitments, avoids much social contact, and is not overly devoted to duty.

Some of his answers are worth noting. Here is what he said:

61. True. I have not lived the right kind of life.
114. True. Often I feel as if there were a tight band about my head.
139. True. Sometimes I feel as if I must injure either myself or someone else.
156. True. I have had periods in which I carried on activities without knowing later what I have been doing.
211. True. I can sleep during the day but not at night.
334. True. Peculiar odors come to me at times.
339. True. Most of the time I wish I were dead.
526. True. The future seems hopeless to me.

It may be worthwhile to discuss those answers with him to find out what he meant by them.

His personality makeup is not truly typical of patients seen by psychiatrists and clinical psychologists; neither is it unusual for that group. He is better organized, more self-controlled, and more systematic than are most patients.

He is a somewhat insecure person. He is somewhat tense and worried. He is a steady person. He uses self-control. He is cautious and careful. He is a rather unhappy person just now. He is in some distress. He feels that he has more than his share of troubles. He is somewhat upset, both now and in the long run, and he is not very good at recognizing and expressing his problems.

He is the sort of person who does things slowly, quietly, and deliberately, and in the conventional ways. He is simple, modest, unassuming, and passive. He doesn't take much initiative. He prefers to wait and see what will happen. He is a much better follower than a leader.

He is a quiet, sentimental, and sensitive person. Throughout his life he has almost always been peaceful and well-behaved. He obeys rules and submits to authorities. He takes his obligations seriously and does his duties conscientiously. Yet he is unhappy and dissatisfied; he worries and broods about things. His restricted and inhibited behavior pattern is an overcontrol used in an effort to contain his anxiety. At heart he is emotional and high-strung. Under stress, when hostility is aroused, he turns it against himself. He blames himself, and feels inferior and inadequate. At such times he becomes anxious and tense, and has trouble sleeping. He feels tired, discouraged, and unhappy. The clinical picture may be a depressive reaction or an obsessive-compulsive reaction.

He is not at all the sort of person that gets bodily symptoms to symbolize his emotional conflicts without organic cause.

Evidence for psychosis or mental illness

He is not at all mentally ill; that is, not at all psychotic. He shows no tendency toward psychosis at all.

Basic trust, confidence, and self-esteem

His attitude is rather pessimistic. He doesn't have much confidence in himself to make a success, nor confidence in others to do well by him. He expects poorly of the future. He is not a person that maintains an optimistic attitude by denying discouragement. He tends to blame himself and feel guilty more than most people, and hence tends to be methodical, conventional, passive, and narrow in interests.

He tells of more feelings of guilt, embarrassment, fear, and worry now, in his present mood, than he usually does.

He shows moderate signs of guilt feeling. He tells of moderate feelings of self-consciousness or embarrassment. He shows signs of having some fears of phobias. He seems to be worrying to some extent. He deals with anxiety by planning and worrying. He is somewhat timid, worrying, indecisive, or neurotic.

Dependency problems

He is a rather dependent person. If you keep seeing him once a week or oftener over a period of time, you can expect that he will come to lean on you for emotional support, advice, and reassurance. He is dependent in a passive way. In his inward feelings he longs to be passively dependent. Comparison of his dependency in action with his dependency urge shows that he strongly uses the defense of reaction formation against dependency. He tends to be aware of his dependency needs.

He is neither clearly demanding nor clearly undemanding.

He is a somewhat indecisive person, but he seems serious, steady, and reliable.

Masochistic dependency and bitterness

He does not seem especially bitter. If it is so, it is very slightly so. He has only a slight tendency, if any, to feel sorry for himself. To some extent, he is a dependent masochist, who does things so as to get people to disappoint him, reject him, or let him down. He shows no special tendency to get into trouble.

Hostility and coping

He is not a particularly hostile person. He is about like the average. He builds some resentment up within himself, but not much. Now let us see what he does with whatever hostility he has.

In general, he is a person who takes things out on himself. In this case, however, there might be other considerations. He takes things out on himself much more than he takes things out on other people. This is something he needs to think about seriously. He is the sort of person who hates to hurt other people and would rather be hurt himself. In his dealings with people, he keeps putting himself at a disadvantage. He lets people take advantage of him. And they do. Sometimes he may be seriously damaged by it, in one way or another. When trouble arises, he takes care not to let it hurt the other person. He lets it hurt him, instead, perhaps without knowing that he is causing his own troubles. In fairness to him, he needs to call a halt to this business. He needs to decide what he wants from life, and then take realistic steps toward getting it.

No matter how he may feel, he tends to be somewhat meek, mild, and timid in dealing with people.

He tends to blame himself. And in certain ways, he takes things out on himself. He turns hostility against himself, making himself discouraged, depressed, moody, and pessimistic. He is unhappy and dissatisfied in life, and he is especially dissatisfied with himself. He thinks badly of himself, and he feels inadequate. He seems to have lost interest in people and in what goes on around him. He seems unresponsive to people. He readily and openly expresses some thoughts and feelings of discouragement. He appears somewhat discouraged and depressed. He turns some blame against himself unconsciously. That may burden him more than he knows. It may give him more feeling of discouragement than he is aware of.

Response to authorities

He shows some tendency to get people to tell him what to do and then resist them. On the whole, he responds submissively to authorities. He expresses mostly submissive feelings.

Compulsive character features

He is systematic, at least to an average degree, if not more. He is not a controlling person.

Hysterical personality features

He is not an especially hysterical personality. His use of dissociation and other hysterical mechanisms is well within the normal limits. He tends to make the worst of his troubles, and emphasizes his distress.

Identifications, ideals, and responsibilites

He is ethical enough. He generally deals fairly with people, and generally respects their rights.

Altogether, his conscience and ego ideal are of average strength, and his conduct for the most part is within normal limits. Nevertheless, he suffers guilt. He suffers more guilt than his deeds seem to account for. Maybe the guilt flows not so much from any deeds of his as from forbidden wishes, perhaps unconscious ones. Maybe his conscience has unrealistic, puritanical, and perfectionistic standards. The guilt is a control mechanism that comes into play late and acts harshly and punitively. It may be that he goes through cycles of breaking rules, suffering guilt, and getting punished. The guilt is a source of his depression, blaming of himself, taking things out on himself, and getting people to disappoint him. Some goals of treatment are to reveal the guilt, to interpret the self-punishment, to reveal the unconscious forbidden wishes, to lessen the guilt and the self-punishment, to make the control mechanisms work more promptly and less harshly, and to interrupt the cycles, if such there be, and put an end to them.

He doesn't seize the chance to make decisions. He would rather wait for somebody else to decide what to do. He doesn't care to dominate a social situation. Socially, he is somewhat introverted. He hesitates to speak out. He is cautious and shy with other people. He is rather hesitant and restrained, and not very sophisticated. He doesn't express himself very well. He is unsure what to do, and he keeps vacillating indecisively.

World of work

Because he is 27 years old, he must have taken some steps already in choosing a career and getting started in its work. But if he is thinking of taking a new job, or of making some change in his life work, it may be up to you, as his counselor, to help him consider how his personality jibes with the requirements of the various kinds of jobs that may be open to him.

At this time, being either somewhat upset or confused, or perhaps only too frank, he gives the impression that he is somewhat lacking in what it takes to do well in most kinds of work. But he can do better than that. In the long run, it may be fairer to say that he has good, normal ability to do work. He can do as well as any average, normal person in most kinds of work. His abilities are higher than his aspirations. Maybe you can encourage him to loosen up and aspire to positions of greater leadership. He does well enough in the personal qualities that make for success at work. Of course, some kinds of working situations fit him better than others.

His strongest point, the one that can help him the most to succeed in his work, is his self-reliance in his work, and ability to use good judgment about it. Within normal range, he seems to use good judgment in his work. He can do well enough in a job that calls on him to take responsibility for going ahead with the work and solving problems for himself, keep working constructively without being supervised, and use sound judgment in making decisions about the work.

Another strong point that can help him in his work is his persistence and willingness to keep working till the job is done.

You will be wise to help him choose a line of work that calls on his strong points. In the right line of work, and in the right working conditions and setting, people will appreciate him for his best qualities.

One of his weak points, something that may handicap him in his work, is some lack of initiative, dominance, and leadership. He is lacking in leadership ability. He is not persuasive. He is not the sort of person to take leadership in a group, dominate it, and plan how to get the job done. If one of the main requirements in his work is to take initiative, take charge of a group and lead it, and persuade people, it may be hard for him.

Another possible drawback, a point that may hamper him in his work, is some lack of readiness to try new ideas. Although within the normal range, he seems not to have much breadth of outlook and interests. He doesn't seem to care for new ideas.

You will be wise to help him choose a line of work that doesn't demand so much along those lines.

You may discuss his weak points with him, see whether he recognizes them, and see whether he feels willing and able to change in this regard or not.

Diagnostic impression

Categorizing a patient with a diagnostic judgment must never be done from the results of psychological tests alone, or from the reports of other laboratory tests alone. In making your diagnostic assessment of this patient, you will rely upon the careful history that you have taken, and upon the shrewd observations that you have made of the patient's behavior in the interview as well as the laboratory results.

Insofar as we can judge from the analysis of the psychological testing alone, the diagnostic label most likely to fit the patient is:

301.81 Personality trait disorder, neurotic personality trends, with elements of passive-aggressive personality, passive-dependent type, and with obsessive-compulsive and depressive features.

Other diagnostic labels which may be worth considering are as follows (they are ordered according to the probability of application to this patient):

301.81 Personality trait disorder, passive-aggressive personality, passive-dependent type, with depressive features.

301.4 Personality trait disorder, compulsive personality, submissive type, in some situational stress.

301.81 Personality trait disorder, masochistic personality, with behavior to get people to make him suffer.

307.3 Transient situational disturbance, adjustment reaction of adult life, in a compulsive personality.

319.0 Questionable validity of test. In spite of anything else that may show up, there are some signs that in certain ways he may have twisted his answers in the direction of looking good. For this reason, we cannot put the usual degree of confidence in the findings.

300.4 Psychoneurosis, depressive reaction.

300.0 Psychoneurosis, anxiety reaction, with depressive and possibly obsessive featues.

300.3 Psychoneurosis, obsessive-compulsive.

318. No diagnosable psychiatric condition. He falls within normal limits, psychologically. He cannot be fitted into any diagnostic category.

Potential for psychotherapy

He is a good prospect for making use of intensive psychotherapy and benefitting from it.

He has emotional problems which he unwittingly makes for himself. He feels troubled and distressed, and hence can be motivated to change himself. The process of gaining insight and self-understanding through psychotherapy is painful. Not everyone has the courage to face the unflattering truth about himself, to learn to recognize the motives and purposes behind his dealings with other people. Fortunately, this patient has what it takes. With the professional help of a skilled psychotherapist he can learn to live a healthier way of life, more satisfying to himself and to those around him.

If you do not already have him in psychotherapy, explain to him what it is, and encourage him to undertake it. If you yourself specialize in psychotherapy, you will probably choose to work with him yourself, if you have the time. If not, arrange for him to see another professional psychotherapist. If he is unable to pay for treatment privately, direct him to the local community mental health center, or to a university hospital outpatient psychiatry clinic, or a university psychological clinic.

The masochistic processes are an asset to treatment. If psychotherapy is undertaken, examples of self-defeating behavior should be pointed out and labeled early and often.

Counseling or social casework may be done if intensive psychotherapy is impossible to arrange.

He may be helped by antidepressant medicines.

Summary

The statements that can be made most clearly about this person are as follows (these statements are generated from the scale scores which are most deviant from 50.0):

He admits his faults willingly. He describes himslef as an unreactive, unenthusiastic person, one who firmly avoids commitments, avoids much social contact, and is not overly devoted to duty.

He is highly inhibited, shy, withdrawn, submissive, and unsociable.

In his inward feelings he longs to be passively dependent.

He does not use denial.

He turns hostility against himself, making himself discouraged, depressed, moody, and pessimistic. He is unhappy and dissatisfied in life, and he is especially dissatisfied with himself. He thinks badly of himself, and he feels inadequate. He seems to have lost interest in people, and lost interest in what goes on around him. He seems unresponsive to people.

He is an inhibited person, and not very self-confident. He is not at all the drinking and carousing type. He is well behaved, conforming, submissive, and perhaps puritanical. He is timid, shy, and self-conscious. He always tries hard to do the right thing, but he worries about it. One thing that bothers him is sex. He feels doubtful about religion; he doesn't have much faith in it. If we must choose between the two categories, he looks more like a neurotic patient than like an alcoholic.

He keeps himself withdrawn from people. He doesn't mingle with people.

Institute of Clinical Analysis MMPI-ICA Report

MI, Multiphasic Index, 115 — moderate to marked elevation.
Probability of significant disturbance: %.

Two separate and distinct methods of appraising emotional conflict are shown on scores above. Either score may suggest a disorder but clinical significance is greater when both are elevated.

MI interpretation

The MI, Multiphasic Index, reflects a marked degree of emotional disturbance. Although the patient is overly confessive and spills out a vast array of symptoms, psychological defenses are functioning better than expected for this pattern.

Summary

Test findings clearly indicate a significant emotional disorder. The dynamics shown place this protocol in an uncertain diagnostic classification.

The subject is markedly confessive to numerous and deviate symptoms, but actual coping ability is difficult to assess because of overemphasis or possible attention-getting motives. If dependency is in fact this extreme, then psychiatric evaluation should be considered as urgent. Even if the condition is not as bad as portrayed, the subject feels a need to appear on the test as mentally ill.

Validity

The patient is very confessive to psychological problems, with strong unconscious, if not conscious, feelings of inadequacy or self-effacement.

Personality description

Dejection of mood is a cardinal symptom. There are marked feelings of self-doubt, discouragement, and a tendency to give up. Unhappiness, brooding, gloom, and despondency are admitted.

Anxiety is greatly internalized associated with subjective distress and somatization. Loss of confidence, repressed hostility, and a negative approach to daily problems are the major dynamics in this disorder.

Suggestions to improve coping

Provide the subject with an opportunity to discuss personal problems and previous failure in life adjustment. This pattern is usually associated with good motivation for therapy.

Special coping problems

Investigate schizoid or dissociative fantasy indications. Hostility is mostly intropunitive or turned inward at this time. Some overt expressions of self-punishment or suicidal tendencies are noted.

Patient's positive traits

Sensitive, conscientious, permissive, peaceable, perfectionistic, self-reflective, and compliant toward authority.

Diagnostic impression (Pattern resemblance to clinical cases)

Depressive reaction.

Symptom review (Critical item number marked by asterisk)

Anxiety . . .
  Anxiety appears moderate.
  Tense and restless.
    Moderate nervousness or tension.
    Moderate autonomic concomitants.
Phobias and Obsessions . . .
  Phobias are moderately likely.

Depression . . .
  A significant degree of depression is signalled.
  Encourage open discussion pertaining to despondency.
  * 339 Most of the time I wish I were dead .... True
Intropunitive . . .
  Somewhat intropunitive.
  There is admission of some feelings of guilt, regret, or unworthiness.
Hostility . . .
  Tends to hold back anger and express it later when self-justified.
  * 139 Sometimes I feel as if I must injure either myself or someone
      else .... True
Emotional Control . . .
  Hostility tends to be accumulated or inhibited from direct expression.
Hyperactivity . . .
  Considerably agitated or restless.
  Dysphoric episodes.
Unusual Thoughts and Experiences . . .
  * 156 I have had periods in which I carried on activities without knowing
      later what I had been doing .... True
  * 334 Peculiar odors come to me at times .... True
  * 345 I often feel as if things were not real .... True
Dreams . . .
  Occasionally.
Defense Mechanisms . . .
  Intellectualization.
  Obsessive-compulsive.
Somatic Expression . . .
  Somatic complaints appear moderate.
    Headache.
    Neckache.
    Precordial distress.
    Sleep disturbance.
    Vasomotor instability
  * 114 Often I feel as if there were a tight band about my head ... True

Veterans Administration MMPI Laboratory

T-code = 2*7//801/3549-6   P-code = /37

  Test-taking attitude seems to reveal help-seeking. The patient's current
state appears to be characterized by marked anxiety.
  Single and pair-wise scale analysis suggests the possibility of the following traits and characteristics. Depression. Lack of optimism. Dysphoric,
worrying, pessimistic. Obsessive trends. Self-punishing. Introjects anger.
Anxious and depressed. Probable feelings of worthlessness and sinfulness.
Tension. Immature, self-centered, and impulsive. Family and social
maladjustments of immature kinds. Anxiety. Obsessive thinking. Dissatisfied with social relationships. No apparent abnormality in energy or
activity level. Markedly withdrawn, shy, and socially isolated.
  The following should be looked for among trait and diagnostic alterna-

tives — schizoid obsessional thinking. Wiggins content scales indicate that the patient's self-report shows the following characteristics to be prominent — depressed, worrying.

Profile is a type which when obtained from medical patients referred for consultation indicates type of maladjustment which warrants a psychiatric formulation and diagnosis as described in the following psychiatric codebook summary paragraph. In general, profile is a type frequent among patients in whom current situational difficulties, with associated anxiety and depression, tend to predominate in the clinical picture except when the depressive state rule indicates a depressive reaction or scales 8 and/or 6 are elevated beyond normal limits but Pd and Ma are not, suggesting psychosis.

Comparison of Interpretations

In spite of the great diversity in format, language, and basis for interpretations, the six computerized interpretations of the sample case (J. A. K.) are remarkably congruent. The general picture emerging from the various reports is the same. Differences that exist are in form, as some reports speak to an aspect of personality and functioning whereas other reports include nothing about that aspect. There is only one clearly contradictory interpretation among the reports. The Psychological Corporation, Caldwell, Institute of Clinical Analysis, and Roche reports all suggest that J. A. K. is likely to report somatic complaints that have no clear organic basis. Whereas the Veterans Administration report makes no statement about somatic complaints, the Behaviordyne report states, "he is not at all the sort of person that gets bodily symptoms to symbolize his emotional conflicts without organic cause."

All six reports agree that the protocol is valid, although several of them point out that J. A. K. was rather revealing and self-critical in his approach to the test. There also is rather clear agreement that J. A. K. has emotional problems serious enough to warrant professional intervention. The reports also are in unanimous agreement in describing J. A. K. as a very uncomfortable individual who is likely to be depressed and anxious. The Caldwell, Institute of Clinical Analysis, and Roche reports suggest a neurotic diagnosis (depressive or anxiety) for J. A. K. The Behaviordyne report offers both personality trait disturbances and neuroses as probable diagnostic labels. Neither the Psychological Corporation nor Veterans Administration reports makes a direct diagnostic statement, but the general interpretation of the protocol by these two services is consistent with a neurotic diagnosis. The Roche and Institute of Clinical Analysis reports also mention the possibility of some unusual qualities in J. A. K's thinking and suggest that they be explored more thoroughly. In this regard, the Caldwell report indicates that some patients with this kind of MMPI pattern are seen as schizoid or as having chronic undifferentiated schizophrenic reactions.

Four of the reports indicate that J. A. K. is likely to have excessive bodily concern and to report somatic symptoms for which there is no clear organic basis. There also is agreement that J. A. K. tends to have a poor self-concept, that he is likely to have problems in making decisions, and that he tends to be rather shy, passive, and withdrawn. Further, they agree that he is likely to avoid close involvement with other people. Whereas he does not have a great deal of anger and resentment, the negative feelings that he does harbor are not expressed and may be turned inward. Three of the reports (Caldwell, Institute of Clinical Analysis, Roche) make clear statements that suicidal thoughts and preoccupations are likely. The Caldwell report includes suggestions for handling this problem if it is supported by other data. The Psychological Corporation report makes no mention of suicidal ideation. Whereas the Behaviordyne and Veterans Administration reports do not state explicitly that suicidal preoccupation is likely, the formulation of the case in both reports would suggest to an experienced clinician that such ideation is likely. Further, both of these services print out the examinee's responses to the critical items, including ones in which the examinee admits that most of the time he wishes he were dead and that he has impulses to harm himself or other people.

The Behaviordyne report is the only one that gives detailed information about the work situation, although the Caldwell report mentions that dissatisfaction with work achievement is a likely focus in psychotherapy. The Caldwell report is the only one that describes the family background typically found for persons with this kind of MMPI protocol. It is suggested that such persons have experienced indirect rejection from one or both parents, that their personal pecularities often have provoked negative reactions from other family members, and that they tended to be teased excessively by siblings. In addition, it is suggested that difficulties in giving love resulted in repeated frustrations of their wishes for emotional closeness with family members and that they often cultivated interests in obscure intellectual subjects, such as religion and philosophy.

Although all of the reports, except for the Veterans Administration one, make some statements about treatment, they differ in the amount of such information included. The Psychological Corporation report simply states that the examinee would like to discuss his emotional problems. The Institute of Clinical Analysis report indicates that the examinee has good motivation for therapy. The Roche report suggests that he is willing to accept therapy, that he is in need of therapy, and that spontaneous recoveries rarely occur for patients with this kind of MMPI protocol. The Behaviordyne report indicates that J. A. K. is a good prospect for intensive psychotherapy and that he is likely to benefit from it. The report also suggests that the therapist should help him to understand the self-defeating nature of his behavior. It also suggests that antidepressant medicine may be helpful. The Caldwell report gives the most comprehensive information about treatment. It indicates that a gradual positive response to psychotherapy is likely. Slowness to relate, immature emotional distortions, and a resistive negative self-image are liabilities in therapy. Persons with this kind of protocol tend to gain intellectual insight without significant changes in behavior. Goals for therapy for J. A. K. include working through of anger and guilt and consideration of his dissatisfaction with work achievement. It is suggested that an older, kindly, understanding, well-adjusted, and motherly female therapist might be most beneficial for J. A. K.

In summary, although the interpretations vary considerably in the amount of information provided about various aspects of the examinee's functioning, there is considerable agreement about the basic formulation of his personality and problems. In addition, the picture emerging from these six reports is quite congruent with the author's interpretation of the protocol (see Chapter 8).

A CONCLUDING CAUTION

As stated earlier in this chapter, the computerized MMPI interpretation services do not constitute an adequate replacement or substitute for the clinical judgment process. The services of a trained and experienced clinician are needed to give meaning to the test data for the unique characteristics of the specific individual who has been tested.

REFERENCES

Altus, W. D., & Tafejian, T. T. MMPI correlates of the California E-F scale. *Journal of Social Psychology*, 1953, *38*, 145-149.

Barron, F. An ego strength scale which predicts response to psychotherapy. *Journal of Consulting Psychology*, 1953, *17*, 327-333.

Barron, F. Ego-strength and the management of aggression. In G. S. Welsh and W. G. Dahlstrom (Eds.), *Basic Readings on the MMPI in Psychology and Medicine*. Minneapolis: University of Minnesota Press, 1956.

Barron, F., & Leary, T. Changes in psychoneurotic patients with and without psychotherapy. *Journal of Consulting Psychology*, 1955, *19*, 239-245.

Baughman, E. E., & Welsh, G. S. *Personality: A Behavioral Science*. Englewood Cliffs, N. J.: Prentice-Hall, 1962.

Black, J. D. The interpretation of MMPI profiles of college women. Unpublished doctoral dissertation, University of Minnesota, 1953.

Block, J. *The Challenge of Response Sets: Unconfounding Meaning, Acquiescence, and Social Desirability in the MMPI*. New York: Appleton-Century-Crofts, 1965.

Block, J., & Bailey, D. Q Sort Item Analyses of a Number of MMPI Scales. Officer Education Research Laboratory, Technical Memorandum, OERL-TM-55-7, 1955.

Boerger, A. R. The utility of some alternative approaches to MMPI scale construction. Unpublished doctoral dissertation, Kent State University, 1975.

Boerger, A. R., Graham, J. R., & Lilly, R. S. Behavioral correlates of single-scale MMPI code types. *Journal of Consulting and Clinical Psychology*, 1974, *42*, 398-402.

Button, A. D. A study of alcoholics with the MMPI. *Quarterly Journal of Studies on Alcohol*, 1956, *17*, 263-281.

Byrne, D. *An Introduction to Personality: Research, Theory, and Applications*. Englewood Cliffs, N. J.: Prentice-Hall, 1974.

Calvin, J. Two dimensions or fifty: factor analytic studies with the MMPI. Unpublished materials, Kent State University, 1974.

Calvin, J. A replicated study of the concurrent validity of the Harris subscales for the MMPI. Unpublished doctoral dissertation, Kent State University, 1975.

Carkhuff, R. R., Barnette, W. L., & McCall, J. N. *The Counselor's Handbook: Scale and Profile Interpretations of the MMPI*. Urbana, Ill.: Parkinson, 1965.

Carson, R. C. Interpretive manual to the MMPI. In J. N. Butcher (Ed.), *MMPI: Research Developments and Clinical Applications*. New York: McGraw-Hill, 1969.

Chu, C. Object cluster analysis of the MMPI. Unpublished doctoral dissertation, University of California, Berkeley, 1966.

Cohler, B. J., Weiss, J. L., & Grunebaum, H.

V. "Short-form" content scales for the MMPI. *Journal of Personality Assessment*, 1974, *38*, 563-572.

Comrey, A. L. A factor analysis of items on the MMPI depression scale. *Educational and Psychological Measurement*, 1957, *17*, 578-585. (a)

Comrey, A. L. A factor analysis of items on the MMPI hypochondriasis scale. *Educational and Psychological Measurement*, 1957, *17*, 566-577. (b)

Comrey, A. L. A factor analysis of items on the MMPI hysteria scale. *Educational and Psychological Measurement*, 1957, *17*, 586-592. (c)

Comrey, A. L. A factor analysis of items on the F scale of the MMPI. *Educational and Psychological Measurement*, 1958, *18*, 621-632. (a)

Comrey, A. L. A factor analysis of items on the MMPI hypomania scale. *Educational and Psychological Measurement*, 1958, *18*, 313-323. (b)

Comrey, A. L. A factor analysis of items on the MMPI paranoia scale. *Educational and Psychological Measurement*, 1958, *18*, 99-107. (c)

Comrey, A. L. A factor analysis of items on the MMPI psychasthenia scale. *Educational and Psychological Measurement*, 1958, *18*, 293-300. (d)

Comrey, A. L. A factor analysis of items on the MMPI psychopathic deviate scale. *Educational and Psychological Measurement*, 1958, *18*, 91-98. (e)

Comrey, A. L., & Margraff, W. A factor analysis of items on the MMPI schizophrenia scale. *Educational and Psychological Measurement*, 1958, *18*, 301-311.

Cuadra, C. A. A scale for control in psychological adjustment (Cn). In G. W. Welsh and W. G. Dahlstrom (Eds.), *Basic Readings on the MMPI in Psychology and Medicine*. Minneapolis: University of Minnesota Press, 1953.

Dahlstrom, W. G. Prediction of adjustment after neurosurgery. *American Psychologist*, 1954, *9*, 353.

Dahlstrom, W. G. Whither the MMPI? In J. N. Butcher (Ed.), *Objective Personality Assessment: Changing Perspectives*. New York: Academic Press, 1972.

Dahlstrom, W. G., & Welsh, G. S. *An MMPI Handbook: A Guide to Clinical Practice and Research*. Minneapolis: University of Minnesota Press, 1960.

Dahlstrom, W. G., Welsh, G. S., & Dahlstrom, L. E. *An MMPI Handbook. Volume I: Clinical Interpretation*. Minneapolis: University of Minnesota Press, 1972.

Dahlstrom, W. G., Welsh, G. S., & Dahlstrom, L. E. *An MMPI Handbook. Volume II: Research Applications*. Minneapolis:

University of Minnesota Press, 1975.

Davis, K. R., & Sines, J. O. An antisocial behavior pattern associated with a specific MMPI profile. *Journal of Consulting and Clinical Psychology,* 1971, *36,* 229–234.

Distler, L. S., May, P. R., & Tuma, A. H. Anxiety and ego strength as predictors of response to treatment in schizophrenic patients. *Journal of Consulting Psychology,* 1964, *28,* 170–177.

Drake, L. E. A social I. E. scale for the MMPI. *Journal of Applied Psychology,* 1946, *30,* 51–54.

Drake, L. E., & Oetting, E. R. *An MMPI Codebook for Counselors.* Minneapolis: University of Minnesota Press, 1959.

Duckworth, J. C., & Duckworth, E. *MMPI Interpretation Manual for Counselors and Clinicians.* Muncie, Ind.: Accelerated Development, Inc., 1975.

Dunbar, J. R., & Rabourn, R. E. A working manual for the MMPI. Unpublished materials, date unknown.

Edwards, A. L. Social desirability and performance on the MMPI. *Psychometrika,* 1964, *29,* 295–308.

Eichman, W. J. Replicated factors on the MMPI with female NP patients. *Journal of Consulting Psychology,* 1961, *25,* 55–60.

Eichman, W. J. Factored scales for the MMPI: A clinical and statistical manual. *Journal of Clinical Psychology,* 1962, *18,* 363–395.

Eichman, W. J. Minnesota Multiphasic Personality Inventory: Computerized scoring and interpreting services. In O. K. Buros (Ed.), *The Seventh Mental Measurements Yearbook.* Vol. I. Highland Park, N. J.: Gryphon Press, 1972. (a)

Eichman, W. J. Minnesota Multiphasic Personality Inventory: MMPI-ICA Computer Report. In O. K. Buros (Ed.), *The Seventh Mental Measurements Yearbook.* Vol. I. Highland Park, N. J.: Gryphon Press, 1972. (b)

Eichman, W. J. Minnesota Multiphasic Personality Inventory: OPTIMUM Psychodiagnostic Consultation Service. In O. K. Buros (Ed.), *The Seventh Mental Measurements Yearbook.* Vol. I. Highland Park, N. J.: Gryphon Press, 1972. (c)

Eichman, W. J. Minnesota Multiphasic Personality Inventory: The Psychological Corporation MMPI Reporting Service. In O. K. Buros (Ed.), *The Seventh Mental Measurements Yearbook.* Vol. I. Highland Park, N. J.: Gryphon Press, 1972. (d)

Eichman, W. J. Minnesota Multiphasic Personality Inventory: Roche MMPI computerized interpretation service. In O. K. Buros (Ed.), *The Seventh Mental Measurements Yearbook.* Vol. I. Highland Park, N. J.: Gryphon Press, 1972. (e)

Ends, E. J., & Page, C. W. Functional relationships among measures of anxiety, ego strength and adjustment. *Journal of Clinical Psychology,* 1957, *13,* 148–150.

Eschenback, A. E., & Dupree, L. The influence of stress on MMPI scale scores. *Journal of Clinical Psychology,* 1959, *15,* 42–45.

Finney, J. C. The MMPI as a measure of character structure as revealed by factor analysis. *Journal of Consulting Psychology,* 1961, *25,* 327–336.

Fowler, R. D. The current status of computer interpretation of psychological tests. *American Journal of Psychiatry,* 1969, *125,* 21–27.

Fowler, R. D., & Coyle, F. A. Overlap as a problem in atlas classification of MMPI profiles. *Journal of Clinical Psychology,* 1968, *24,* 435.

Fowler, R. D., & Coyle, F. A. Collegiate normative data on MMPI content scales. *Journal of Clinical Psychology,* 1969, *25,* 62–63.

Fowler, R. D., Teel, S. K., & Coyle, F. A. The measurement of alcoholic response to treatment by Barron's ego strength scale. *Journal of Psychology,* 1967, *67,* 65–68.

Friedman, S. H. Psychometric effects of frontal and parietal lobe brain damage. Unpublished doctoral dissertation, University of Minnesota, 1950.

Getter, H., & Sundland, D. M. The Barron ego strength scale and psychotherapy outcome. *Journal of Consulting Psychology,* 1962, *26,* 195.

Gilberstadt, H. *Comprehensive MMPI Code Book for Males.* Minneapolis: MMPI Research Laboratory, Veterans Administration Hospital, Report 1B 11-5, 1970.

Gilberstadt, H., & Duker, J. *A Handbook for Clinical and Actuarial MMPI Interpretation.* Philadelphia: Saunders, 1965.

Gocka, E. American Lake norms for 200 MMPI scales. Unpublished materials, 1965.

Gocka, E., & Holloway, H. Normative and Predictive Data on the Harris and Lingoes Subscales for a Neuropsychiatric Population. Technical Report No. 7, Veterans Administration Hospital, American Lake, Washington, 1963.

Goldberg, L. R. Diagnosticians vs. diagnostic signs: the diagnosis of psychosis vs. neurosis from the MMPI. *Psychological Monographs,* 1965, *79,* 9 (whole no. 602).

Goldberg, L. R. Parameters of personality inventory construction: A comparison of prediction strategies and tactics. *Multivariate Behavioral Research Monographs,* 1972, *7,* (2).

Good, P. K., & Brantner, J. P. *The Physician's Guide to the MMPI.* Minneapolis: University of Minnesota Press, 1961.

Gottesman, I. I. More construct validation of the ego-strength scale. *Journal of Consulting Psychology,* 1959, *23,* 342–346.

Gough, H. G. A new dimension of status: I.

Development of a personality scale. *American Sociological Review*, 1948, *13*, 401–409. (a)

Gough, H. G. A new dimension of status: II. Relationship of the St scale to other variables. *American Sociological Review*, 1948, *13*, 534–537. (b)

Gough, H. G. A new dimension of status: III. Discrepancies between the St scale and "objective status." *American Sociological Review*, 1949, *14*, 275–281.

Gough, H. G. The F minus K dissimulation index for the MMPI. *Journal of Consulting Psychology*, 1950, *14*, 408–413.

Gough, H. G. Studies of social intolerance: II. A personality scale for anti-Semitism. *Journal of Social Psychology*, 1951, *33*, 247–255. (a)

Gough, H. G. Studies of social intolerance: III. Relationship of the Pr scale to other variables. *Journal of Social Psychology*, 1951, *33*, 257–262. (b)

Gough, H. G. Brief descriptive and interpretational summary of scales of the Minnesota Multiphasic Personality Inventory. Unpublished materials, 1954.

Gough, H. G., McClosky, H., & Meehl, P. E. A personality scale for dominance. *Journal of Abnormal and Social Psychology*, 1951, *46*, 360–366.

Gough, H. G., McClosky, H., & Meehl, P. E. A personality scale for social responsibility. *Journal of Abnormal and Social Psychology*, 1952, *47*, 73–80.

Gough, H. G., McKee, M. G., & Yandell, R. J. Adjective Check List Analyses of a Number of Selected Psychometric and Assessment Variables. Officer Education Research Laboratory, Technical Memorandum, OERL-TM-5S-10, 1955.

Graham, J. R., Schroeder, H. E., & Lilly, R. S. Factor analysis of items on the Social Introversion and Masculinity-Femininity scales of the MMPI. *Journal of Clinical Psychology*, 1971, *27*, 367–370.

Grayson, H. M. *A Psychological Admissions Testing Program and Manual*. Los Angeles: Veterans Administration Center, Neuropsychiatric Hospital, 1951.

Guthrie, G. M. Common characteristics associated with frequent MMPI profile types. *Journal of Clinical Psychology*, 1952, *8*, 141–145.

Gynther, M. D., Altman, H., & Sletten, I. W. Replicated correlates of MMPI two-point types: the Missouri Actuarial System. *Journal of Clinical Psychology*, 1973, Monograph Supplement no. 39.

Gynther, M. D., Altman, H., & Warbin, W. Interpretation of uninterpretable Minnesota Multiphasic Personality Inventory Profiles. *Journal of Consulting and Clinical Psychology*, 1973, *40*, 78–83.

Gynther, M. D., & Brillant, P. J. The diagnostic utility of Welsh's A-R categories. *Journal of Projective Techniques and Personality Assessment*, 1968, *32*, 572–574.

Hanvik, L. J. Some psychological dimensions of low back pain. Doctoral dissertation, University of Minnesota, 1949.

Hanvik, L. J. MMPI profiles in patients with low back pain. *Journal of Consulting Psychology*, 1951, *15*, 350–353.

Harris, R., & Christiansen, C. Prediction of response to brief psychotherapy. *Journal of Psychology*, 1946, *21*, 269–284.

Harris, R., & Lingoes, J. Subscales for the Minnesota Multiphasic Personality Inventory. Mimeographed materials, The Langley Porter Clinic, 1955.

Harris, R., & Lingoes, J. Subscales for the Minnesota Multiphasic Personality Inventory. Mimeographed materials, The Langley Porter Clinic, 1968.

Hase, H. D., & Goldberg, L. R. Comparative validity of different strategies of constructing personality inventory scales. *Psychological Bulletin*, 1967, *67*, 231–248.

Hathaway, S. R. A coding system for MMPI profiles. *Journal of Consulting Psychology*, 1947, *11*, 334–337.

Hathaway, S. R. Scales 5 (masculinity-femininity), 6 (paranoia), and 8 (schizophrenia). In G. S. Welsh and W. G. Dahlstrom (Eds.), *Basic Readings on the MMPI in Psychology and Medicine*. Minneapolis: University of Minnesota Press, 1956.

Hathaway, S. R. Personality inventories. In B. B. Wolman (Ed.), *Handbook of Clinical Psychology*. New York: McGraw-Hill, 1965.

Hathaway, S. R., & Briggs, P. F. Some normative data on new MMPI scales. *Journal of Clinical Psychology*, 1957, *13*, 364–368.

Hathaway, S. R., & McKinley, J. C. A multiphasic personality schedule (Minnesota): I. Construction of the schedule. *Journal of Psychology*, 1940, *10*, 249–254.

Hathaway, S. R., & McKinley, J. C. A multiphasic personality schedule (Minnesota): III. The measurement of symptomatic depression. *Journal of Psychology*, 1942, *14*, 73–84.

Hathaway, S. R., & McKinley, J. C. *The Minnesota Multiphasic Personality Inventory Manual*. New York: Psychological Corporation, 1967.

Hawkinson, J. R. A study of the construct validity of Barron's ego strength scale with a state mental hospital population. *Dissertation Abstracts International*, 1962, *22*, 4081.

Henrichs, T. F. Objective configural rules for discriminating MMPI profiles in a psychiatric population. *Journal of Clinical Psychology*, 1964, *20*, 157–159.

Henrichs, T. F. A note on the extension of MMPI configural rules. *Journal of Clinical Psychology*, 1966, *22*, 51–52.

Hilgard, E. R., Jones, L. V., & Kaplan, S. J. Conditioned discrimination as related to anxiety. *Journal of Experimental Psychology*, 1951, *42*, 94–99.

Himelstein, P. Further evidence of the ego strength scale as a measure of psychological health. *Journal of Consulting Psychology*, 1964, *28*, 90–91.

Hoffman, H., Loper, R. G., & Kammeier, M. L. Identifying future alcoholics with MMPI alcoholism scales. *Quarterly Journal of Studies on Alcohol*, 1974, *35*, 490–498.

Holmes, D. S. Male-female differences in MMPI ego strength: an artifact. *Journal of Consulting Psychology*, 1967, *31*, 408–410.

Hovey, H. B. Brain lesions and five MMPI items. *Journal of Consulting Psychology*, 1964, *28*, 78–79.

Hovey, H. B., & Lewis, E. G. *Semiautomatic Interpretation of the MMPI*. Brandon, Vt.: Clinical Psychology Publishing Co., 1967.

Huff, F. W. Use of actuarial description of abnormal personality in a mental hospital. *Psychological Reports*, 1965, *17*, 224.

Jackson, D. N. The dynamics of structured tests: 1971. *Psychological Review*, 1971, *78*, 239–249.

Jensen, A. R. Authoritarian attitudes and personality maladjustment. *Journal of Abnormal and Social Psychology*, 1957, *54*, 161–170.

Kammeier, M. L., Hoffman, H., & Loper, R. G. Personality characteristics of alcoholics as college freshmen and at time of treatment. *Quarterly Journal of Studies on Alcohol*, 1973, *34*, 390–399.

Kent, G. H. *Series of Emergency Scales*. New York: Psychological Corporation, 1946.

Kleinmuntz, B. An extension of the construct validity of the ego strength scale. *Journal of Consulting Psychology*, 1960, *24*, 463–464.

Kleinmuntz, B. Minnesota Multiphasic Personality Inventory: Roche MMPI computerized interpretation service. In O. K. Buros (Ed.), *The Seventh Mental Measurements Yearbook*. Vol. I. Highland Park, N. J.: Gryphon Press, 1972.

Knapp, R. R. A reevaluation of the validity of MMPI scales of dominance and responsibility. *Educational and Psychological Measurement*, 1960, *20*, 381–386.

Koss, M. P., & Butcher, J. N. A comparison of psychiatric patients' self-report with other sources of clinical information. *Journal of Research in Personality*, 1973, *7*, 225–236.

Kostlan, A. A method for the empirical study of psychodiagnosis. *Journal of Consulting Psychology*, 1954, *18*, 83–88.

Lachar, D. The MMPI: *Clinical Assessment and Automated Interpretation*. Los Angeles: Western Psychological Services, 1974.

Lewandowski, D., & Graham, J. R. Empirical correlates of frequently occurring two-point code types: a replicated study. *Journal of Clinical Psychology*, 1972, *39*, 467–472.

Lewinsohn, P. M. Dimensions of MMPI change. *Journal of Clinical Psychology*, 1965, *21*, 37–43.

Lingoes, J. MMPI factors of the Harris and Weiner subscales. *Journal of Consulting Psychology*, 1960, *24*, 74–83.

Loper, R. G., Kammeier, M. L., & Hoffman, H. MMPI characteristics of college freshmen males who later became alcoholics. *Journal of Abnormal Psychology*, 1973, *82*, 159–162.

Lorr, M. A test of 7 MMPI factors. *Multivariate Behavioral Research*, 1968, special issue, 151–156.

MacAndrew, C. The differentiation of male alcoholic out-patients from nonalcoholic psychiatric patients by means of the MMPI. *Quarterly Journal of Studies on Alcohol*, 1965, *26*, 238–246.

Marks, P. A., & Seeman, W. *Actuarial Description of Abnormal Personality*. Baltimore: Williams & Wilkins, 1963.

Marks, P. A., Seeman, W., & Haller, D. L. *The Actuarial Use of the MMPI with Adolescents and Adults*. Baltimore: Williams & Wilkins, 1974.

Matarazzo, J. D. *Wechsler's Measurement and Appraisal of Adult Intelligence*. Baltimore: Williams & Wilkins, 1972.

McKinley, J. C., & Hathaway, S. R. A multiphasic personality schedule (Minnesota): II. A differential study of hypochondriasis. *Journal of Psychology*, 1940, *10*, 255–268.

McKinley, J. C., & Hathaway, S. R. The MMPI: V. Hysteria, hypomania, and psychopathic deviate. *Journal of Applied Psychology*, 1944, *28*, 153–174.

McKinley, J. C., Hathaway, S. R., & Meehl, P. E. The MMPI: VI. The K scale. *Journal of Consulting Psychology*, 1948, *12*, 20–31.

Meehl, P. E. *Research Results for Counselors*. St. Paul, Minn.: State Department of Education, 1951.

Meehl, P. E. Wanted—a good cookbook. *American Psychologist*, 1956, *11*, 263–272.

Meehl, P. E., & Dahlstrom, W. G. Objective configural rules for discriminating psychotic from neurotic MMPI profiles. *Journal of Consulting Psychology*, 1960, *24*, 375–387.

Meehl, P. E., & Hathaway, S. R. The K factor as a suppressor variable in the MMPI. *Journal of Applied Psychology*, 1946, *30*, 525–564.

Meier, M. J., & French, L. A. Caudality scale change following unilateral temporal lobectomy. *Journal of Clinical Psychology*, 1964, *20*, 464–467.

Meikle, S., & Gerritse, R. MMPI cookbook pattern frequencies in a psychiatric unit. *Journal of Clinical Psychology*, 1970, *26*, 82–84.

Messick, S., & Jackson, D. N. Acquiescence

and the factorial interpretation of the MMPI. *Psychological Bulletin*, 1961, *58*, 299–304.

Mezzich, J. E., Damarin, F. L., & Erickson, J. R. Comparative validity of strategies and indices of differential diagnosis of depressive states from other psychiatric conditions using the MMPI. *Journal of Consulting and Clinical Psychology*, 1974, *42*, 691–698.

Navran, L. A. A rationally derived MMPI scale to measure dependence. *Journal of Consulting Psychology*, 1954, *18*, 192.

Nelson, J. W. Dependency as a construct: an evaluation and some data. *Dissertation Abstracts*, 1959, *19*, 2149–2150.

Olmstead, D. W., & Monachesi, E. D. A validity check on MMPI scales of responsibility and dominance. *Journal of Abnormal and Social Psychology*, 1956, *53*, 140–141.

Panton, J. The response of prison inmates to MMPI subscales. *Journal of Social Therapy*, 1959, *5*, 233–237.

Payne, F. D., & Wiggins, J. S. MMPI profile types and the self-report of psychiatric patients. *Journal of Abnormal Psychology*, 1972, *79*, 1–8.

Pearson, J. S., & Swenson, W. M. *A User's Guide to the Mayo Clinic Automated MMPI Program.* New York: Psychological Corporation, 1967.

Pepper, L. J., & Strong, P. N. Judgmental subscales for the Mf scale of the MMPI. Unpublished materials, Hawaii Department of Health (Honolulu), 1958.

Persons, R. W., & Marks, P. A. The violent 4-3 personality type. *Journal of Consulting and Clinical Psychology*, 1971, *36*, 189–196.

Peterson, D. R. Predicting hospitalization of psychiatric outpatients. *Journal of Abnormal and Social Psychology*, 1954, *49*, 260–265.

Pruitt, P. W., & Van deCastle, R. L. Dependency measures and welfare chronicity. *Journal of Consulting Psychology*, 1962, *26*, 559–560.

Quay, H. The performance of hospitalized psychiatric patients on the ego-strength scale of the MMPI. *Journal of Clinical Psychology*, 1955, *11*, 403–405.

Rosen, A. Diagnostic differentiation as a construct validity indication for the MMPI ego strength scale. *Journal of General Psychology*, 1963, *69*, 65–68.

Schubert, H. J. P. A wide-range MMPI manual. Unpublished materials, 1973.

Serkownek, K. Subscales for Scales 5 and 0 of the Minnesota Multiphasic Personality Inventory. Unpublished materials, 3134 Whitehorn Road, Cleveland Heights, Ohio 44118, 1975.

Sherriffs, A. C., & Boomer, D. S. Who is penalized by the penalty for guessing? *Journal of Educational Psychology*, 1954, *45*, 81–90.

Simmett, E. R. The relationship between the ego strength scale and rated in-hospital improvement. *Journal of Clinical Psychology*, 1962, *18*, 46–47.

Sines, L. K. The relative contribution of four kinds of data to accuracy in personality assessment. *Journal of Consulting Psychology*, 1959, *23*, 483–492.

Spence, J. T., & Spence, K. W. The motivational components of manifest anxiety: Drive and drive stimuli. In C. D. Spielberger (Ed.), *Anxiety and Behavior.* New York: Academic Press, 1966.

Spiegel, D. E. SPI and MMPI predictors of psychopathology. *Journal of Projective Techniques and Personality Assessment*, 1969, *33*, 265–273.

Spielberger, C. D. The effects of anxiety on complex learning and academic achievement. In C. D. Spielberger (Ed.), *Anxiety and Behavior.* New York: Academic Press, 1966. (a)

Spielberger, C. D. Theory and research on anxiety. In C. D. Spielberger (Ed.), *Anxiety and Behavior.* New York: Academic Press, 1966. (b)

Stein, K. B. The TSC scales: The outcome of a cluster analysis of the 550 MMPI items. In P. McReynolds (Ed.), *Advances in Psychological Assessment.* Vol. I. Palo Alto, Calif.: Science and Behavior Books, 1968.

Stricker, G. A comparison of two MMPI prejudice scales. *Journal of Clinical Psychology*, 1961, *17*, 43.

Sullivan, D. L., Miller, C., & Smelser, W. Factors in length of stay and progress in psychotherapy. *Journal of Consulting Psychology*, 1958, *22*, 1–9.

Sundberg, N. D., & Bachelis, W. D. The fakability of two measures of prejudice: the California F scale and Gough's Pr scale. *Journal of Abnormal and Social Psychology*, 1956, *52*, 140–142.

Tafejian, T. R. The E-F scale, the MMPI, and Gough's Pr scale. *American Psychologist*, 1951, *6*, 501.

Taft, R. The validity of the Barron ego-strength scale and the Welsh anxiety index. *Journal of Consulting Psychology*, 1957, *21*, 247–249.

Tamkin, A. S. An evaluation of the construct validity of Barron's ego-strength scale. *Journal of Consulting Psychology*, 1957, *13*, 156–158.

Tamkin, A. S., & Klett, C. J. Barron's ego-strength scale: a replication of an evaluation of its construct validity. *Journal of Consulting Psychology*, 1957, *21*, 412.

Taulbee, E. S., & Sisson, B. D. Configural analysis of MMPI profiles of psychiatric groups. *Journal of Consulting Psychology*, 1957, *21*, 413–417.

Taylor, J. A. The relationship of anxiety to

the conditioned eyelid response. *Journal of Experimental Psychology,* 1951, *41,* 81–92.

Taylor, J. A. A personality scale of manifest anxiety. *Journal of Abnormal and Social Psychology,* 1953, *48,* 285–290.

Taylor, J. B., Ptacek, M., Carithers, M., Griffin, C., & Coyne, L. Rating scales as measures of clinical judgment. III: Judgments of the self on personality inventory scales and direct ratings. *Educational and Psychological Measurement,* 1972, *32,* 543–557.

Terman, L. M., & Miles, C. C. *Sex and Personality: Studies in Masculinity and Femininity.* New York: McGraw-Hill, 1936.

Tryon, R. C. Unrestricted cluster and factor analysis with application to the MMPI and Holzinger-Harman problems. *Multivariate Behavioral Research,* 1966, *1,* 229–244.

Tryon, H. C., & Bailey, D. (Eds.). *Users' Manual of the BC TRY System of Cluster and Factor Analysis.* (Taped version) Berkeley: University of California Computer Center, 1965.

Warn, L. J. A comparative investigation of dependency in epilepsy, paraplegia and tuberculosis. Unpublished doctoral dissertation, University of California, Los Angeles, 1958.

Welsh, G. S. An extension of Hathaway's MMPI profile coding system. *Journal of Consulting Psychology,* 1948, *12,* 343–344.

Welsh, G. S. Factor dimensions A and R. In G. S. Welsh and W. G. Dahlstrom (Eds.), *Basic Reading on the MMPI in Psychology and Medicine.* Minneapolis: University of Minnesota Press, 1956.

Welsh, G. S. MMPI profiles and factors A and R. *Journal of Clinical Psychology,* 1965, *21,* 43–47.

Welsh, G. S., & Dahlstrom, W. G. (Eds.), *Basic Readings on the MMPI in Psychology and Medicine.* Minneapolis: University of Minnesota Press, 1956.

Wiener, D. N. Subtle and obvious keys for the MMPI. *Journal of Consulting Psychology,* 1948, *12,* 164–170.

Wiggins, J. S. Substantive dimensions of self-report in the MMPI item pool. *Psychological Monographs,* 1966, *80,* 22 (whole no. 630).

Wiggins, J. S. Content dimensions in the MMPI. In J. N. Butcher (Ed.), *MMPI: Research Developments and Clinical Applications.* New York: McGraw-Hill, 1969.

Wiggins, J. S. Content scales: basic data for scoring and interpretation. Unpublished materials, 1971.

Wiggins, J. S., Goldberg, L. R., & Applebaum, M. MMPI content scales: Interpretive norms and correlations with other scales. *Journal of Consulting and Clinical Psychology,* 1971, *37,* 403–410.

Wiggins, J. S., & Vollmar, J. The content of the MMPI. *Journal of Clinical Psychology,* 1959, *15,* 45–47.

Williams, H. L. The development of a caudality scale for the MMPI. *Journal of Clinical Psychology,* 1952, *8,* 293–297.

Wirt, R. D. Further validation of the ego-strength scale. *Journal of Consulting Psychology,* 1955, *20,* 123–124.

Wirt, R. D. Actuarial prediction. *Journal of Consulting Psychology,* 1956, *20,* 123–124.

Zuckerman, M., Levitt, E. E., & Lubin, B. Concurrent and construct validity of direct and indirect measures of dependency. *Journal of Consulting Psychology,* 1961, *25,* 316–323.

appendices

appendix A

SUMMARY OF MMPI ABBREVIATED FORMS

1. The Mini-Mult
   a. Number of Items: 71
   b. Scales Scored: L, F, K, 1, 2, 3, 4, 6, 7, 8, 9
   c. Item Presentation: Oral Interrogative (yes/no response format)
   d. Availability: Test items, scoring procedures, and a table for converting Mini-Mult raw scores to standard raw scores are available from American Documentation Institute. Order Document 9949 from ADI Auxiliary Publications Project, Photoduplication Service, Library of Congress, Washington, D. C. 20540. Remit in advance $1.25 for photocopies or $1.25 for microfilm, and make checks payable to Chief, Photoduplication Service, Library of Congress.
   e. Reliability: Test-retest = .63–.88
   f. Validity: Correlations between Mini-Mult scores and standard scores are reasonably high (.20–.96) for psychiatric patient samples, but the correlations are considerably lower for other kinds of samples (e.g., delinquent adolescents, normal college students, college counselees, alcoholics, reformatory inmates, parents of disturbed children, etc.). When individual Mini-Mult and standard MMPI profile pairs are compared, for such indices as highest scale or two scales in the profile, little agreement is found.
   g. Recommendation: Although the Mini-Mult may be useful for comparing groups of subjects, particularly if they are psychiatric patients, it is the opinion of the author that the instrument should not be used to generate inferences about individual subjects.
   h. References:

   Armentrout, J. A. Correspondence of the MMPI and Mini-Mult in a college population. *Journal of Clinical Psychology*, 1970, *26*, 493–495.

   Armentrout, J. A., & Rouzer, D. L. Utility of the Mini-Mult with adolescents. *Journal of Consulting and Clinical Psychology*, 1970, *34*, 450.

   Finch, A. J., Edwards, G. L., & Griffin, J. L. Utility of the Mini-Mult with parents of emotionally disturbed children. *Journal of Personality Assessment*, 1975, *39*, 146–150.

   Gaines, L. S., Abrams, M. H., Toel, P., & Miller, L. M. Comparison of the MMPI and the Mini-Mult with alcoholics. *Journal of Consulting and Clinical Psychology*, 1974, *42*, 619.

   Gayton, W. F., Bishop, J. S., Citrin, M. M., & Bassett, J. S. An investigation of the Mini-Mult validity scales. *Journal of Personality Assessment*, 1975, *39*, 511–513.

   Gayton, W. F., Ozmon, K. L., & Wilson, W. T. Investigation of a written form of the Mini-Mult. *Psychological Reports*, 1972, *30*, 275–278.

   Gayton, W. F., & Wilson, W. T. Utility of the Mini-Mult in a child guidance setting. *Journal of Personality Assessment*, 1971, *36*, 569–575.

Goldenholtz, N. Correspondence of the MMPI and the Mini-Mult with normal college students and college counselees. Unpublished master's thesis, Kent State University, 1972.

Graham, J. R., & Schroeder, H. E. Abbreviated Mf and Si scales for the MMPI. *Journal of Personality Assessment*, 1972, *36*, 436–439.

Hartford, T., Lubetkin, B., & Alpert, G. Comparison of the standard MMPI and the Mini-Mult in a psychiatric outpatient clinic. *Journal of Consulting and Clinical Psychology*, 1972, *39*, 242–245.

Hedberg, A. G., Campbell, L. M., Weeks, S. R., & Powell, J. A. The use of the MMPI (Mini-Mult) to predict alcoholics' response to a behavioral treatment program. *Journal of Clinical Psychology*, 1975, *31*, 271–274.

Hobbs, T. R. Scale equivalence and profile similarity of the Mini-Mult and the MMPI in an outpatient clinic. *Journal of Clinical Psychology*, 1974, *30*, 349–350.

Hobbs, T. R., & Fowler, R. D. Reliability and scale equivalence of the Mini-Mult and MMPI. *Journal of Consulting and Clinical Psychology*, 1974, *42*, 89–92.

Hoffman, N. G., & Butcher, J. N. Clinical limitations of three Minnesota Multiphasic Personality Inventory short forms. *Journal of Consulting and Clinical Psychology*, 1975, *43*, 32–39.

Huisman, R. W. Correspondence between Mini-Mult and standard MMPI scale scores in patients with neurological disease. *Journal of Consulting and Clinical Psychology*, 1974, *42*, 149.

Kincannon, J. C. Prediction of the standard MMPI scale scores from 71 items: the Mini-Mult. *Journal of Consulting and Clinical Psychology*, 1968, *32*, 319–325.

Lacks, P. Further investigation of the Mini-Mult. *Journal of Consulting and Clinical Psychology*, 1970, *35*, 126–127.

Lacks, P. B., & Powell, B. J. The Mini-Mult as a personnel screening technique: a preliminary report. *Psychological Reports*, 1970, *27*, 909–910.

McLachlan, J. F. C. Test-retest stability of long and short MMPI scales over two years. *Journal of Clinical Psychology*, 1974, *30*, 189–191.

Mlott, S. The Mini-Mult and its use with adolescents. *Journal of Clinical Psychology*, 1973, *29*, 376–377.

Newton, J. A comparison of studies of the Mini-Mult. *Journal of Clinical Psychology*, 1971, *27*, 489–490.

Palmer, A. B. A comparison of the MMPI and Mini-Mult in a sample of state mental hospital patients. *Journal of Clinical Psychology*, 1973, *29*, 484–485.

Percell, L. P., & Delk, J. L. Relative usefulness of three forms of the Mini-Mult with college students. *Journal of Consulting and Clinical Psychology*, 1971, *27*, 489–490.

Platt, J. J., & Scura, W. C. Validity of the Mini-Mult with female reformatory inmates. *Journal of Clinical Psychology*, 1972, *28*, 528–529.

Pulvermacher, G. D., & Bringmann, W. G. The Mini-Mult used with French-Canadian college students. *Psychological Reports*, 1971, *29*, 134.

Rybolt, G. A., & Lambert, J. A. Correspondence of the MMPI and Mini-Mult with psychiatric inpatients. *Journal of Clinical Psychology*, 1975, *31*, 279–280.

Simono, R. B. Comparison of the standard MMPI and the Mini-Mult in a university counseling center. *Educational and Psycho-*

logical Measurement, 1975, *35,* 401–404.

Thornton, L. S., Finch, A. J., & Griffin, J. L. The Mini-Mult with criminal psychiatric patients. *Journal of Personality Assessment,* 1975, *39,* 394–396.

Trybus, R., & Havitt, C. The Mini-Mult in a non-psychiatric population. *Journal of Clinical Psychology,* 1972, *28,* 371.

2. The Midi-Mult
   a. Number of Items: 86
   b. Scales Scored: L, F, K, 1, 2, 3, 4, 6, 7, 8, 9
   c. Item Presentation: Printed Statements (true/false response format)
   d. Availability: Test items, directions of scoring, and regression equations to convert short-form raw scores to standard raw score equivalents are available from the National Auxiliary Publications Service. Order Document no. 01411 from the National Auxiliary Publications Service of the American Society for Information Science, c/o CCM Information Services, Inc., 909 3rd Avenue, New York, New York 10022. Remit in advance $5.00 for photocopies or $2.00 for microfiche and make checks payable to: Research and Microfilm Publications, Inc.
   e. Reliability: None Reported
   f. Validity: Correlations between Midi-Mult scores and standard scores are reasonably high for medical patients (.81–.94), college students (.52–.84), and psychiatric inpatients (.44–.82). Agreement between the two forms concerning validity of the protocols ranges from 63% to 98%. Congruence for other configural indices (highest scale, two highest scales, Meehl-Dahlstrom Rules, etc.) was not great (41%–58%).
   g. Recommendation: The Midi-Mult is somewhat superior to the Mini-Mult in comparing groups of normal subjects on individual scales.

However, the lack of congruence between individual profile pairs leads this author to conclude that the instrument should not be used for generating inferences about individual subjects.

   h. References:
      Dean, E. F. A lengthened Mini: the Midi-Mult. *Journal of Clinical Psychology,* 1972, *28,* 68–71.

      Gilroy, F. D., & Steinbacher, R. Extension of the Midi-Mult to a college population. *Journal of Personality Assessment,* 1973, *37,* 263–266.

      Griffin, J. L., Finch, A. J., Edwards, G. L., & Kendall, P. C. MMPI/Midi-Mult correspondence with parents of emotionally disturbed children. *Journal of Clinical Psychology,* 1976, *32,* 54–56.

      Newmark, C., Cook, L., & Greer, W. Application of the Midi-Mult to psychiatric inpatients. *Journal of Clinical Psychology,* 1973, *29,* 481–484.

      Newmark, C. S., Newmark, L., & Faschingbauer, T. R. Utility of three abbreviated MMPI's with psychiatric outpatients. *Journal of Nervous and Mental Disease,* 1974, *159,* 438–443.

3. Faschingbauer's Abbreviated MMPI (FAM)
   a. Number of Items: 166
   b. Scales Scored: L, F, K, 1, 2, 3, 4, 5, 6, 7, 8, 9, 0
   c. Item Presentation: Printed Statements (true/false response format)
   d. Availability: Items and a table for converting FAM raw scores into standard raw scores are available from Thomas R. Faschingbauer, Highland Hospital Division, Duke University Medical Center, Asheville, North Carolina 28802.
   e. Reliability: Test-retest = .42–.95
   f. Validity:
      (1) Correlations between standard MMPI scores and corresponding scores derived from the

FAM have ranged from .55 to .92 for samples of psychiatric inpatients, psychiatric outpatients, hospitalized adolescents, and normal college students.

(2) Means based on standard MMPI scores and FAM scores have been quite similar.

(3) Decisions concerning profile validity and degree of pathology have been similar for individual pairs of profiles.

(4) The agreement concerning single scale and two-point code types has been quite variable. For example, agreement concerning the single scale elevation has ranged from 40% to 83%.

(5) No significant differences have been found between the accuracy of interpretations based on the FAM and those based on the standard MMPI.

g. Recommendation: The FAM appears to be as good as or better than the Mini-Mult and the Midi-Mult in prediction of group results. In addition, the FAM seems useful in decisions concerning degree of pathology and diagnosis. However, the lack of definitive evidence concerning congruence of profile types leads this author to conclude that the FAM is not an acceptable substitute for the standard MMPI when individual profiles are interpreted in a traditional manner.

h. References:

Faschingbauer, T. R. A 166-item written short form of the group MMPI: the FAM. *Journal of Consulting and Clinical Psychology*, 1974, *42*, 645–655.

Hoffman, N. G., & Butcher, J. N. Clinical limitations of three Minnesota Multiphasic Personality Inventory short forms. *Journal of Clinical and Consulting Psychology*, 1975, *43*, 32–39.

Newmark, C. S., Boas, B., & Messerry, T. An abbreviated MMPI for use with college students. *Psychological Reports*, 1974, *34*, 631–634.

Newmark, C. S., Conger, A. J. & Faschingbauer, T. R. The interpretive validity and effective test length functioning of an abbreviated MMPI relative to the standard MMPI. *Journal of Clinical Psychology*, 1976, *32*, 27–32.

Newmark, C. S., Cook, L., Clarke, M., & Faschingbauer, T. R. Application of Faschingbauer's Abbreviated MMPI to psychiatric inpatients. *Journal of Consulting and Clinical Psychology*, 1973, *41*, 416–421.

Newmark, C. S., Galen, R., & Gold, K. Efficacy of an abbreviated MMPI as a function of type of administration. *Journal of Consulting Psychology*, 1975, *31*, 639–642.

Newmark, C. S., & Galen, L. Sensitivity of the Faschingbauer Abbreviated MMPI to hospitalized adolescents. *Journal of Abnormal Child Psychology*, 1974, *4*, 299–306.

Newmark, C. S., Newmark, L., & Faschingbauer, T. R. Utility of three abbreviated MMPI's with psychiatric outpatients. *Journal of Nervous and Mental Disease*, 1974, *159*, 438–443.

Newmark, C. S., Owen, M., Newmark, L., Cook, L., & Faschingbauer, T. R. Comparison of three abbreviated MMPIs for psychiatric patients and normals. *Journal of Personality Assessment*, 1975, *39*, 261–270.

4. The Maxi-Mult

a. Number of Items: 94

b. Scales Scored: L, F, K, 1, 2, 3, 4, 5, 6, 7, 8, 9, 0

c. Item Presentation: Printed Statements (true/false response format)

d. Availability: Items are taken from Kincannon's Mini-Mult (1968), Dean's Midi-Mult (1972), and the abbreviated Mf and Si scales of Graham and Schroeder (1972). In addition, 12 items are based on a study by McLachlan (1974). Scoring criteria are available from John F. C. McLachlan, 175 Brentcliffe Road, Toronto M4G 3Z1, Canada.

e. Reliability: Test-retest = .37–.80

f. Validity: Correlations between Maxi-Mult scores and standard MMPI scores ranged from .00 to .91. No data are available concerning comparisons of individual profile pairs.

g. Conclusions: With the exceptions of scales L and 5, especially with females, the Maxi-Mult scales tend to be reliable and to correspond well with standard MMPI scales. It is this author's opinion that until additional data are available concerning profile similarity, the Maxi-Mult scales should not be used with individual clinical cases.

h. References:

Dean, E. F. A lengthened Mini: the Midi-Mult. *Journal of Clinical Psychology,* 1972, *28,* 68–71.

Elsie, R. D., & McLachlan, J. F. C. Reliability of the Maxi-Mult and scale equivalence with the MMPI. *Journal of Clinical Psychology,* 1976, *32,* 67–69.

Graham, J. R., & Schroeder, H. E. Abbreviated Mf and Si Scales for the MMPI. *Journal of Personality Assessment,* 1972, *36,* 436–439.

Kincannon, J. C. Prediction of the standard MMPI scales from 71 items. *Journal of Consulting and Clinical Psychology,* 1968, *36,* 436–439.

McLachlan, J. F. C. Test-retest stability of long and short MMPI scales over two years. *Journal of Clinical Psychology,* 1974, *30,* 189–191.

5. The MMPI-168

a. Number of Items: 168

b. Scales Scored: L, F, K, 1, 2, 3, 4, 5, 6, 7, 8, 9, 0

c. Item Presentation: Printed Statements (true/false response format)

d. Availability: The first 168 items in either the booklet form or Form R may be used and are scored using standard scoring templates. A table to be used for determining standard raw scores from abbreviated raw scores is presented by Overall, Higgins, and deSchweinitz (1975).

e. Reliability: None Reported

f. Validity:

(1) Correlations between standard MMPI scores and corresponding scores derived from the MMPI-168 for psychiatric patients, medical patients, and normal college students have ranged from .77 to .97.

(2) Means based on standard MMPI scores and MMPI-168 scores have been remarkably similar.

(3) Decisions concerning profile validity and degree of pathology have been quite similar for individual pairs of profiles.

(4) The agreement concerning single scale and two-point code types has been about 75% for psychiatric patients and about 64% for medical patients.

(5) Utilizing external criterion measures, no significant differences have been found between the standard MMPI and the MMPI-168 in ability to discriminate between psychiatric patients and college students or among 10 major psychiatric diagnostic categories.

g. Conclusions: The MMPI-168 is the most promising abbreviated form currently available. The MMPI-168 seems to be equivalent to the standard MMPI in terms of both group and individual comparisons. In addition, there is evidence that the MMPI-168 has validity independent of the standard instrument. However, until further evidence becomes available concerning the usefulness of the MMPI-168 in a variety of settings, this author believes that this abbreviated form should be used with caution.

h. References:

Hedlund, J. L. The use of MMPI short forms with psychiatric patients. *Journal of Consulting and Clinical Psychology*, 1975, *43*, 924.

Hoffman, N. G., & Butcher, J. N. Clinical limitations of three Minnesota Multiphasic Personality Inventory short forms. *Journal of Consulting and Clinical Psychology*, 1975, *43*, 32–39.

Hunter, S., Overall, J. E., & Butcher, J. N. Factor structure of the MMPI in a psychiatric population. *Multivariate Behavioral Research*, 1974, *9*, 293–302.

Newmark, C. S., Falk, R., & Finch, A. J. Interpretive accuracy of abbreviated MMPIs. *Journal of Personality Assessment*, 1976, *40*, 266–268.

Newmark, C. S., Newmark, L., & Cook, L. The MMPI-168 with psychiatric patients. *Journal of Clinical Psychology*, 1975, *31*, 61–64.

Newmark, C. S., & Raft, D. Using an abbreviated MMPI as a screening device for medical patients. *Psychosomatics*, 1976, *17*, 45–48.

Overall, J. E., & Gomez-Mont, F. The MMPI-168 for psychiatric screening. *Educational and Psychological Measurement*, 1974, *34*, 315–319.

Overall, J. E., Higgins, W., & deSchweinitz, A. Comparison of differential diagnostic discrimination for abbreviated and standard MMPI. *Journal of Clinical Psychology*, 1976, *32*, 237–245.

Overall, J. E., Butcher, J. N., & Hunter, S. Validity of the MMPI-168 for psychiatric screening. *Educational and Psychological Measurement*, 1975, *35*, 393–400.

Overall, J. E., Hunter, S., & Butcher, J. N. Factor structure of the MMPI-168 in a psychiatric population. *Journal of Consulting and Clinical Psychology*, 1973, *41*, 284–286.

appendix   B

COMPOSITION OF FREQUENTLY SCORED RESEARCH SCALES*

A — Anxiety (Welsh, 1954)
  True: 32, 41, 67, 76, 94, 138, 147, 236, 259, 267, 278, 301, 305, 321, 337, 343, 344, 345, 356, 359, 374, 382, 383, 384, 389, 396, 397, 411, 414, 418, 431, 443, 465, 499, 511, 518, 544, 555
  False: 379
R — Repression (Welsh, 1954)
  True: None
  False: 1, 6, 9, 12, 39, 51, 81, 112, 126, 131, 140, 145, 154, 156, 191, 208, 219, 221, 271, 272, 281, 282, 327, 406, 415, 429, 440, 445, 447, 449, 450, 451, 462, 468, 472, 502, 516, 529. 550, 556
MAS — Manifest Anxiety scale (Taylor, 1953)
  True: 13, 14, 23, 31, 32, 43, 67, 86, 125, 142, 158, 186, 191, 217, 238, 241, 263, 301, 317, 321, 322, 335, 337, 340, 352, 361, 397, 418, 424, 431, 439, 442, 499, 506, 530, 549, 555
  False: 7, 18, 107, 163, 190, 230, 242, 264. 287, 371. 407. 523. 528
Es — Ego Strength (Barron, 1953)
  True: 2, 36, 51, 95, 109, 153, 174, 181, 187, 192, 208, 221, 231, 234, 253, 270, 355, 367, 380, 410, 421, 430, 458, 513, 515
  False: 14, 22, 32, 33, 34, 43, 48, 58, 62, 82, 94, 100, 132, 140, 189, 209, 217, 236, 241, 244, 251, 261, 341, 344, 349, 359, 378, 384, 389, 420, 483, 488, 489, 494, 510, 525, 541, 544, 548, 554, 555, 559, 561
Lb — Low Back Pain (Hanvik, 1949)
  True: 67, 111, 127, 238, 346
  False: 3, 45, 98, 109, 148, 153, 180, 190,

230, 267, 321, 327, 378, 394, 429, 483, 502, 504, 516, 536
Ca — Caudality (Williams, 1952)
  True: 28, 39, 76, 94, 142, 147, 159, 180, 182, 189, 236, 239, 273, 313, 338, 343, 361, 389, 499, 512, 544, 549, 551, 560
  False: 8, 46, 57, 69, 163, 188, 242, 407, 412, 450, 513, 523
Dy — Dependency (Navran, 1954)
  True: 19, 21, 24, 41, 63, 67, 70, 82, 86, 98, 100, 138, 141, 158, 165, 180, 189, 201, 212, 236, 239, 259, 267, 304, 305, 321, 337, 338, 343, 357, 361, 362, 375, 382, 383, 390, 394, 397, 398, 408, 443, 487, 488, 489, 509, 531, 549, 554, 564
  False: 9, 79, 107, 163, 170, 193, 264, 369
Do — Dominance (Gough, McClosky, & Meehl, 1951)
  True: 64, 229, 255, 270, 368, 432, 523
  False: 32, 61, 82, 86, 94, 186, 223, 224, 240, 249, 250, 267, 268, 304, 343, 356, 395, 419, 483, 558, 562
Re — Social Responsibility (Gough, Mc-Closky, & Meehl, 1952)
  True: 58, 111, 173, 221, 294, 412, 501, 552
  False: 6, 28, 30, 33, 56, 116, 118, 157, 175, 181, 223, 224, 260, 304, 419, 434, 437, 468, 469, 471, 472, 529, 553, 558
Pr — Prejudice (Gough, 1951)
  True: 47, 84, 93, 106, 117, 124, 136, 139, 157, 171, 186, 250, 280, 304, 307, 313, 319, 323, 338, 349, 373, 395, 406, 411, 435, 437, 469, 485, 543
  False: 78, 176, 221
St — Social Status (Gough, 1948)
  True: 78, 118, 126, 149, 199, 204, 229, 237, 289, 430, 441, 452, 491, 513, 521
  False: 136, 138, 180, 213, 249, 267, 280, 297, 304, 314, 324, 352, 365, 378, 388, 427, 448, 480, 488

* Source: W. G. Dahlstrom & G. S. Welsh, *An MMPI Handbook: A Guide to Use in Clinical Practice and Research*. The University of Minnesota Press, Minneapolis. Copyright 1960 by the University of Minnesota. Reproduced with permission.

Cn – Control (Cuadra, 1953)
True: 6, 20, 30, 56, 67, 105, 116, 134, 145, 162, 169, 181, 225, 236, 238, 285, 296, 319, 337, 382, 411, 418, 436, 446, 447, 460, 529, 555
False: 58, 80, 92, 96, 111, 167, 174, 220, 242, 249, 250, 291, 313, 360, 378, 439, 444, 483, 488, 489, 527, 548

appendix C

T-score conversions for frequently scored research scales[a]

Raw score	Males												Females										
	A	R	MAS	Es	Lb	Ca	Dy	Do	Re	Pr	St	Cn	A	R	MAS	Es	Lb	Ca	Dy	Do	Re	Pr	St
68				87												94							
67				86												92							
66				85												91							
65				83												89							
64				82												87							
63				80												86							
62				78												84							
61				77												83							
60				75												81							
59				74												80							
58				72												78							
57				70			91									76			84				
56				69			90									75			83				
55				67			89									73			82				
54				66			88									72			81				
53				64			87									70			80				
52				62			86									69			79				
51				61			85									67			78				
50			99	59			84					115			99	65			77				
49			98	58			83					112			98	64			76				
48			96	56			81					109			96	62			75				
47			95	54			80					107			95	61			74				
46			94	53			79					104			94	59			73				
45			92	51			78					102			92	58			72				
44			91	49			77					99			91	56			71				
43			90	48			76					97			90	54			69				
42			88	46			75					94			88	53			68				
41			87	45			74					91			87	51			67				
40		101	85	43			73					89		102	85	50			66				
39	84	99	84	41			72					86	78	100	84	48			65				
38	82	97	83	40			70					84	77	98	83	47			64				
37	81	95	81	38			69					81	76	95	81	45			63				
36	80	93	80	37		99	68					79	75	93	80	43		95	62				

Raw Score	Males												Females											
	A	R	MAS	Es	Lb	Ca	Dy	Do	Re	Pr	St	Cn	A	R	MAS	Es	Lb	Ca	Dy	Do	Re	Pr	St	Cn
35	79	91	78	35		98	67					76	74	91	78	42		93	61					74
34	77	89	77	33		96	66				86	73	73	88	77	41		91	60				86	72
33	76	86	76	32		94	65				84	71	71	86	76	39		89	59				84	69
32	75	84	74	30		92	64		78	88	82	68	70	84	74	37		87	58		78	88	82	66
31	74	82	73	29		90	63		76	86	80	66	69	81	73	36		85	57		75	86	80	64
30	72	80	71	27		88	62		74	84	78	63	68	79	71	34		84	56		72	84	78	61
29	71	78	70	25		86	61		71	82	75	61	67	76	70	32		82	55		70	82	75	58
28	70	76	69	24		84	59	87	69	80	73	58	66	74	69	31		80	54	87	67	80	73	56
27	69	74	67	22		83	58	85	66	78	71	55	64	72	67	29		78	53	85	64	78	71	53
26	67	72	66	20	120	81	57	82	64	76	69	53	63	69	66	28	120	76	51	82	62	76	69	51
25	66	70	65	19	116	79	56	79	62	75	66	50	62	67	65	26	116	74	50	79	59	75	66	48
24	65	68	63	17	112	77	55	76	59	73	64	48	61	65	63	24	112	72	49	76	57	73	64	45
23	64	66	62	16	108	75	54	73	57	71	62	45	60	62	62	23	108	71	48	73	54	71	62	43
22	62	63	60	14	104	73	53	70	54	69	60	43	58	60	60	21	104	69	47	70	51	69	60	40
21	61	61	59	12	99	71	52	68	52	67	58	40	57	58	59	20	99	67	46	68	49	67	58	38
20	60	59	58		95	69	51	65	50	65	55	38	56	55	58	18	95	65	45	65	46	65	55	35
19	59	57	56		91	68	50	62	47	63	53	35	55	53	56	17	91	63	44	62	43	63	53	32
18	57	55	55		87	66	48	59	45	62	51	32	54	51	55	15	87	61	43	59	41	62	51	30
17	56	53	53		83	64	47	56	42	60	49	30	53	48	53	14	83	60	42	56	38	60	49	27
16	55	51	52		78	62	46	53	40	58	46	27	51	46	52	12	78	58	41	53	35	58	46	25
15	54	49	51		74	60	45	51	37	56	44	25	50	44	51		74	56	40	51	33	56	44	22
14	52	47	49		70	58	44	48	35	54	42	22	49	41	49		70	54	39	48	30	54	42	19
13	51	45	48		66	56	43	45	33	52	40	20	48	39	48		66	52	38	45	28	52	40	17
12	50	43	46		62	55	42	42	30	51	38	17	47	36	46		62	50	37	42	25	51	38	14
11	49	40	45		57	53	41	39	28	49	35	14	46	34	45		57	49	36	39	22	49	35	11
10	47	38	44		53	51	40	37	25	47	33	12	44	32	44		53	47	35	37	20	47	33	9
9	46	36	42		49	49	39	34	23	45	31	9	43	29	42		49	45	34	34		45	31	6
8	45	34	41		45	47	37	31	21	43	29	7	42	27	41		45	43	32	31		43	29	4
7	44	32	40		41	45	36	28	18	41	27	4	41	25	40		41	41	31	28		41	27	1
6	42	30	38		36	43	35	25		39	24	2	40	22	38		36	39	30	25		39	24	
5	41	28	37		32	41	34	22		38	22		38	20	37		32	38	29	22		38	22	
4	40	26	35		28	40	33	20		36	20		37	18	35		28	36	28	20		36	20	
3	38	24	34		24	38	32			34	18		36	15	34		24	34	27			34	18	
2	37	22	33		20	36	31			32	15		35	13	33		20	32	26			32	15	
1	36	20	31			34	30			30	13		34	11	31			30	25			30	13	
0	35	17	30			32	29			28	11		33		30			28	24			28	11	

[a] Source: W. G. Dahlstrom, G. S. Welsh, & L. E. Dahlstrom, *An MMPI Handbook, Vol. I*. The University of Minnesota Press, Minneapolis. Copyright 1960, 1972 by the University of Minnesota. Reproduced with permission.

appendix D

COMPOSITION OF HARRIS SUBSCALES*

Scale 2 – Depression

D₁ – Subjective Depression
  True: 32, 41, 43, 52, 67, 86, 104, 138,
      142, 158, 159, 182, 189, 236, 259
  False: 2, 8, 46, 57, 88, 107, 122, 131,
      152, 160, 191, 207, 208, 242, 272,
      285, 296
D₂ – Psychomotor Retardation
  True: 41, 52, 182, 259
  False: 8, 30, 39, 57, 64, 89, 95, 145, 207,
      208, 233
D₃ – Physical Malfunctioning
  True: 130, 189, 193, 288
  False: 2, 18, 51, 153, 154, 155, 160
D₄ – Mental Dullness
  True: 32, 41, 86, 104, 159, 182, 259, 290
  False: 8, 9, 46, 88, 122, 178, 207
D₅ – Brooding
  True: 41, 67, 104, 138, 142, 158, 182,
      236
  False: 88, 107

Scale 3 – Hysteria

Hy₁ – Denial of Social Anxiety
  True: None
  False: 141, 172, 180, 201, 267, 292
Hy₂ – Need for Affection
  True: 253
  False: 26, 71, 89, 93, 109, 124, 136, 162,
      234, 265, 289
Hy₃ – Lassitude-Malaise
  True: 32, 43, 76, 189, 238
  False: 2, 3, 8, 9, 51, 107, 137, 153, 160,
      163
Hy₄ – Somatic Complaints
  True: 10, 23, 44, 47, 114, 186
  False: 7, 55, 103, 174, 175, 188, 190,
      192, 230, 243, 274

* Source: W. G. Dahlstrom, G. S. Welsh, &
L. E. Dahlstrom, *An MMPI Handbook, Vol. I.*
The University of Minnesota Press, Minneap-
olis. Copyright 1960, 1972 by the University of
Minnesota. Reproduced with permission.

Hy₅ – Inhibition of Aggression
  True: None
  False: 6, 12, 30, 128, 129, 147, 170

Scale 4 – Psychopathic Deviate

Pd₁ – Familial Discord
  True: 21, 42, 212, 216, 224, 245
  False: 96, 137, 235, 237, 527
Pd₂ – Authority Problems
  True: 38, 59, 118, 520
  False: 37, 82, 141, 173, 289, 294, 429
Pd₃ – Social Imperturbability
  True: 64, 479, 520, 521
  False: 82, 141, 171, 180, 201, 267, 304,
      352
Pd₄ₐ – Social Alienation
  True: 16, 24, 35, 64, 67, 94, 110, 127,
      146, 239, 244, 284, 305, 368, 520
  False: 20, 141, 170
Pd₄ᵦ – Self-Alienation
  True: 32, 33, 61, 67, 76, 84, 94, 102,
      106, 127, 146, 215, 368
  False: 8, 107

Scale 6 – Paranoia

Pa₁ – Persecutory Ideas
  True: 16, 24, 35, 10, 121, 123, 127, 151,
      157, 202, 275, 284, 291, 293, 338,
      364
  False: 347
Pa₂ – Poignancy
  True: 24, 158, 299, 305, 317, 341, 365
  False: 111, 268
Pa₃ – Naiveté
  True: 314
  False: 93, 109, 117, 124, 313, 316, 319,
      348

Scale 8 – Schizophrenia

Sc₁ₐ – Social Alienation
  True: 16, 21, 24, 35, 52, 121, 157, 212,
      241, 282, 305, 312, 324, 325, 352,
      364
  False: 65, 220, 276, 306, 309

Sc_{1B} — Emotional Alienation
  True: 76, 104, 202, 301, 339, 355, 360, 363
  False: 8, 196, 322
Sc_{2A} — Lack of Ego Mastery, Cognitive
  True: 32, 33, 159, 168, 182, 335, 345, 349, 356
  False: 178
Sc_{2B} — Lack of Ego Mastery, Conative
  True: 32, 40, 41, 76, 104, 202, 259, 301, 335, 339, 356
  False: 8, 196, 322
Sc_{2C} — Lack of Ego Mastery, Defective Inhibition
  True: 22, 97, 156, 194, 238, 266, 291, 303, 352, 354, 360
  False: None
Sc_3 — Bizarre Sensory Experiences
  True: 22, 33, 47, 156, 194, 210, 251, 273, 291, 332, 334, 341, 345, 350
  False: 103, 119, 187, 192, 281, 330

Scale 9 — Hypomania

Ma_1 — Amorality
  True: 143, 250, 271, 277, 298
  False: 289
Ma_2 — Psychomotor Acceleration
  True: 13, 97, 100, 134, 181, 228, 238, 266, 268
  False: 111, 119
Ma_3 — Imperturbability
  True: 167, 222, 240
  False: 105, 148, 171, 180, 267
Ma_4 — Ego Inflation
  True: 11, 59, 64, 73, 109, 157, 212, 232, 233
  False: None

appendix E

T-score conversions for Harris subscales[a]

Raw score	D1	D2	D3	D4	D5	Hy1	Hy2	Hy3	Hy4	Hy5	Pd1	Pd2	Pd3	Pd4A	P
							Males								
32	122														
31	119														
30	117														
29	114														
28	111														
27	108														
26	105														
25	102														
24	99														
23	96														
22	93														
21	91														
20	88														
19	85														
18	82														95
17	79								106						91
16	76								102						88
15	73	103		114				104	98						84
14	70	98		109				100	94						81
13	67	92		104				95	91						77
12	65	87		100			79	91	87					68	74
11	62	81	104	95			75	87	83		103	92		64	70
10	59	76	98	90	92		71	83	79		98	86	60	66
9	56	70	91	85	87		66	79	75		92	80	56	63
8	53	65	84	80	82		62	74	71		86	74	52	59
7	50	59	77	75	76		58	70	67	82	80	67	48	56
6	47	54	70	70	71	64	54	66	63	75	74	61	44	52
5	44	48	63	65	65	59	50	62	59	68	69	55	40	49
4	41	43	56	60	60	53	46	57	55	60	63	49	35	45
3	39	37	49	55	54	47	42	53	51	53	57	43	31	42
2	36	32	42	50	49	42	38	49	47	46	51	37	27	38
1	33	26	35	45	44	36	34	45	43	39	45	30	23	35
0	30	21	29	40	38	31	30	41	39	31	39	24	19	31

[a] Source: W. G. Dahlstrom, G. S. Welsh, & L. E. Dahlstrom, *An MMPI Handbook*, Vol. I. The Universi Minnesota Press, Minneapolis. Copyright 1960, 1972 by the University of Minnesota. Reproduced with per sion.

PPENDIX E – CONTINUED

Raw score	D1	D2	D3	D4	D5	Hy1	Hy2	Hy3	Hy4	Hy5	Pd1	Pd2	Pd3	Pd4A	Pd4B
							Females								
32	109														
31	106														
30	104														
29	101														
28	99														
27	96														
26	94														
25	91														
24	89														
23	86														
22	84														
21	81														
20	79														
19	76														
18	74														96
17	71								93						92
16	69								89						89
15	66	97		110				97	86					85	93
14	64	92		106				93	83					81	90
13	61	86		101				90	79					78	86
12	59	81		96			81	86	76				69	74	82
11	56	76	99	91			77	82	73		103	106	66	70	78
10	54	71	93	87	88		73	78	69		98	98	62	67	74
9	51	66	87	82	83		69	74	66		92	91	58	63	70
8	49	61	80	77	77		64	70	63		86	84	54	59	67
7	46	56	74	72	72		60	67	59	74	80	76	50	56	63
6	44	51	67	68	66	65	56	63	56	67	74	69	47	52	59
5	41	45	61	63	61	59	51	59	53	60	69	62	43	49	55
4	39	40	55	58	55	54	47	55	49	54	63	54	39	45	51
3	36	35	48	54	50	48	43	51	46	47	57	47	35	41	47
2	34	30	42	49	45	43	39	47	43	41	51	40	31	38	44
1	31	25	36	44	39	38	34	44	39	34	45	32	28	34	40
0	29	20	29	39	34	32	30	40	36	27	39	25	24	30	36

APPENDIX E — CONTINUED

Raw score	Pa1	Pa2	Pa3	Sc1A	Sc1B	Sc2A	Sc2B	Sc2C	Sc3	Ma1	Ma2	Ma3
						Males						
32												
31												
30												
29												
28												
27												
26												
25												
24												
23												
22												
21												
20				120					121			
19				116					117			
18				111					113			
17	117			107					109			
16	113			103					105			
15	108			99					101			
14	104			94			115		97			
13	99			90			110		93			
12	95			86			105		89			
11	90			82			99	112	85		102	
10	86			77	118	103	94	106	81		95	
9	82	95	76	73	109	97	88	99	77		87	
8	77	88	71	69	101	91	83	93	73		80	77
7	73	81	66	65	92	85	77	86	69		73	71
6	68	75	61	60	83	78	72	80	65	81	66	65
5	64	68	56	56	74	72	66	73	60	74	59	59
4	59	62	51	52	66	66	61	67	56	67	52	53
3	55	55	46	48	57	60	55	60	52	59	45	47
2	50	49	41	44	48	53	50	54	48	52	38	42
1	46	42	36	39	39	47	45	47	44	45	31	36
0	41	36	31	35	31	41	39	41	40	37	24	30

PPENDIX E—CONTINUED

aw score	Pa1	Pa2	Pa3	Sc1A	Sc1B	Sc2A	Sc2B	Sc2C	Se3	Ma1	Ma2	Ma3	Ma4
						Females							
32													
31													
30													
29													
28													
27													
26													
25													
24													
23													
22													
21													
20				117					118				
19				113					114				
18				109					110				
17	124			105					106				
16	119			101					102				
15	114			97					98				
14	110			93			110		94				
13	105			88			105		91				
12	100			84			100		87				
11	95			80			95	102	83		98		
10	90			76	120	104	90	96	79		92		
9	85	97	78	72	111	98	85	91	75		85		88
8	80	90	73	68	103	91	80	85	71		79	81	82
7	75	83	68	64	94	85	74	80	67		73	75	76
6	71	76	62	60	85	79	69	74	63	89	66	69	70
5	66	69	57	55	76	72	64	69	59	81	60	63	64
4	61	62	52	51	67	66	59	63	55	72	53	57	58
3	56	55	47	47	58	60	54	58	51	64	47	51	52
2	51	49	42	43	50	53	49	52	47	55	41	45	46
1	46	42	37	39	41	47	44	46	43	47	34	39	40
0	41	35	32	35	32	41	39	41	39	38	28	33	34

appendix F

ITEM OVERLAP FOR HARRIS SUBSCALES AND COMREY FACTORS

Scale 2—Depression (D)

Harris Subscales

D1. Subjective Depression
D2. Psychomotor Retardation
D3. Physical Malfunctioning
D4. Mental Dullness
D5. Brooding

Comrey Factors

  I. Neuroticism
  II. Cynicism
  IV. Religious Fervor
  V. Poor Physical Health
  VI. Euphoria
 VII. Repression
  IX. Hostility
  XI. Depression
XIV. Tearfulness

	D1 (30)	D2 (15)	D3 (11)	D4 (15)	D5 (10)
I (28)	23	6	3	14	7
II (3)	0	2	0	0	0
IV (3)	0	1	0	0	0
V (12)	3	0	5	1	0
VI (3)	2	0	0	0	0
VII (4)	1	2	0	0	0
IX (6)	1	3	1	2	0
XI (5)	4	1	0	4	2
XIV (1)	1	0	0	0	1

Scale 3—Hysteria (Hy)

Harris Subscales

Hy1. Denial of Social Anxiety
Hy2. Need for Affection
Hy3. Lassitude-Malaise
Hy4. Somatic Complaints
Hy5. Inhibition of Aggression

Comrey Factors

  I. Poor Physical Health
  II. Shyness
 III. Cynicism
  V. Headaches
  IX. Neuroticism

	Hy1 (6)	Hy2 (12)	Hy3 (15)	Hy4 (17)	Hy5 (7)
I (15)	0	0	8	7	0
II (9)	5	1	0	0	2
III (5)	0	4	0	0	0
V (10)	0	0	1	8	0
IX (10)	0	0	8	2	0

Scale 4—Psychopathic Deviate (Pd)

Harris Subscales

Pd1. Familial Discord
Pd2. Authority Problems
Pd3. Social Imperturbability
Pd4A. Social Alienation

Comrey Factors

  I. Neuroticism
  II. Paranoia
 III. Psychopathic Personality
 IV. Shyness

Pd4B. Self-Alienation

    V. Delinquency
    VI. Euphoria
    VIII. Antisocial Behavior
    XII. Family Dissension

	Pd1 (11)	Pd2 (11)	Pd3 (12)	Pd4A (18)	Pd4B (15)
I (13)	2	0	1	5	7
II (7)	1	0	0	5	1
III (3)	0	1	0	1	0
IV (7)	1	1	5	1	1
V (3)	1	2	0	0	0
VI (3)	0	0	0	0	0
VIII (2)	0	1	0	0	1
XII (6)	4	1	0	0	0

Scale 6 – Paranoia (Pa)

Harris Subscales
  Pa1. Persecutory Ideas
  Pa2. Poignancy
  Pa3. Naivete

Comrey Factors
    I. Imaginary Persecution
    II. Neuroticism
    III. Cynicism
    V. Anti-Social Behavior
    VI. Hysteria
    XI. Rigidity
    XIII. Actual Persecution
    XV. Real Persecution

	Pa1 (17)	Pa2 (9)	Pa3 (9)
I (10)	9	1	0
II (7)	2	0	0
III (5)	0	0	5
V (1)	0	0	0
VI (3)	0	1	0
XI (3)	0	0	1
XIII (5)	4	0	0
XV (5)	5	1	0

Scale 8 – Schizophrenia (Sc)

Harris Subscales
  Sc1A. Social Alienation
  Sc1B. Emotional Alienation
  Sc2A. Lack of Ego Mastery, Cognitive
  Sc2B. Lack of Ego Mastery, Conative
  Sc2C. Lack of Ego Mastery,
     Defective Inhibition
  Sc3.   Bizarre Sensory Experiences

Comrey Factors
    I. Paranoia
    II. Poor Concentration
    III. Poor Physical Health
    IV. Psychotic Tendencies
    V. Rejection
    VI. Withdrawal
    VII. Father Identification
    VIII. Sex Concern
    IX. Repression
    X. Unnamed
    XI. Mother Identification
    XII. Age

	Sc1A(21)	Sc1B(11)	Sc2A(10)	Sc2B(14)	Sc2C(11)	Sc3(20)
I (10)	4	1	0	1	1	1
II (8)	0	1	2	5	0	0
III (7)	0	0	0	0	1	7
IV (7)	1	2	1	0	0	4
V (6)	3	0	0	0	0	0
VI (7)	1	3	0	2	1	1
VII (2)	1	0	0	0	0	0
VIII (4)	0	0	0	0	0	0
IX (2)	1	0	0	0	1	0
X (7)	0	1	2	0	1	3
XI (3)	1	0	0	0	0	0
XII (2)	1	0	0	0	0	0

Scale 9 – Hypomania (Ma)

Harris Subscales
Ma1. Amorality
Ma2. Psychomotor Acceleration
Ma3. Imperturbability
Ma4. Ego Inflation

Comrey Factors
I. Shyness
II. Bitterness
III. Acceptance of Taboos
IV. Poor Reality Contact
V. Thrill Seeking
VI. Age
VII. Social Dependency
VIII. Psychopathic Personality
X. High Water Consumption
XI. Hospitalization
XII. Sex
XIII. Hypomania
XIV. Agitation
XV. Defensiveness

	Ma1 (6)	Ma2 (11)	Ma3 (8)	Ma4 (9)
I (5)	0	0	4	1
II (2)	1	0	0	1
III (4)	2	0	1	0
IV (4)	0	1	0	0
V (5)	1	3	0	0
VI (3)	0	1	1	0
VII (3)	1	1	0	0
VIII (2)	1	0	1	0
X (3)	0	0	0	1
XI (2)	1	0	0	0
XII (2)	0	0	0	1
XIII (7)	0	2	0	3
XIV (6)	0	4	0	0
XV (2)	0	0	1	1

appendix G

COMPOSITION OF SCALE 5 AND SCALE 0 SUBSCALES*

Mf1 – Narcissism-Hypersensitivity
    True: 25, 89, 117, 179, 214, 217, 226,
        239, 278, 282, 297, 299
    False: 79, 133, 187, 198, 262, 264
Mf2 – Stereotypic Feminine Interests
    True: 4, 70, 74, 77, 78, 87, 92, 132, 140,
        149, 204, 261, 295, 300
    False: None
Mf3 – Denial of Stereotypic Masculine
Interests
    True: None
    False: 1, 81, 144, 176, 219, 221, 223, 283
Mf4 – Heterosexual Discomfort-Passivity
    True: 69
    False: 19, 80, 231
Mf5 – Introspective-Critical
    True: 204
    False: 92, 99, 115, 249, 254, 264
Mf6 – Socially Retiring
    True: None
    False: 89, 99, 112, 116, 117, 126, 140,
        203, 229
Si1 – Inferiority-Personal Discomfort
    True: 32, 67, 82, 138, 147, 171, 172,

        180, 201, 236, 267, 278, 292, 304,
        321, 336, 359, 377, 383, 411, 455,
        549, 564
    False: 57, 309, 353, 371
Si2 – Discomfort with Others
    True: 377, 427, 469, 473, 487, 505
    False: 357, 449, 450, 462, 479, 481, 521,
        547
Si3 – Staid-Personal Rigidity
    True: None
    False: 33, 91, 99, 143, 208, 229, 231,
        254, 400, 415, 440, 446, 449, 450,
        469, 505
Si4 – Hypersensitivity
    True: 25, 32, 126, 138, 236, 278, 391,
        427, 487, 549
    False: None
Si5 – Distrust
    True: 117, 124, 147, 278, 316, 359, 383,
        398, 411, 436, 482
    False: 481
Si6 – Physical-Somatic Concerns
    True: 33, 236, 332
    False: 119, 193, 262, 281, 309, 449, 451

* Source: Serkownek, 1975.

appendix H

T-score conversions for scale 5 and scale 0 subscales[a]

Raw score	Males						Females					
	Si1	Si2	Si3	Si4	Si5	Si6	Si1	Si2	Si3	Si4	Si5	Si6
27	131						126					
26	127						122					
25	123						118					
24	118						114					
23	114						109					
22	110						105					
21	105						101					
20	101						97					
19	96						92					
18	92						88					
17	88						84					
16	83		88				80		82			
15	79		82				76		76			
14	75	113	77				71	110	70			
13	70	106	72				67	104	64			
12	66	100	66		97		63	97	58		99	
11	61	94	61		90		59	91	53		92	
10	57	87	55	103	84	122	54	85	47	91	86	119
9	53	81	50	95	77	114	50	79	41	84	79	110
8	48	75	45	88	71	105	46	73	35	77	73	102
7	44	68	39	80	64	96	42	66	29	70	66	94
6	40	62	34	72	58	87	37	60	23	63	60	85
5	35	55	28	65	52	79	33	54	17	56	53	77
4	31	49	23	57	45	70	29	48	12	49	47	69
3	26	43	18	50	39	62	25	42	6	42	41	60
2	22	36	12	42	32	53	20	35	0	35	34	52
1	18	30	7	35	26	44	16	29	0	28	28	44
0	13	24	1	28	20	36	12	23	0	21	21	35

[a] Source: Serkownek (1975).

APPENDIX H—CONTINUED

	Mf1	Mf2	Mf3	Mf4	Mf5	Mf6	Mf1	Mf2	Mf3	Mf4	Mf5	Mf6
18	122						115					
17	116						108					
16	111						103					
15	105						97					
14	100	121					92	84				
13	94	115					86	78				
12	89	108					81	72				
11	83	101					75	66				
10	78	95					70	60				
9	72	88				77	64	54				81
8	67	81	88			70	59	48	66			73
7	61	74	81		81	63	53	42	58		82	66
6	56	68	73		73	56	48	36	49		73	58
5	50	61	66		64	49	43	30	40		64	52
4	45	54	58	70	55	42	37	24	31	68	55	44
3	39	48	51	58	46	35	32	18	22	53	46	37
2	34	41	43	46	37	28	26	12	13	38	37	30
1	28	34	35	33	29	21	21	6	5	23	29	22
0	23	27	28	21	20	14	15	0	0	8	20	15

appendix I

COMPOSITION OF WIGGINS CONTENT SCALES*

SOC – Social Maladjustment
   True: 52, 171, 172, 180, 201, 267, 292,
      304, 377, 384, 453, 455, 509
   False: 57, 91, 99, 309, 371, 391, 449,
      450, 479, 482, 502, 520, 521, 547
DEP – Depression
   True: 41, 61, 67, 76, 94, 104, 106, 158,
      202, 209, 210, 217, 259, 305, 337,
      338, 339, 374, 390, 396, 413, 414,
      487, 517, 518, 526, 543
   False: 8, 79, 88, 207, 379, 407
FEM – Feminine Interests
   True: 70, 74, 77, 78, 87, 92, 126, 132,
      140, 149, 203, 261, 295, 463, 538,
      554, 557, 562
   False: 1, 81, 219, 221, 223, 283, 300,
      423, 434, 537, 552, 563
MOR – Poor Morale
   True: 84, 86, 138, 142, 244, 321, 357,
      361, 375, 382, 389, 395, 397, 398,
      411, 416, 418, 431, 531, 549, 555
   False: 122, 264
REL – Religious Fundamentalism
   True: 58, 95, 98, 115, 206, 249, 258,
      373, 483, 488, 490
   False: 491
AUT – Authority Conflict
   True: 59, 71, 93, 116, 117, 118, 124,
      250, 265, 277, 280, 298, 313, 316,
      319, 406, 436, 437, 446
   False: 294
PSY – Psychoticism
   True: 16, 22, 24, 27, 33, 35, 40, 48, 50,
      66, 73, 110, 121, 123, 127, 136,

      151, 168, 184, 194, 197, 200, 232,
      275, 278, 284, 291, 293, 299, 312,
      317, 334, 341, 345, 348, 349, 350,
      364, 400, 420, 433, 448, 476, 511,
      551
   False: 198, 347, 464
ORG – Organic Symptoms
   True: 23, 44, 108, 114, 156, 159, 161,
      186, 189, 251, 273, 332, 335, 541,
      560
   False: 46, 68, 103, 119, 154, 174, 175,
      178, 185, 187, 188, 190, 192, 243,
      274, 281, 330, 405, 496, 508, 540
FAM – Family Problems
   True: 21, 212, 216, 224, 226, 239, 245,
      325, 327, 421, 516
   False: 65, 96, 137, 220, 527
HOS – Manifest Hostility
   True: 28, 39, 80, 89, 109, 129, 139, 145,
      162, 218, 269, 282, 336, 355, 363,
      368, 393, 410, 417, 426, 438, 447,
      452, 468, 469, 495, 536
   False: None
PHO – Phobias
   True: 166, 182, 351, 352, 360, 365, 385,
      388, 392, 473, 480, 492, 494, 499,
      525, 553
   False: 128, 131, 169, 176, 287, 353, 367,
      401, 412, 522, 539
HYP – Hypomania
   True: 13, 134, 146, 181, 196, 228, 234,
      238, 248, 266, 268, 272, 296, 340,
      342, 372, 381, 386, 409, 439, 445,
      465, 500, 505, 506
   False: None
HEA – Poor Health
   True: 10, 14, 29, 34, 72, 125, 279, 424,
      519, 544
   False: 2, 18, 36, 51, 55, 63, 130, 153,
      155, 163, 193, 214, 230, 462, 474,
      486, 533, 542

* Source: J. S. Wiggins, Substantive dimensions of self-report in the MMPI item pool. *Psychological Monographs*, 1966, *80* (22, whole no. 630). Copyright 1966 by the American Psychological Association. Reprinted by permission.

appendix J

T-score conversions for Wiggins content scales[a]

Raw score	SOC	DEP	FEM	MOR	REL	AUT	PSY	ORG	FAM	HOS	PHO	HYP	HEA
							Females						
43							120						
42							118						
41							116						
40							114						
39							112						
38							110						
37							108						
36							106	114					
35							104	112					
34							102	109					
33		98					100	107					
32		96					98	105					
31		94					96	103					
30		92	80				94	101					
29		90	77				92	98					
28		88	74				90	96					106
27	83	86	71				88	94		90	91		104
26	81	84	68				86	92		87	89		101
25	79	82	65				84	90		85	86	82	99
24	77	80	62				82	87		83	84	79	96
23	75	78	59	76			80	85		81	82	76	94
22	73	76	56	74			78	83		79	80	74	91
21	71	74	53	72			76	81		77	77	71	89
20	69	72	51	70		82	74	79		75	75	69	86
19	67	70	48	68		79	72	77		72	73	66	83
18	65	68	45	66		77	70	74		70	70	63	81
17	63	66	42	64		74	68	72		68	68	61	78
16	61	64	39	62		71	66	70	98	66	66	58	76
15	59	62	36	60		69	64	68	94	64	64	56	73
14	57	60	33	58		66	63	66	90	62	61	53	71
13	55	58	30	56		63	61	63	86	59	59	50	68
12	53	56	27	54	68	61	59	61	82	57	57	48	65
11	52	54	24	52	64	58	57	59	78	55	55	45	63
10	50	53	21	50	60	55	55	57	74	53	52	43	60
9	48	51	18	48	57	53	53	55	70	51	50	40	58
8	46	49	15	46	53	50	51	52	66	49	48	37	55
7	44	47	13	44	49	47	49	50	62	47	45	35	53
6	42	45	10	42	46	45	47	48	58	44	43	32	50
5	40	43	07	40	42	42	45	46	54	42	41	30	48
4	38	41	04	38	38	39	43	44	50	40	39	27	45
3	36	39	01	36	35	36	41	42	46	38	36	24	42
2	34	37		34	31	34	39	39	42	36	34	22	40
1	32	35		32	27	31	37	37	38	34	32	19	37
0	30	33		30	24	28	35	35	34	31	30	17	35

[a] Source: Wiggins, 1971.

Raw score	SOC	DEP	FEM	MOR	REL	AUT	PSY	ORG	FAM	HOS	PHO	HYP	HEA
							Males						
48							119						
47							117						
46							116						
45							114						
44							112						
43							110						
42							109						
41							107						
40							105						
39							104						
38							102						
37							100						
36							98						
35							97	120					
34							95	117					
33		101					93	115					
32		99					91	113					
31		97					90	110					
30		95	108				88	108					
29		93	105				86	106					
28		91	102				85	103					110
27	88	89	100				83	101		86	107		107
26	86	87	97				81	98		84	104		105
25	84	85	94				79	96		82	102	80	102
24	82	83	91				78	94		79	99	77	99
23	80	81	89	80			76	91		77	96	75	97
22	78	79	86	78			74	89		75	94	73	94
21	76	77	83	76			72	87		73	91	71	92
20	74	75	80	74		76	71	84		71	88	68	89
19	72	73	77	72		74	69	82		69	86	66	87
18	70	71	75	70		71	67	80		67	83	64	84
17	67	69	72	68		69	65	77		65	80	62	81
16	65	68	69	66		66	64	75	103	63	78	59	79
15	63	66	66	64		64	62	73	99	61	75	57	76
14	61	64	64	62		61	60	70	94	59	72	55	74
13	59	62	61	60		59	59	68	90	57	70	53	71
12	57	60	58	58	69	56	57	66	86	55	67	50	68
11	55	58	55	56	65	54	55	63	81	53	64	48	66
10	53	56	52	54	62	51	53	61	77	51	62	46	63
9	51	54	50	52	59	49	52	59	73	49	59	44	61
8	49	52	47	50	56	46	50	56	68	47	56	41	58
7	47	50	44	48	52	44	48	54	64	45	54	39	55
6	45	48	41	46	49	41	46	52	60	43	51	37	53
5	43	46	39	44	46	39	45	49	56	41	48	34	50
4	40	44	36	42	42	36	43	47	51	39	46	32	48
3	38	42	33	40	39	34	41	45	47	37	43	30	45
2	36	40	30	38	36	31	40	42	43	35	40	28	42
1	34	38	27	36	32	29	38	40	38	33	38	25	40
0	32	36	25	34	29	26	36	37	34	31	35	23	37

appendix K

COMPOSITION OF TRYON, STEIN, AND CHU CLUSTER SCALES*

I – Social Introversion versus Interpersonal Poise and Outgoingness

> True: 52, 86, 138, 171, 172, 180, 201, 267, 292, 304, 317, 321, 371, 377, 509
>
> False: 57, 79, 264, 309, 353, 415, 449, 479, 482, 521, 547

II – Body Symptoms versus Lack of Physical Complaints

> True: 10, 14, 23, 29, 44, 47, 62, 72, 108, 114, 125, 161, 189, 191, 263, 544
>
> False: 2, 3, 18, 36, 51, 55, 68, 103, 153, 160, 163, 175, 190, 192, 230, 243, 330

III – Suspicion and Mistrust versus Absence of Suspicion

> True: 71, 89, 112, 136, 244, 265, 278, 280, 284, 316, 319, 348, 368, 383, 390, 404, 406, 426, 436, 438, 447, 455, 469, 507, 558
>
> False: None

---

* Source: K. B. Stein, The TSC scales: the outcome of a cluster analysis of the 550 MMPI items. In P. McReynolds (Ed.), *Advances in Psychological Assessment,* Volume I. Palo Alto, California: Science and Behavior Books, 1968. Copyright 1968 by Science and Behavior Books Inc. Reproduced with permission.

IV – Depression and Apathy versus Positive and Optimistic Outlook

> True: 41, 61, 67, 76, 84, 104, 142, 168, 236, 259, 301, 339, 357, 361, 384, 396, 397, 411, 414, 418, 487, 526, 549
>
> False: 8, 46, 88, 107, 379

V – Resentment and Aggression versus Lack of Resentment and Aggression

> True: 28, 39, 94, 97, 106, 129, 139, 145, 147, 148, 162, 234, 336, 375, 381, 382, 416, 443, 468, 536
>
> False: None

VI – Autism and Disruptive Thoughts versus Absence of Such Disturbances

> True: 15, 31, 33, 40, 100, 134, 241, 297, 329, 342, 345, 349, 356, 358, 359, 374, 389, 425, 459, 511, 545, 559, 560
>
> False: None

VII – Tension, Worry, Fears versus Absence of Such Complaints

> True: 13, 22, 32, 43, 102, 158, 166, 182, 186, 217, 238, 303, 322, 335, 337, 338, 340, 351, 360, 365, 388, 431, 439, 442, 448, 473, 492, 494, 499, 506, 543, 555
>
> False: 131, 152, 242, 407

appendix L

T-score conversions for Tryon, Stein, and Chu cluster scales[a]

Raw score	Male							Female					
	I	II	III	IV	V	VI	VII	I	II	III	IV	V	VI
36							113						
35							111						
34							109						
33		150					107		111				
32		146					104		108				
31		143					102		106				
30		139					100		104				
29		136					98		102				
28		133		116			96		100		98		
27		129		113			94		97		96		
26	91	126		111			92	79	95		94		
25	89	123	80	108			90	77	93	89	92		
24	87	119	78	105			88	76	91	87	90		
23	85	116	76	103		104	86	74	89	85	87		101
22	83	113	74	100		101	84	72	86	83	85		98
21	81	109	73	97	92	98	82	70	84	81	83	89	95
20	79	106	71	94	90	95	79	69	82	78	81	86	92
19	77	103	69	92	87	92	77	67	80	76	79	83	89
18	75	99	68	89	85	89	75	65	78	74	77	81	86
17	73	96	66	86	82	86	73	63	75	72	75	78	83
16	71	93	64	83	80	83	71	62	73	70	73	76	80
15	69	89	62	81	77	80	69	60	71	68	70	73	77
14	67	86	61	78	75	77	67	58	69	65	68	71	74
13	65	83	59	75	72	74	65	57	67	63	66	68	71
12	63	79	57	73	70	72	63	55	64	61	64	65	68
11	61	76	55	70	67	69	61	53	62	59	62	63	65
10	59	73	54	67	65	66	59	51	60	57	60	60	63
9	57	69	52	64	62	63	57	50	58	55	58	58	60
8	55	66	50	62	59	60	54	48	56	52	55	55	57
7	53	63	49	59	57	57	52	46	53	50	53	53	54
6	51	59	47	56	54	54	50	44	51	48	51	50	51
5	49	56	45	54	52	51	48	43	49	46	49	47	48
4	47	53	43	51	49	48	46	41	47	44	47	45	45
3	45	49	42	48	47	45	44	39	44	41	45	42	42
2	43	46	40	45	44	42	42	38	42	39	43	40	39
1	41	43	38	43	42	39	40	36	40	37	41	37	36
0	39	40	36	41	40	36	38	34	38	35	39	34	33

[a] These T-scores were calculated on the basis of means and standard deviations reported by S (1968).

appendix M

GRAYSON CRITICAL ITEMS*

20 (310) My sex life is satisfactory. (F)

27   Evil spirits possess me at times. (T)

33 (323) I have had very peculiar and strange experiences. (T)

37 (302) I have never been in trouble because of my sex behavior (F)

44   Much of the time my head seems to hurt all over. (F)

48   When I am with people I am bothered by hearing very queer things. (T)

66   I see things or animals or people around me that others do not see. (T)

69   I am very strongly attracted by members of my own sex. (T)

74   I have often wished I were a girl. (Or if you are a girl) I have never been sorry that I am a girl. (T/F)

85   Sometimes I am strongly attracted by the personal articles of others such as shoes, gloves, etc., so that I want to handle or steal them though I have no use for them. (T)

114   Often I feel as if there were a tight band about my head. (T)

121   I believe I am being plotted against. (T)

123   I believe I am being followed. (T)

133   I have never indulged in any unusual sex practices. (F)

139   Sometimes I feel as if I must injure either myself or someone else. (T)

146   I have the wanderlust and am never happy unless I am roaming or traveling about. (T)

151   Someone has been trying to poison me. (T)

---

* NOTE – Numbers in parentheses indicate number of items second time they appear in the booklet; T or F in parentheses indicates the critical direction. Source: Grayson, 1951.

156   I have had periods in which I carried on activities without knowing later what I had been doing. (T)

168   There is something wrong with my mind. (T)

179   I am worried about sex matters. (T)

182   I am afraid of losing my mind. (T)

184   I commonly hear voices without knowing where they come fromm (T)

200   There are persons who are trying to steal my thoughts and ideas. (T)

202   I believe I am a condemned person. (T)

205   At times it has been impossible for me to keep from stealing or shoplifting something. (T)

209   I believe my sins are unpardonable. (T)

215   I have used alcohol excessively. (T)

251   I have had blank spells in which my activities were interrupted and I did not know what was going on around me. (T)

275   Someone has control over my mind. (T)

291   At one or more times in my life I felt that someone was making me do things by hypnotizing me. (T)

293   Someone has been trying to influence my mind. (T)

334   Peculiar odors come to me at times. (T)

337   I feel anxiety about something or someone almost all the time. (T)

339   Most of the time I wish I were dead. (T)

345   I often feel as if things were not real. (T)

349   I have strange and peculiar thoughts. (T)

350   I hear strange things when I am alone. (T)

354   I am afraid of using a knife or anything very sharp or pointed. (T)

appendix N

COMPOSITION OF STANDARD VALIDITY AND CLINICAL SCALES[a]

L Scale
True: NONE
False: 15, 30, 45, 60, 75, 90, 105, 120, 135, 150, 165, 195, 225, 255, 285

F Scale
True: 14, 23, 27, 31, 34, 35, 40, 42, 48, 49, 50, 53, 56, 66, 85, 121, 123, 139, 146, 151, 156, 168, 184, 197, 200, 202, 205, 206, 209, 210, 211, 215, 218, 227, 245, 246, 247, 252, 256, 269, 275, 286, 291, 293
False: 17, 20, 54, 65, 75, 83, 112, 113, 115, 164, 169, 177, 185, 196, 199, 220, 257, 258, 272, 276

K Scale
True: 96
False: 30, 39, 71, 89, 124, 129, 134, 138, 142, 148, 160, 170, 171, 180, 183, 217, 234, 267, 272, 296, 316, 322, 374, 383, 397, 398, 406, 461, 502

Scale 1 — Hypochondriasis (Hs)
True: 23, 29, 43, 62, 72, 108, 114, 125, 161, 189, 273
False: 2, 3, 7, 9, 18, 51, 55, 63, 68, 103, 130, 153, 155, 163, 175, 188, 190, 192, 230, 243, 274, 281

Scale 2 — Depression (D)
True: 5, 13, 23, 32, 41, 43, 52, 67, 86, 104, 130, 138, 142, 158, 159, 182, 189, 193, 236, 259
False: 2, 8, 9, 18, 30, 36, 39, 46, 51, 57, 58, 64, 80, 88, 89, 95, 98, 107, 122, 131, 145, 152, 153, 154, 155, 160, 178, 191, 207, 208, 233, 241, 242, 248, 263, 270, 271, 272, 285, 296

Scale 3 — Hysteria (Hy)
True: 10, 23, 32, 43, 44, 47, 76, 114, 179, 186, 189, 238, 253

False: 2, 3, 6, 7, 8, 9, 12, 26, 30, 51, 55, 71, 89, 93, 103, 107, 109, 124, 128, 129, 136, 137, 141, 147, 153, 160, 162, 163, 170, 172, 174, 175, 180, 188, 190, 192, 201, 213, 230, 234, 243, 265, 267, 274, 279, 289, 292

Scale 4 — Psychopathic Deviate (Pd)
True: 16, 21, 24, 32, 33, 35, 38, 42, 61, 67, 84, 94, 102, 106, 110, 118, 127, 215, 216, 224, 239, 244, 245, 284
False: 8, 20, 37, 82, 91, 96, 107, 134, 137, 141, 155, 170, 171, 173, 180, 183, 201, 231, 235, 237, 248, 267, 287, 289, 294, 296

Scale 5 — Masculinity-Femininity (Mf), Male
True: 4, 25, 69, 70, 74, 77, 78, 87, 92, 126, 132, 134, 140, 149, 179, 187, 203, 204, 217, 226, 231, 239, 261, 278, 282, 295, 297, 299
False: 1, 19, 26, 28, 79, 80, 81, 89, 99, 112, 115, 116, 117, 120, 133, 144, 176, 198, 213, 214, 219, 221, 223, 229, 249, 254, 260, 262, 264, 280, 283, 300

Scale 5 — Masculinity-Feminity (Mf), Female
True: 4, 25, 70, 74, 77, 78, 87, 92, 126, 132, 133, 134, 140, 149, 187, 203, 204, 217, 226, 239, 261, 278, 282, 295, 299
False: 1, 19, 26, 28, 69, 79, 80, 81, 89, 99, 112, 115, 116, 117, 120, 144, 176, 179, 198, 213, 214, 219, 221, 223, 229, 231, 249, 254, 260, 262, 264, 280, 283, 297, 300

Scale 6 — Paranoia (Pa)
True: 15, 16, 22, 24, 27, 35, 110, 121, 123, 127, 151, 157, 158, 202, 275, 284, 291, 293, 299, 305, 317, 338, 341, 364, 365
False: 93, 107, 109, 111, 117, 124, 268, 281, 294, 313, 316, 319, 327, 347, 348

[a] Source: W. G. Dahlstrom, G. S. Welsh, L. E. Dahlstrom, *An MMPI Handbook, Vol. I.* The University of Minnesota Press, Minneapolis. Copyright 1960, 1972 by the University of Minnesota. Reproduced with permission.

Scale 7 — Psychasthenia (Pt)
    True: 10, 15, 22, 32, 41, 67, 76, 86, 94,
          102, 106, 142, 159, 182, 189, 217,
          238, 266, 301, 304, 305, 317, 321,
          336, 337, 340, 342, 343, 344, 346,
          349, 351, 352, 356, 357, 358, 359,
          360, 361
    False: 3, 8, 36, 122, 152, 164, 178, 329,
          353
Scale 8 — Schizophrenia (Sc)
    True: 15, 16, 21, 22, 24, 32, 33, 35, 38,
          40, 41, 47, 52, 76, 97, 104, 121,
          156, 157, 159, 168, 179, 182, 194,
          202, 210, 212, 238, 241, 251, 259,
          266, 273, 282, 291, 297, 301, 303,
          305, 307, 312, 320, 324, 325, 332,
          334, 335, 339, 341, 345, 349, 350,
          352, 354, 355, 356, 360, 363, 364
    False: 8, 17, 20, 37, 65, 103, 119, 177,
          178, 187, 192, 196, 220, 276, 281,

306, 309, 322, 330
Scale 9 — Hypomania (Ma)
    True: 11, 13, 21, 22, 59, 64, 73, 97, 100,
          109, 127, 134, 143, 156, 157, 167,
          181, 194, 212, 222, 226, 228, 232,
          233, 238, 240, 250, 251 263, 266,
          268, 271, 277, 279, 298
    False: 101, 105, 111, 119, 120, 148, 166,
          171, 180, 267, 289
Scale 0 — Social Introversion (Si)
    True: 32, 67, 82, 111, 117, 124, 138,
          147, 171, 172, 180, 201, 236, 267,
          278, 292, 304, 316, 321, 332, 336,
          342, 357, 377, 383, 398, 411, 427,
          436, 455, 473, 487, 549, 564
    False: 25, 33, 57, 91, 99, 119, 126, 143,
          193, 208, 229, 231, 254, 262, 281,
          296, 309, 353, 359, 371, 391, 400,
          415, 440, 446, 449, 450, 451, 462,
          469, 479, 481, 482, 505, 521, 547

appendix O

PRACTICE MMPI PROFILES

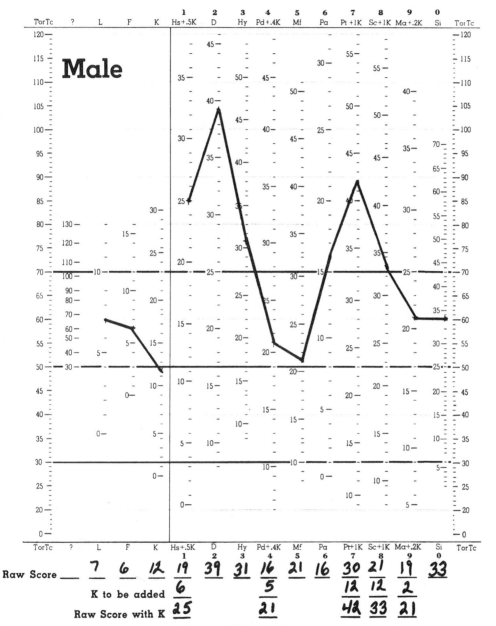

Practice MMPI Profile A

	1	2	3	4	5	6	7	8	9	0
	Hs+.5K	D	Hy	Pd+.4K	Mf	Pa	Pt+1K	Sc+1K	Ma+.2K	Si
Raw Score										

Raw Score ___ 7 6 12 19 39 31 16 21 16 30 21 19 33

K to be added 6   5   12 12 2

Raw Score with K 25   21   42 33 21

Sex, male; age, 40; race, white; marital status, married; education, college graduate (engineering); occupation, business executive.

Source: J. D. Matarazzo, *Wechsler's Measurement and Appraisal of Adult Intelligence.* Baltimore: Williams & Wilkins, 1972, p. 496. Copyright 1972 by Williams & Wilkins. Reproduced with permission.

MMPI profile sheet copyright 1948 by the Psychological Corporation. Reproduced by permission granted in test catalog.

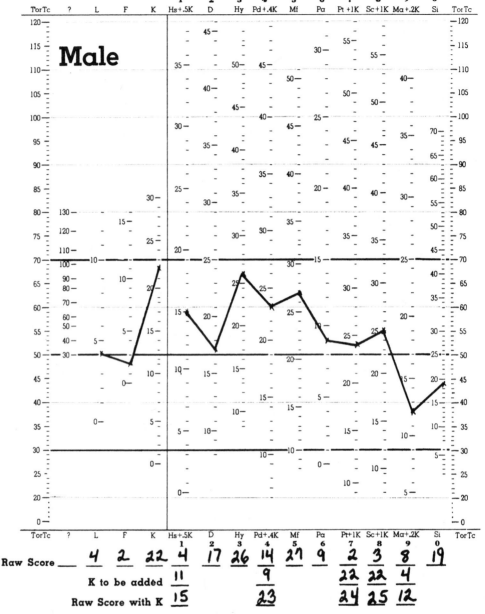

TorTc	?	L	F	K	1 Hs+.5K	2 D	3 Hy	4 Pd+.4K	5 Mf	6 Pa	7 Pt+1K	8 Sc+1K	9 Ma+.2K	0 Si	TorTc
Raw Score	4	2	22	4	17	26	14	27	9	2	3	8	19		
K to be added				11				9			22	22	4		
Raw Score with K				15			23				24	25	12		

Practice MMPI Profile B

Sex, male; age, 24; race, white; marital status, single; education, high school graduate; occupation, highway patrol applicant.

Source: J. D. Matarazzo, *Wechsler's Measurement and Appraisal of Adult Intelligence*. Baltimore: Williams & Wilkins, 1972, p. 505. Copyright 1972 by Williams & Wilkins. Reproduced with permission.

MMPI profile sheet copyright 1948 by the Psychological Corporation. Reproduced by permission granted in test catalog.

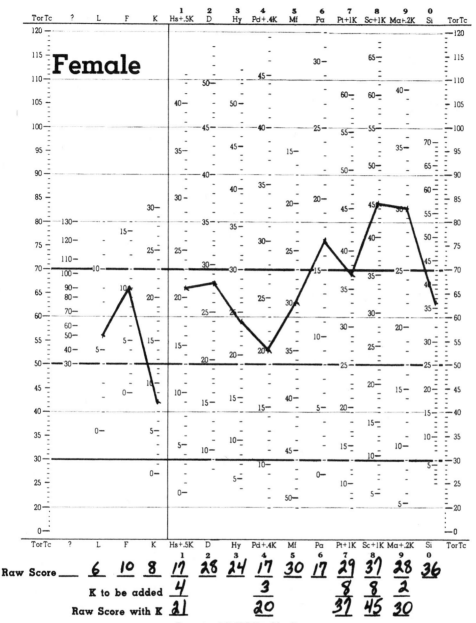

TorTc	?	L	F	K	1 Hs+.5K	2 D	3 Hy	4 Pd+.4K	5 Mf	6 Pa	7 Pt+1K	8 Sc+1K	9 Ma+.2K	0 Si

Female

Practice MMPI Profile C

Raw Score ___ 6 10 8 17 28 24 17 30 17 29 37 28 36

K to be added 4 ___ 3 ___ 8 8 2

Raw Score with K 21 ___ 20 ___ 37 45 30

Sex, female; age, 38; race, white; marital status, married; education, high school graduate; occupation, medical technician.

Source: J. D. Matarazzo, *Wechsler's Measurement and Appraisal of Adult Intelligence.* Baltimore: Williams & Wilkins, 1972, p. 419. Copyright 1972 by Williams & Wilkins. Reproduced with permission.

MMPI profile sheet copyright 1948 by the Psychological Corporation. Reproduced by permission granted in test catalog.

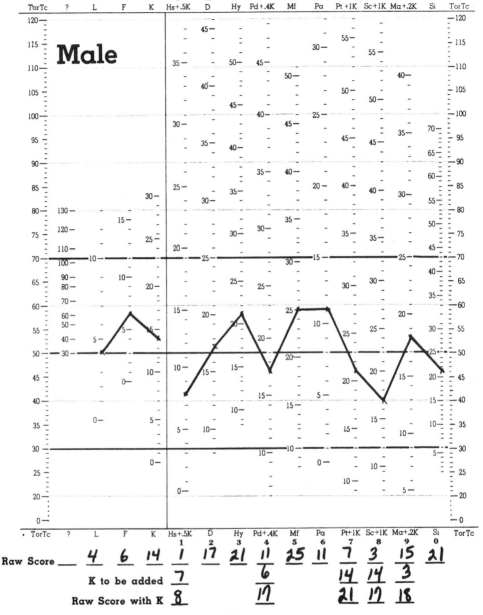

Raw Score		4	6	14	1	17	21	11	25	11	7	3	15	21
K to be added				7				6			14	14	3	
Raw Score with K				8			17				21	17	18	

Practice MMPI Profile D

Sex, male; age, 37; race, white; marital status, married; education, junior college graduate; occupation, business executive.

Source: J. D. Matarazzo, *Wechsler's Measurement and Appraisal of Adult Intelligence.* Baltimore: Williams & Wilkins, 1972, p. 500. Copyright 1972 by Williams & Wilkins. Reproduced with permission.

MMPI profile sheet copyright 1948 by the Psychological Corporation. Reproduced by permission granted in test catalog.

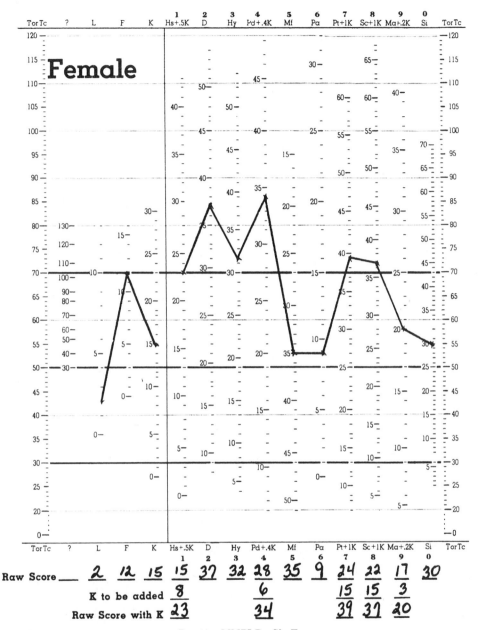

Raw Score	?	L	F	K	Hs+.5K (1)	D (2)	Hy (3)	Pd+.4K (4)	Mf (5)	Pa (6)	Pt+1K (7)	Sc+1K (8)	Ma+.2K (9)	Si (0)
Raw Score	2	12	15	15	15	37	32	28	35	9	24	22	17	30
K to be added					8			6			15	15	3	
Raw Score with K					23			34			39	37	20	

Practice MMPI Profile E

Sex, female; age, 29; race, white; marital status, married; education, college graduate (nursing); occupation, housewife.

Source: W. G. Dahlstrom, Whither the MMPI? In J. N. Butcher (Ed.), *Objective Personality Assessment: Changing Perspectives*. New York: Academic Press, 1972, p. 95. Copyright 1972 by Academic Press. Reproduced with permission.

MMPI profile sheet copyright 1948 by the Psychological Corporation. Reproduced by permission granted in test catalog.

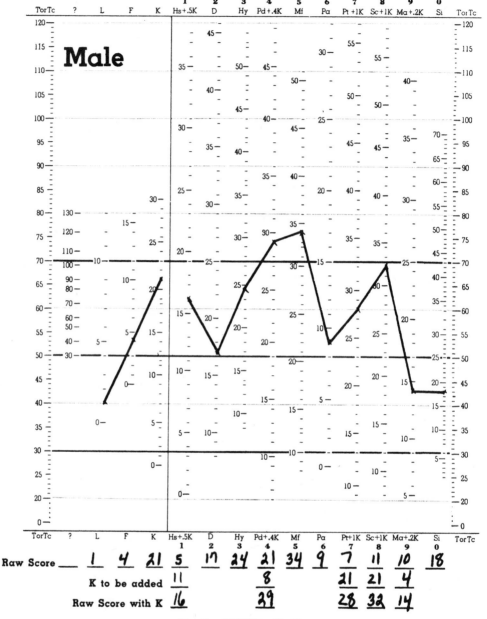

Raw Score		1	4	21	5	17	24	21	34	9	7	11	10	18
K to be added					11			8			21	21	4	
Raw Score with K					16			29			28	32	14	

Practice MMPI Profile F

Sex, male; age, 22; race, white; marital status, single; education, college senior; occupation, student.

Source: E. E. Baughman & G. S. Welsh, *Personality: A Behavioral Science*. Englewood Cliffs, N. J.: Prentice-Hall, 1962, p. 529. Copyright 1962 by Prentice-Hall, Inc. Reproduced with permission.

MMPI profile sheet copyright 1948 by the Psychological Corporation. Reproduced by permission granted in test catalog.

INDEX